Review of Immunology

Review of Immunology

Andrew H. Lichtman, MD, PhD

Associate Professor of Pathology
Harvard Medical School
Brigham and Women's Hospital
Boston, Massachusetts

Rajeev Malhotra, MD

Massachusetts General Hospital
Clinical Fellow
Harvard Medical School
Boston, Massachusetts

Viviany R. Taqueti, BA

Harvard Medical School
Boston, Massachusetts

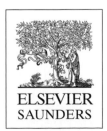

ELSEVIER
SAUNDERS

ELSEVIER
SAUNDERS

The Curtis Center
170 S Independence Mall W 300E
Philadelphia, Pennsylvania 19106

REVIEW OF IMMUNOLOGY
Copyright © 2005, Elsevier Inc.

ISBN 0-7216-0343-2

NOTICE

Library of Congress Cataloging-in-Publication Data

Lichtman, Andrew H.
    Review of immunology / Andrew H. Lichtman, Rajeev Malhotra, Viviany R. Taqueti.—1st ed.
        p. ; cm.
    ISBN 0-7216-0343-2
    1. Immunology—Examinations, questions, etc.   2. Immunity—Examinations, questions, etc.
 3. Immunologic diseases—Examinations, questions, etc.   I. Malhotra, Rajeev.   II. Taqueti, Viviany R.
III. Title.
    [DNLM: 1. Immunity—immunology—Examination Questions.   2. Immunologic Diseases—
immunology—Examination Questions. QW 518.2 L699r 2005]
    QR182.6.L535 2005
    616.07'9'076—dc22

                                                                    2004051482

Acquisitions Editor: William R. Schmitt
Developmental Editor: Carla Holloway
Publishing Services Manager: Tina Rebane
Project Manager: Norm Stellander
Designer: Gene Harris

Printed in China

Last digit is the print number: 9 8 7 6 5 4 3 2 1

To
The students, whose curiosity inspires the best teaching. (AHL)
Mom, Dad, Alka, and Abha, for their unending love and support. (RM)
My teachers. (VRT)

Preface

This book encompasses a systematic review of introductory immunology in the format of multiple choice questions and discussions of the correct and incorrect answers. The organization of the questions parallels the content of Abbas and Lichtman: *Cellular and Molecular Immunology* (CMI5) and Abbas and Lichtman: *Basic Immunology: Functions and Disorders of the Immune System* (BI2). The intended users of this book are students in introductory immunology courses in college, medical school, or other health professional schools, as well as medical students preparing for the USMLE.

The format of the questions includes single best answer multiple choice and matching from extended lists. Some questions have clinical vignettes typical of the USMLE, but many of the questions about basic aspects of the immune system do not incorporate clinical information directly. Unlike the current USMLE format, many of the questions require choosing the one wrong answer among four correct answers. This reflects our belief in the pedagogic value of having students read more correct answer choices than incorrect ones. There are several questions that incorporate images from *Cellular and Molecular Immunology, Basic Immunology: Functions and Disorders of the Immune System,* and *Robbins Pathologic Basis of Disease.*

We believe this book will be most useful if the student first reads a chapter in the primary textbooks and then attempts to answer the questions in the corresponding review book chapter. A careful reading of the answer discussions should indicate the topics that do or do not require further study. The answer discussions cover both the correct and incorrect choices. Each answer is referenced to Abbas and Lichtman: *Cellular and Molecular Immunology* (CMI5) and, for most questions, Abbas and Lichtman: *Basic Immunology: Functions and Disorders of the Immune System* (BI2). It is our hope that students and teachers will find that this book facilitates the learning of immunology and enhances the educational value of the textbooks.

Most importantly, this book reflects our belief that asking the interesting and piercing questions in any research arena is just as important as finding answers to those questions. Immunology is a dynamic field with applications in essentially all subspecialties of medicine. By asking probing questions, immunology students and researchers have facilitated numerous advancements in our understanding and treatment of disease. Therefore, we hope that students will take away from this book not only a better understanding of immunologic concepts, but also a skill and enthusiasm for asking questions of their own.

Andrew H. Lichtman
Rajeev Malhotra
Viviany R. Taqueti

Acknowledgments

Several individuals provided important roles in the writing and production of this book. William Schmitt, Jason Malley, and Carla Holloway at Elsevier have been helpful colleagues throughout the process. Susan Kelley performed highly skilled editorial assistance, and her efforts were essential to ensure consistency and clarity of the quality of the questions. We are grateful to Harvard Medical students who contributed ideas for questions, including Sarah Henrickson, Paul Dieffenbach, Neil Wagle, and Payal Kohli.

Contents

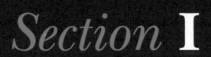

Section I

Introduction to Immunology

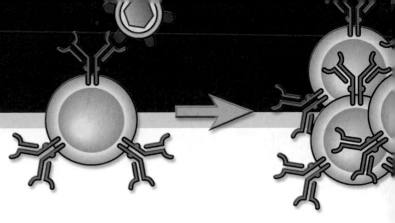

Chapter 1

General Properties of Immune Responses

Cellular and Molecular Immunology, 5/E: Chapter 1—General Properties of Immune Responses

Basic Immunology, 2/E: Chapter 1— Introduction to the Immune System

1. The principal function of the immune system is:
   A. Defense against cancer
   B. Repair of injured tissues
   C. Defense against microbial infections
   D. Prevention of inflammatory diseases
   E. Protection against environmental toxins

2. Which of the following infectious diseases was prevented by the first successful vaccination?
   A. Polio
   B. Tuberculosis
   C. Smallpox
   D. Tetanus
   E. Rubella

3. A previously healthy 8-year-old boy is infected with an upper respiratory tract virus for the first time. During the first few hours of infection, which one of the following events occurs?
   A. The adaptive immune system responds rapidly to the virus and keeps the viral infection under control.
   B. The innate immune system responds rapidly to the viral infection and keeps the viral infection under control.
   C. Passive immunity mediated by maternal antibodies limits the spread of infection.
   D. B and T lymphocytes recognize the virus and stimulate the innate immune response.
   E. The virus causes malignant transformation of respiratory mucosal epithelial cells, and the malignant cells are recognized by the adaptive immune system.

4. Which of the following is a unique property of the adaptive immune system?

   A. Highly diverse repertoire of specificities for antigens
   B. Self-nonself discrimination
   C. Recognition of microbial structures by both cell-associated and soluble receptors
   D. Protection against viral infections
   E. Responses that have the same kinetics and magnitude on repeated exposure to the same microbe

5. Antibodies and T lymphocytes are the respective mediators of which two types of immunity?

   A. Innate and adaptive
   B. Passive and active
   C. Specific and nonspecific
   D. Humoral and cell-mediated
   E. Adult and neonatal

6. A standard treatment of animal bite victims, when there is a possibility that the animal was infected with the rabies virus, is administration of human immunoglobulin preparations containing anti–rabies virus antibodies. Which type of immunity would be established by this treatment?

   A. Active humoral immunity
   B. Passive humoral immunity
   C. Active cell-mediated immunity
   D. Passive cell-mediated immunity
   E. Innate immunity

7. At 15 months of age, a child received a measles-mumps-rubella vaccine (MMR). At age 22, she is living with a family in Mexico that has not been vaccinated and she is exposed to measles. Despite the exposure, she does not become infected. Which of the following properties of the adaptive immune system is best illustrated by this scenario?

   A. Specificity
   B. Diversity
   C. Specialization
   D. Memory
   E. Nonreactivity to self

8. A vaccine administered in the autumn of one year may protect against the prevalent strain of influenza virus that originated in Hong Kong that same year, but it will not protect against another strain of influenza virus that originated in Russia. This phenomenon illustrates which property of the adaptive immune system?

   A. Specificity
   B. Amnesia
   C. Specialization
   D. Cultural diversity
   E. Self-tolerance

9. The two major functional classes of effector T lymphocytes are:

   A. Helper T lymphocytes and cytotoxic T lymphocytes
   B. Natural killer cells and cytotoxic T lymphocytes
   C. Memory T cells and effector T cells
   D. Helper cells and antigen-presenting cells
   E. Cytotoxic T lymphocytes and target cells

10. Which of the following cell types is required for all humoral immune responses?

    A. Natural killer cells
    B. Dendritic cells
    C. Cytolytic T lymphocytes
    D. B lymphocytes
    E. Helper T lymphocytes

11. During a humoral immune response to a newly encountered bacterial infection, B cells are first stimulated to proliferate and then secrete antibodies specific for the bacterium. The antibodies may then bind to the bacteria and facilitate ingestion of the microbes by phagocytic cells. In what phase of the humoral immune response does the binding of secreted antibodies to bacteria occur?

    A. Recognition phase
    B. Activation phase
    C. Effector phase
    D. Homeostatic phase
    E. Memory phase

12. Which of the following statements is consistent with the process of clonal selection?

    A. The specificity of a lymphocyte antigen receptor changes to accommodate the structure of an antigen that binds to it.
    B. Many different antigen receptors with different specificities are expressed on each lymphocyte.
    C. Lymphocytes do not express antigen receptors on their cell surfaces until after exposure to antigen.
    D. The diversity of the lymphocyte repertoire for antigens is very small before exposure to antigen but increases significantly after antigen exposure.
    E. The diversity of the lymphocyte repertoire for antigens is very large before exposure to antigen, with millions of different clones of lymphocytes, each having a different specificity.

13. Which of the following best describes clonal expansion in adaptive immune responses?

    A. Increased number of different lymphocyte clones, each clone specific for a different antigen during the course of an infection
    B. Increased number of different lymphocyte clones, each clone specific for a different antigen during development of the immune system, before exposure to antigen
    C. Increased number of lymphocytes with identical specificities, all derived from a single lymphocyte due to nonspecific stimuli from the innate immune system
    D. Increased number of lymphocytes with identical specificities, all derived from a single lymphocyte stimulated by a single antigen
    E. Increased size of the lymphocytes of a single clone due to antigen-induced activation of the cells

14. The estimated number of distinct structures that can be recognized by the mammalian adaptive immune system is

    A. 1-10
    B. 10^2-10^3
    C. 10^3-10^5
    D. 10^7-10^9
    E. ∞

15. Which of the following statements best describes the "two-signal requirement" for naive lymphocyte activation?

    A. Lymphocytes must recognize two different antigens to become activated.
    B. Lymphocytes must recognize the same antigen at two sequential times to become activated.
    C. Lymphocytes must recognize antigen and respond to another signal generated by microbial infection to become activated.
    D. Both naive B and naive T lymphocytes must simultaneously recognize antigen for either to be activated.
    E. When lymphocytes recognize antigen, the antigen receptors must activate two-signal transduction pathways to become activated.

16. In addition to T cells, which cell type is required for initiation of all T cell–mediated immune responses?

    A. Effector cells
    B. Memory cells
    C. Natural killer cells
    D. Antigen-presenting cells
    E. B lymphocytes

Answers

1. (C) The immune system has evolved in the setting of selective pressures imposed by microbial infections. Although immune responses to cancer may occur, the concept that "immunosurveillance" against cancer is a principal function of the immune system is controversial. Repair of injured tissues may be a secondary consequence of the immune responses and inflammation. Although the immune system has regulatory features that are needed to prevent excessive inflammation, prevention of inflammatory diseases is not a primary function. The immune system can protect against microbial toxins, but it generally does not offer protection against toxins of nonbiologic origin.
   CMI5 3; BI2 1-2

2. (C) In 1798, Edward Jenner reported the first intentional successful vaccination, which was against smallpox in a boy, using material from the cowpox pustules of a milkmaid. In 1980, smallpox was reported to be eradicated worldwide by a vaccination program. Effective vaccines against tetanus toxin, rubella virus, and poliovirus were developed in the 20th century and are widely used. There

is no effective vaccine against *Mycobacterium tuberculosis*.
CMI5 4; BI2 2

3. (B) The innate immune response to microbes develops within hours of infection, well before the adaptive immune response. B and T lymphocytes are components of the adaptive immune response, and they would not be able to respond to a newly encountered virus before the innate immune response. An 8-year-old boy would no longer have maternal antibodies from transplacental passive transfer and is unlikely to be breast-feeding, which is another potential source of maternal antibodies. Malignant transformation takes months or years to develop.
CMI5 4-5; BI2 3-4

4. (A) Highly diverse repertoires of specificities for antigens are found only in T and B lymphocytes, which are the central cellular components of the adaptive immune system. Both the innate and the adaptive immune systems use cell-associated and soluble receptors to recognize microbes, display some degree of self-nonself discrimination, and protect against viruses. On repeated exposure to the same microbe, the adaptive immune response becomes more rapid and of greater magnitude; this is the manifestation of memory.
CMI5 9-11; BI2 3-4

5. (D) Both B and T lymphocytes are principal components of adaptive immunity. B lymphocytes produce antibodies, which are the recognition and effector molecules of humoral immune responses to extracellular pathogens. T cells recognize and promote eradication of intracellular pathogens in cell-mediated immunity. Passive and active immunity both can be mediated by either B or T lymphocytes. *Specific immunity* is another term for adaptive immunity. Both B and T lymphocytes participate in adult adaptive immunity but are still developing in the neonatal period.
CMI5 6-8; BI2 6-8

6. (B) Humoral immunity is mediated by antibodies. The transfer of protective antibodies made by one or more individuals into another individual is a form of passive humoral immunity. Active immunity to an infection develops when an individual's own immune system responds to the microbe. Cell-mediated immunity is mediated by T lymphocytes, not antibodies, and innate immunity is not mediated by either antibodies or T lymphocytes.
CMI5 7; BI2 4-5

7. (D) Protection against infections after vaccination is due to immunologic memory of the adaptive immune system. Memory is manifested as a more rapidly developing and vigorous response on repeat exposure to an antigen compared with the first exposure. Specificity and diversity are properties related to the range of antigenic structures recognized by the immune system, and specialization is

the ability of the adaptive immune system to use distinct effector mechanisms for distinct infections.
CMI5 9-10; BI2 5

8. (A) Adaptive immune responses are highly specific for distinct molecular structures, which may be present in a vaccine and be produced by one strain of virus but not by a closely related strain. Amnesia, although generally not used in immunology, implies lack of memory, but the efficacy of the vaccine against the Hong Kong strain implies it has induced memory. The same effector mechanisms would be required to combat different strains of influenza, and therefore failure of a vaccine to protect against two different strains of virus is not related to specialization of effector functions.
CMI5 9-10; BI2 6-8

9. (A) T cells can be classified into effector subsets that perform different effector functions. Most effector T cells are either helper T lymphocytes, which promote macrophage and B cell responses to infections, or cytotoxic T lymphocytes, which directly kill infected cells. Natural killer cells are not T lymphocytes. Antigen-presenting cells usually are not T cells. Memory T cells are not effector T cells.
CMI5 11; BI2 9-14

10. (D) Humoral immune responses are antibody-mediated immune responses, and all antibodies are made by B lymphocytes and by no other cell type.
CMI5 6; BI2 9-14

11. (C) The effector phase of an immune response occurs when cells or molecules eliminate the microbe or microbial toxin. In a humoral immune response, the effector phase includes secretion of antibody, binding of the antibody to the microbe or toxin, and subsequent antibody-dependent elimination of the microbe or toxin. The recognition phase is the initial binding of the antigen by the naive lymphocyte. The activation phase includes proliferation and differentiation of lymphocytes in response to antigen recognition. The homeostatic phase follows the effector phase, during which the response wanes. In the memory phase, memory B cells and antibodies secreted by long-lived antibody-secreting cells are "waiting" for a repeat exposure to the microbe.
CMI5 12-13; BI2 8-9

12. (E) The clonal selection hypothesis accurately predicted that individuals possess large numbers of different clones of lymphocytes before antigen exposure, with cells in each clone expressing antigen receptors with a single identical specificity, but with different specificities from other clones. Thus, the diversity of the lymphocyte repertoire is very large even before antigen exposure. These receptors are expressed before antigen exposure, and their specificities generally do not change in response to antigen.
CMI5 12-14; BI2 6-7

13. (D) Clonal expansion occurs during the activation phase of an adaptive immune response. A single lymphocyte is stimulated to divide by antigen, and the progeny go through several rounds of division until there are many lymphocytes, all with identical specificities, all derived from one cell. The number of different clones is not influenced by antigen exposure. Expansion does not refer to the size of the cells, although activated lymphocytes are larger than their naive precursors.
CMI5 13; BI2 6-9

14. (D) Although the theoretical number of antigen specificities of the adaptive immune system is higher, estimates of the actual number of different antibody and T cell antigen receptor specificities are in the range of 10^7-10^9. This number is large enough to accommodate most of the diversity in molecular structures that the microbial world is capable of producing.
CMI5 13; BI2 6-7

15. (C) Naive lymphocytes will not become activated by antigen alone (signal 1). In addition, they require "costimulatory" signals (signal 2), which are either microbial products or molecules on host cells induced by microbial infection. The molecules that provide signal 2 bind to receptors on the lymphocytes that are distinct from the clonally distributed antigen receptors. Each lymphocyte cannot generally recognize more than one antigen. Although lymphocyte activation may require recognition of antigen molecules by more than one antigen receptor, the two-signal requirement does not refer to this. There is no general requirement for both T and B cells to recognize the same antigen for activation of either to occur. The two-signal requirement does not refer to antigen receptor–associated signal transduction pathways.
CMI5 14-15; BI2 9

16. (D) T cell–mediated immune responses are initiated when naive T cells are activated. Antigen-presenting cells, such as dendritic cells, are required to display antigens (peptide-MHC molecule complexes) for naive T cell recognition and to express costimulatory molecules also needed for T cell activation. Memory cells, cytotoxic T cells, and B lymphocytes are not involved in the initial activation of naive T lymphocytes.
CMI5 11; BI2 14

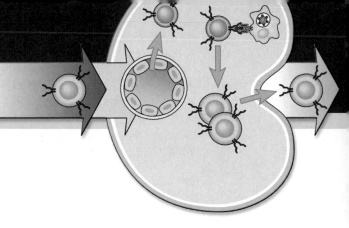

Chapter 2

Cells and Tissues of the Immune System

Cellular and Molecular Immunology, 5/E: Chapter 2—Cells and Tissues of the Immune System

Basic Immunology, 2/E: Chapter 1—Introduction to the Immune System and Chapter 2—Innate Immunity

1. Which type of white blood cell is most numerous in normal human blood?

   A. Basophil
   B. Lymphocyte
   C. Monocyte
   D. Neutrophil
   E. Eosinophil

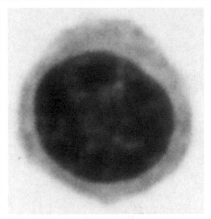 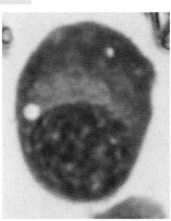 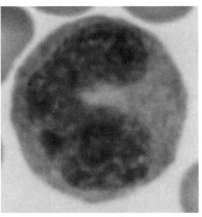

1   2   3

2. The cells labeled 1, 2, and 3 shown in the figure above are:

   A. 1, plasma cell; 2, monocyte; 3, resting lymphocyte
   B. 1, monocyte; 2, plasma cell; 3, resting lymphocyte
   C. 1, plasma cell; 2, resting lymphocyte; 3, monocyte
   D. 1, resting lymphocyte; 2, monocyte; 3, plasma cell
   E. 1, resting lymphocyte; 2, plasma cell; 3, monocyte

3. Each of the following is a characteristic of resting small lymphocytes EXCEPT:

    A. They are in G_0 stage of the cell cycle.
    B. They are larger than erythrocytes.
    C. They have a high nuclear-cytoplasmic ratio.
    D. They secrete immunoglobulins.
    E. They express membrane-bound antigen receptors.

4. Which of the following cell types do NOT have clonally distributed antigen receptors?

    A. Natural killer cells
    B. Cytotoxic T lymphocytes
    C. Naive B cells
    D. Helper T lymphocytes
    E. Memory B cells

5. In the blood of a healthy individual, the most abundant type of lymphocyte is the:

    A. CD4$^+$ T cell
    B. CD8$^+$ T cell
    C. B cell
    D. Natural killer cell
    E. Plasma cell

6. A 52-year-old man who receives radiation therapy and cytotoxic drugs for treatment of cancer sustains significant damage to his bone marrow. Which of the following changes will most likely occur?

    A. Decreased production of B lymphocytes but not T lymphocytes
    B. Decreased production of T lymphocyte but not B lymphocytes
    C. Decreased production of neutrophils and monocytes but not B or T lymphocytes
    D. Decreased production of B lymphocytes and T lymphocytes
    E. Normal production of all blood cells due to compensatory extramedullary hematopoiesis

7. In DiGeorge syndrome, the thymus fails to develop. Which of the following characterizes the immunodeficiency state in this syndrome?

    A. Deficiency in monocytes and tissue macrophages
    B. Defect in naive B cell activation and antibody production in response to bacterial polysaccharides
    C. Deficiency in T lymphocytes and associated defects in cell-mediated immunity
    D. Normal numbers of naive T cells that cannot be activated by antigen
    E. Deficiency in B cell maturation

8. T cell antigen receptor expression is required for all of the following EXCEPT:

    A. Development of mature T lymphocytes from bone marrow precursors
    B. Maintenance of the pool of naive T lymphocytes in peripheral lymphoid organs
    C. Activation of effector T lymphocytes at sites of infection by antigen

    D. Activation of naive T lymphocytes in the lymph node by antigen
    E. Activation of antigen-presenting cells by microbes

9. Which of the following statements about memory cells is NOT true?

    A. Memory cells can survive for several years.
    B. Memory cells are responsible for the more rapid and enhanced responses to antigen upon secondary exposure, as compared with primary responses.
    C. Memory cells can be distinguished from naive cells by the expression of certain cell surface molecules.
    D. Memory cells continuously produce effector cytokines.
    E. Many memory cells express adhesion molecules that favor their migration to peripheral sites of infection.

10. Each of the following molecules is more highly expressed by human effector T cells than by human naive T lymphocytes EXCEPT:

    A. High-affinity IL-2 receptors
    B. L-selectin
    C. CD44
    D. VLA-4 (CD29CD49d)
    E. CD45RO

11. Which of the following is a typical property of memory B cells but not naive B cells?

    A. Surface IgG expression
    B. Surface IgD expression
    C. Surface IgM expression
    D. High expression of CXCR5
    E. Active antibody secretion

12. Mononuclear phagocytes participate in adaptive immune responses in each of the following ways EXCEPT:

    A. Antigen presentation to T lymphocytes
    B. Activation by helper T cells to kill ingested microbes
    C. Production of proinflammatory cytokines
    D. Ingestion of microbes opsonized by antibodies
    E. Antigen-specific killing of virus-infected cells

13. Tissue macrophages are derived from which type of circulating blood cell?

    A. Polymorphonuclear leukocyte
    B. Small lymphocyte
    C. Monocyte
    D. Basophil
    E. Lymphoblast

14. Which statement about follicular dendritic cells (FDCs) is true?

    A. They are the most efficient antigen-presenting cells for naive T lymphocytes.
    B. They are abundant in the hair follicles of the scalp, where they serve as part of the cutaneous immune system.

C. They are mostly derived from bone marrow precursors.

D. They are present in germinal centers of lymph nodes, where they display antigens for B cell recognition.

E. They are specialized neurons involved in nervous system regulation of immune responses.

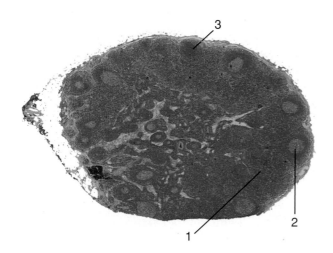

15. The three features of a lymph node labeled 1, 2, and 3 in the figure above are

A. 1, germinal center; 2, T cell zone; 3, primary follicle

B. 1, T cell zone; 2, germinal center; 3, primary follicle

C. 1, primary follicle; 2, germinal center; 3, T cell zone

D. 1, primary follicle; 2, T cell zone; 3, germinal center

E. 1, T cell zone; 2, primary follicle; 3, germinal center

16. Which of the following is the generative lymphoid organ for T lymphocytes?

A. Bone marrow

B. Spleen

C. Lymph node

D. Thymus

E. Tonsil

17. A 5-year-old boy with recurrent infections is discovered to have a genetic defect that impairs B cell maturation. Which of the following abnormalities is most likely to be found in this patient?

A. Small thymus

B. Absence of follicles in lymph nodes and spleen

C. Enlarged tonsils

D. Diminished parafollicular zones in lymph nodes

E. Hypocellular bone marrow

18. A genetic deficiency in the chemokine receptor CCR7 would result in which of the following abnormalities?

A. Reduced numbers of T cells and dendritic cells in lymph nodes

B. Absence of primary follicles in lymph nodes

C. Reduced blood neutrophil count

D. Absence of follicular dendritic cells in lymph node follicles

E. Thin thymic cortex

Questions 19-23

Match each of the descriptions in questions 19-23 with the appropriate name (A-M) of an anatomic feature of lymphoid tissues.

A. Periarteriolar lymphoid sheath

B. Thymic medulla

C. Thymic cortex

D. Parafollicular cortex of lymph node

E. Hematopoietic bone marrow

F. Afferent lymphatic

G. Efferent lymphatic

H. Marginal zone

I. Red pulp of spleen

J. White pulp of spleen

K. Epidermis

L. Dermis

M. Peyer's patch

19. Location of most T lymphocytes in the spleen (   )

20. Vessels that drain lymph away from a lymph node (   )

21. Site of least mature T cell precursors in the thymus (   )

22. Location of Langerhans cells (   )

23. Lymphoid aggregate of the mucosal immune system (   )

24. In naive T cell recirculation, entry of the cells into peripheral lymph nodes occurs through which specialized vessel?

A. Efferent lymphatic

B. Thoracic duct

C. Central artery

D. High endothelial venule

E. Sinusoid

Questions 25-29

For each description of a molecule involved in lymphocyte migration in questions 25-29, choose the lettered description (A-I) that most closely matches it.

A. Peripheral lymph node addressin

B. Intercellular adhesion molecule-1 (ICAM-1)

C. Very late activation antigen-4 (VLA-4)

D. E-selectin

E. P-selectin ligand

F. CCR7

G. CXCR5

H. MadCAM-1

I. Vascular cell adhesion molecule-1 (VCAM-1)

25. This molecule binds SLC and ELC and is involved in naive T cell migration into interfollicular zones of lymph nodes. (   )

26. The expression of this molecule is induced on endothelial cells in inflamed tissues, and it mediates rolling of T cells along the endothelial surface. ( )

27. This molecule is expressed on activated endothelium, is a member of the immunoglobulin superfamily, and binds to β1 integrins on activated T cells. ( )

28. This vascular addressin binds to integrins on T cells and mediates their homing to intestinal mucosa. ( )

29. This receptor is expressed on naive B cells and promotes their migration into lymph node follicles. ( )

Answers

1. (D) The neutrophil (polymorphonuclear leukocyte, neutrophilic granulocyte) is the most abundant white blood cell (~1.8-7.7 × 10^3/mm^3). The basophil is the least abundant.
   CMI5 17; BI2 10

2. (E) Resting lymphocytes can be found in blood and tissues and may be naive or memory cells. They are 8 to 10 mm in diameter and have a large nucleus with dense nuclear chromatin and little visible cytoplasm. Plasma cells, which are differentiated antibody-secreting B lymphocytes, are found in tissues. They are larger than resting lymphocytes and have eccentric nuclei with heterogeneous chromatin staining and abundant cytoplasm with a distinct perinuclear halo. Monocytes are the circulating precursors of tissue macrophages. They are 10 to 15 μm in diameter and have a typically bean-shaped nucleus and abundant cytoplasm.
   CMI5 19, 23, 25; BI2 10

3. (D) Small resting lymphocytes may be either naive lymphocytes or memory cells. Only activated B lymphocytes or their derivative plasma cells secrete antibodies.
   CMI5 17-18; BI2 9-10

4. (A) Natural killer cells, specialized cells with lymphocyte-like morphology, do not express clonally distributed antigen receptors (i.e., they do not express immunoglobulin or T cell antigen receptors). Cytotoxic T lymphocytes, naive B cells, helper T lymphocytes, and memory B cells are all forms of lymphocytes and do express clonally distributed antigen receptors.
   CMI5 17

5. (A) Seventy to 85 percent of blood lymphocytes are T cells, and there are usually about twice as many CD4$^+$ T cells as CD8$^+$ T cells.
   CMI5 19; BI2 9-12

6. (D) Hematopoietic precursor cells that give rise to both B and T lymphocyte lineages are located in the bone marrow. Neutrophils and monocytes would also be reduced. Although blood cell production (hematopoiesis) may occur in non–bone marrow sites (extramedullary sites), such as liver, when bone marrow is damaged, full compensation for bone marrow loss is not usually achieved, and even extramedullary hematopoiesis is impaired by irradiation and cytotoxic drugs.
   CMI5 26-27; BI2 12

7. (C) The thymus is the principal site for production of mature T lymphocytes. Therefore, lack of a thymus results in a global defect in T cell–mediated immunity. There would not be a specific defect in naive T cell activation, but rather a lack of naive T cells. Monocytes and macrophages are produced independently of the thymus or mature T cells. B cell maturation is not dependent on T cells. Although B cell responses to protein antigens depend on helper T cells, B cells specific for polysaccharides can be activated and produce antibodies independently of T cells.
   CMI5 20-26

8. (E) Dendritic cells, macrophages, and other antigen-presenting cells express receptors for and become activated by commonly encountered microbial molecules, independently of T cells. T cell development into naive T cells, long-term maintenance of pools of naive T cells, and activation of both naive and effector T cells by antigen all require expression of the T cell antigen receptor.
   CMI5 20-26; BI2 12-14

9. (D) Memory cells are functionally quiescent and do not produce effector molecules such as antibodies or cytokines. They may survive for years in this state, identifiable by certain cell surface markers, including adhesion molecules that favor migration to peripheral sites of infection. On re-exposure to antigen, they can mediate rapid adaptive immune responses.
   CMI5 23-24; BI2 19

10. (B) L-selectin typically is most highly expressed on naive T cells and mediates homing of these cells into lymph nodes through high endothelial venules. High-affinity IL-2 receptors are expressed on recently activated effector T cells. CD44 and VLA-4 are adhesion molecules most highly expressed on activated effector T cells, mediating homing into peripheral inflammatory sites. CD45RO is an isoform of CD45 that is expressed more abundantly on memory T cells than on naive T cells, whereas CD45RA is more abundantly expressed on naive T cells.
    CMI5 24; BI2 18-19, 109

11. (A) Surface IgG expression requires prior Ig-isotype switching. Memory B cells may express surface IgG because they may be derived from B cells that have undergone activation, differentiation, and isotype switching. Naive B cells express only surface IgD and IgM. CXCR5 is a chemokine receptor that is expressed on naive B cells and

promotes their migration into follicles. Memory B cells are quiescent and do not actively secrete antibodies.
CMI5 23-24; BI2 79-80

12. (E) Macrophages are not capable of antigen-specific killing of virus-infected cells. They ingest and kill extracellular microbes, and they may be activated by antigen-specific helper T cells. Macrophages do function as antigen-presenting cells, produce inflammatory cytokines such as IL-1 and TNF, and express Ig Fc receptors that allow them to ingest and kill antibody-opsonized microbes.
CMI5 25-26; BI2 25-30

13. (C) Blood monocytes migrate into tissues and become macrophages.
CMI5 25; BI2 26

14. (D) Follicular dendritic cells (FDCs) are residents of the germinal centers of B cell follicles in the spleen and lymph nodes. They display antigens on their surface during selection of B cells expressing high-affinity antibodies. FDCs are not the same cells as dendritic cells that present antigen to T cells, and most are not derived from bone marrow precursors. FDCs are neither present in hair follicles, nor are they neurons.
CMI5 26; BI2 14-15, 138

15. (B) The T cell zone (parafollicular cortex) is the region between follicles where T cells and dendritic cells are concentrated. Germinal centers are lighter-staining areas within follicles where B cells undergo proliferation and affinity maturation during humoral immune responses. Primary follicles are spherical collections of resting or naive B cells.
CMI5 28-30; BI2 15-17

16. (D) Generative lymphoid organs are the organs where lymphocytes first express antigen receptors and attain functional maturity. Although T cell precursors arise in the bone marrow, these precursors migrate to the thymus, where maturation takes place. In contrast, B cells mature in the bone marrow. Spleen, lymph node, and tonsil are secondary lymphoid organs populated by mature B and T cells.
CMI5 26-32; BI2 11-12

17. (B) The follicles of the spleen and lymph nodes are largely made up of mature B lymphocytes. Thus, if this patient lacks mature B cells, he will lack follicles. The thymus is the site of T cell maturation, which should not be affected by a defect in B cell maturation. Tonsils, which normally contain many B cells, should be small, not enlarged, in this patient. The parafollicular zones of lymph nodes are sites where T cells are abundant and should be of normal size in this patient. Most bone marrow is composed of nonlymphoid hematopoietic elements, so a defect in B cell maturation should not influence the cellularity. Furthermore, with multiple infections, the patient may have increased production of neutrophils, resulting in hypercellular marrow.
CMI5 26-31; BI2 15-17

18. (A) CCR7 is a chemokine receptor expressed on naive T cells and dendritic cells. This receptor binds chemokines produced in the parafollicular zones of lymph nodes. T cell and dendritic cell migration into lymph nodes is dependent on CCR7, and therefore a deficiency in CCR7 expression would result in reduced numbers of these cells in lymph nodes. Primary follicles contain mainly naive B cells, and migration of B cells into the follicles is not dependent on CCR7 expression. CCR7 is not involved in migration of neutrophils into or out of the blood, of follicular dendritic cells into lymphoid follicles, or of T cell precursors into the thymic cortex.
CMI5 29-30, 36-37

19. (A) The periarteriolar lymphoid sheath surrounds the central arteries in the spleen and is the T cell zone in this organ.
CMI5 31-32; BI2 17

20. (G) Efferent lymphatic vessels drain lymph away from lymph nodes; afferent vessels drain lymph into lymph nodes.
CMI5 28-30; BI2 16

21. (C) Bone marrow–derived T cell precursors first enter the thymic cortex and migrate into the medulla as they become more mature.
CMI5 27-28

22. (K) Langerhans cells are immature dendritic cells located in the epidermis of the skin.
CMI5 32; BI2 43-44

23. (M) Peyer's patches are B cell–rich lymphoid aggregates located in the submucosa of the small intestine.
CMI5 33-34; BI2 15

24. (D) The high endothelial venule is a specialized vessel in the lymph node paracortex that expresses adhesion molecules that mediate the binding and transmigration of naive T cells into lymph node tissue. The efferent lymphatic is a route of exit of T cells from the lymph node. The thoracic duct is a major site of drainage of lymph back into the blood circulation. A central artery is a vessel in the spleen around which are T cell lymphoid aggregates (periarteriolar lymphoid sheath). Sinusoids are blood channels in the spleen lined by fenestrated endothelium and phagocytic cells.
CMI5 34-36; BI2 18-19

25. (F) SLC and ELC are the chemokines that bind to CCR7 on naive T lymphocytes and dendritic cells, and direct their migration into lymph nodes.
CMI5 29-30, 36-37

26. (D) E-selectin expression is induced on endothelial cells by cytokines and microbial products, and

it mediates rolling interactions of T cells and other leukocytes.
CMI5 36-38; BI2 25,109

27. (B) Intercellular adhesion molecule-1 (ICAM-1) on endothelial cells binds to the integrin LFA-1 on activated T cells.
CMI5 36-38; BI2 109

28. (H) MadCAM-1 is expressed on vessels in the intestine and binds to $\alpha4\beta1$ integrins on gut-homing T cells.
CMI5 33, 38

29. (G) CXCR5 is a chemokine receptor on naive B cells that binds chemokines made in lymphoid follicles.
CMI5 30

Section II

Recognition of Antigens

Chapter 3

Antibodies and Antigens

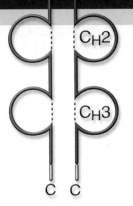

Cellular and Molecular Immunology, 5/E: Chapter 3—Antibodies and Antigens

Basic Immunology, 2/E: Chapter 4—Antigen Recognition in the Adaptive Immune System

1. The three major families of antigen-binding molecules in the adaptive immune system are:
   A. Toll-like receptors, MHC molecules, and antibodies
   B. MHC molecules, integrins, and antibodies
   C. Antibodies, T cell receptors, and selectins
   D. Antibodies, T cell receptors, and MHC molecules
   E. MHC molecules, antibodies, and Fc receptors

2. Which of the following statements about antibodies is NOT true?
   A. They serve as membrane-bound antigen receptors on the surface of B cells.
   B. In secreted form, they serve as effector molecules that facilitate the elimination of microbes or toxins.
   C. They are specific for proteins and polysaccharides exclusively.
   D. They bind antigen with average higher affinity than do T cell receptors.
   E. They are present in most biologic fluids in the body.

3. Detection of antibodies specific for a particular microbe is commonly used as evidence of prior infection by that microbe. To obtain these antibodies, blood is collected into tubes and allowed to clot. Antibodies are found in the fraction of the blood that remains fluid after clotting. What is this fluid fraction called?

A. Plasma
B. Serum
C. Lymph
D. Water
E. Urine

4. Each of the following accurately describes most monoclonal antibody preparations EXCEPT:

   A. Single antigen specificity
   B. Production by a B cell hybridoma
   C. Single isotype
   D. Monovalent antibodies, with one antigen-binding site
   E. Known antigen specificity

5. All of the following accurately describe the basic symmetric core structure of an antibody molecule EXCEPT:

   A. Two heavy chains and two light chains
   B. Covalent bonds between heavy chains
   C. Spatial separation of variable regions from constant regions
   D. Covalent bonds between light chains
   E. Ig domains in both heavy and light chains

6. Which one of the following statements does NOT accurately describe the antigen-binding regions of antibody molecules?

   A. The variable regions of heavy and light chains are at the C termini of the polypeptide chains.
   B. The greatest amino acid variability among different antibody molecules is present in the complementarity-determining regions.
   C. The antigen-binding sites are formed by juxtaposition of variable regions of one heavy chain and one light chain.
   D. The variable regions of both light and heavy chains are composed of one immunoglobulin (Ig) domain.
   E. There are six hypervariable loops in each antigen-binding site of an antibody molecule.

7. The structure of which portion of an antibody defines its isotype?

   A. The variable regions of the light chains
   B. The variable regions of the heavy chains
   C. The constant regions of the heavy chains
   D. The J chain
   E. The complementarity-determining regions

8. Which of the following is the major significance of isotypic differences between antibodies?

   A. Some isotypes are more likely to be autoreactive than others.
   B. Isotypes reflect allelic variants of heavy chain genes, and each individual in a population will express only a subset of isotypes.
   C. Only certain isotypes of antibodies are radioactive.

D. Function and bodily distribution of antibodies are determined by isotype.
E. The antigen specificity of antibodies is determined by the isotype.

Questions 9-13

Match each of the descriptions in questions 9-13 with the correct lettered antibody isotype (A-E). (Answers may be used more than once.)

   A. IgA
   B. IgD
   C. IgE
   D. IgG
   E. IgM

9. The secreted form of this isotype forms pentamers around a J chain (   )

10. The most abundant Ig isotype in the blood (   )

11. The isotype only found in membrane-bound form on naive B cells (   )

12. The isotype found predominantly in mucosal secretions (   )

13. The isotype most closely associated with immediate hypersensitivity (allergic) disease (   )

14. The strength of binding between a single antigen-binding site of an Ig molecule and an antigen, which is quantitatively expressed as the dissociation constant, is called:

    A. Avidity
    B. Stickiness
    C. Velcrocity
    D. Affinity
    E. Complementarity

15. Which of the following changes in antibodies made by a single clone of B cells does NOT occur during an immune response?

    A. Single amino acid substitutions (point mutations) in the variable regions
    B. Change from κ to λ light chain isotype
    C. Change from IgM to IgG isotype
    D. Increases in affinity of antibody for antigen
    E. Change from membrane-bound to secreted Ig

Questions 16-20

Match each description in questions 16-20 with the appropriate lettered term (A-I).

    A. Conformational determinant
    B. Linear determinant
    C. Neoantigenic determinant
    D. Hinge region
    E. Immunocomplex
    F. Fab
    G. Fc
    H. Tail piece
    I. Hapten

16. A proteolytic fragment of an antibody molecule that contains an intact antigen-binding site (   )

17. A three-dimensional shape, formed by a portion of a macromolecule, to which an antibody binds (   )

18. A small chemical group recognized by an antibody that is attached to a larger macromolecule (   )

19. The proteolytic fragment of an antibody molecule that contains the heavy chain constant region (   )

20. A region of an antibody molecule that permits bivalent binding of antibodies to pairs of surface epitopes varying in distance from one another (   )

21. All of the following molecules are members of the Ig superfamily EXCEPT:

    A. IgG
    B. T cell antigen receptor
    C. Lymphocyte function–associated antigen-1 (LFA-1)
    D. Class I MHC molecules
    E. Intercellular adhesion molecules-1 (ICAM-1)

22. Which of the following statements about Ig heavy chain isotypes is NOT true?

    A. Differences between isotypes are mostly found in the constant regions of the heavy chains.
    B. IgG and IgA isotypes each include more than one subtype.
    C. Ig molecules of different isotypes differ in their ability to bind to cell surface Ig receptors on cells.
    D. The antigen-binding sites of Ig molecules of two different isotypes can be structurally identical.
    E. Each heavy chain isotype exclusively associates with only one light chain isotype.

23. Antibody proteins from one individual can be immunogens that stimulate anti-Ig humoral responses when injected into another individual of the same or another species. Some anti-Ig antibodies recognize determinants unique to the antibodies produced by a single clone of B cells. These determinants are called

    A. Allotopes
    B. Isotypes
    C. Idiotopes
    D. Rheumatoid factors
    E. Conformational determinants

Questions 24-27

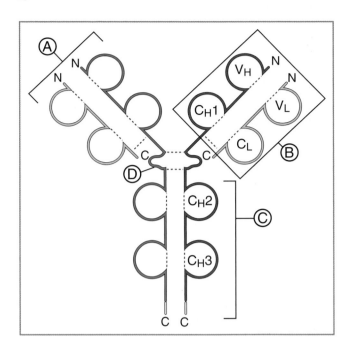

For each region of an antibody molecule described in questions 24-27, match the lettered (A-D) label from the schematic diagram above.

24. Fc (   )

25. Fab (   )

26. Hinge (   )

27. Antigen-binding site (   )

Answers

1. (D) Antibodies and T cell receptors are the clonally distributed antigen receptors made by B and T lymphocytes, respectively. MHC molecules bind peptide fragments of protein antigens for recognition by T cells. Integrins and selectins serve intercellular adhesive functions. Fc receptors are membrane-bound receptors that bind antibodies. Toll-like receptors recognize microbial products in innate immunity.
   CMI5 44; BI2 64-65

2. (C) Antibodies may be specific for all classes of molecules including protein, polysaccharides, and lipids.
   CMI5 43-44; BI2 65

3. (B) Clots form from the cellular elements of blood, including platelets, and a meshwork of cross-linked coagulation proteins. The acellular fluid phase that is left after clotting is called serum, which contains most of the soluble protein elements of whole blood, except clotting factors.

Plasma is the acellular fluid fraction of unclotted blood, and it does contain all of the soluble protein components of whole blood, including antibodies. Lymph is extracellular fluid derived from blood; it may contain antibodies. Urine is the fluid filtrate of blood exclusively produced and excreted by the kidneys. It normally does not contain antibodies.
CMI5 44

4. (D) Monoclonal antibodies are, by definition, identical antibodies of a single isotype and antigen specificity, produced by a single clone of cells. They are usually produced in vitro by clonal B cell hybridomas and are structurally normal, with at least two antigen-binding sites and a known specificity. Tumors of B lymphocytes (e.g., myelomas) may produce monoclonal antibodies, usually of unknown specificity, or often single chains of antibody molecules.
CMI5 45-47; BI2 69-70

5. (D) Although each light chain of an antibody molecule is covalently linked to a heavy chain by a disulfide bond, the light chains are not linked to one another.
CMI5 48; BI2 66-67

6. (A) The variable regions are at the N termini of the heavy and light chains.
CMI5 48-49; BI2 66-67

7. (C) Isotypes are defined by the structure of the constant regions of the heavy chains, which are the portions of antibody molecules that interact with Ig receptors on cells and complement proteins. There are no characteristics of the variable regions of heavy and light chains that are typical of any particular isotype. The J chain is an invariant protein that serves to bind subunits of IgA or IgM together. The complementarity-determining regions are the hypervariable loops of the variable regions of heavy and light chains.
CMI5 51-53; BI2 68-69

8. (D) Isotypic differences reflect structural differences in the constant regions of heavy chains, which are the regions that interact with Ig receptors on cells and with complement proteins. Therefore, the transport of antibodies between body compartments, the clearance of antibodies by phagocytic cells, and the functions of antibodies related to phagocytosis of antibody-bound antigens or activation of complement vary from one isotype to another. The specificity of antibodies for either foreign or self antigens is a function of the variable regions and not the isotype. Although there are some allelic variants of each isotype, all normal individuals produce all the Ig isotypes. Isotypes should not be confused with elemental isotopes, some of which are radioactive.
CMI5 51-54; BI2 68-69

9. (E) IgM is secreted as a J chain–linked pentamer.
CMI5 44, 53; BI2 69

10. (D) The blood IgG concentration is about 3.5 mg/mL and includes four subtypes (IgG1 to IgG4).
CMI5 51-54; BI2 69

11. (B) IgD is not secreted and is found only on the surface of naive B cells. Its function is not well understood.
CMI5 53; BI2 69

12. (A) IgA accounts for almost two thirds of the 3 g of antibody produced each day by an adult, most of which is produced in the gastrointestinal mucosa.
CMI5 51-54; BI2 69

13. (C) Most IgE that is secreted is bound to mast cells, and it plays a role in the activation of mast cells during allergic reactions.
CMI5 53, 433-452; BI2 69, 193-207

14. (D) The affinity of antibody molecules for antigens, expressed as the dissociation constant, ranges from 10^{-7} to 10^{-11} M. Avidity, which is the overall strength of attachment of an antibody molecule to antigen, is a function of both affinity and the number of binding sites. A pentameric IgM molecule with 10 binding sites will generally have higher avidity than a monomeric IgG molecule with two binding sites. *Velcrocity* and *stickiness* are not immunologic terms. *Complementarity* refers to the fit between antigen-binding site and antigen but implies nothing about strength of binding.
CMI5 60; BI2 68

15. (B) The Ig light chain isotype is fixed by genetic events during B cell development and cannot change in mature B cells during an immune response. Single amino acid changes occur during antibody responses to protein antigens and may lead to increases in affinity of the antibodies produced. Heavy chain isotype switching from IgM to other isotypes, as well as transition from production of membrane-bound to secreted forms of antibody, are normal occurrences during humoral immune responses.
CMI5 61-63; BI2 68, 133-139

16. (F) Fab fragments, derived from enzymatic cleavage of Ig molecules, are composed of one intact light chain covalently linked to the N-terminal region of one heavy chain and include a single intact antigen-binding site.
CMI5 55-57

17. (A) Conformational determinants will usually be destroyed by physicochemical disruption of macromolecules, such as by denaturation or proteolysis of proteins.
CMI5 58-59; BI2 68

18. (I) Although haptens can be recognized by antibodies, they are not, by themselves, able to stimulate an antibody response (i.e., they are not immunogens). Antibody responses to haptens can

be induced when the hapten is attached to a macro-molecule, called a carrier.
CMI5 58

19. (G) The Fc fragment, generated by proteolytic cleavage of an antibody molecule, is composed of the C-terminal end of the heavy chain and lacks the antigen-binding region. This region of an intact Ig molecule, which can interact with Ig receptors and complement, is called the Fc region.
CMI5 55-57; BI2 66-67

20. (D) The hinge region, located between the two N-terminal Ig domains of the heavy chains of most isotypes, is flexible, permitting variations in the distance between the two antigen-binding sites.
CMI5 54-55; BI2 67

21. (C) Lymphocyte function–associated antigen-1 (LFA-1) is a member of the integrin family; it does not contain an Ig domain.
CMI5 50-51; BI2 89,108

22. (E) Either light chain isotype (κ or λ) can associate with any of the heavy chain isotypes. Isotypes are defined by the amino acid sequences of the constant regions of the heavy chains. Furthermore, the IgG isotype has four subtypes and the IgA isotype has two subtypes. Each Ig isotype may perform distinct functions based on differences in binding to cell surface Fc receptors. During heavy chain isotype switching, the antigen-binding variable region of antibodies produced by a B cell clone remains unchanged and therefore antibodies of two different isotypes can share identical antigen-binding sites.
CMI5 51-54; BI2 66-68

23. (C) Idiotopes are formed by the hypervariable regions of antibody molecules, which are encoded by unique genetic sequences found only in single B cell clones or by invariant variable region sequences found in antibodies produced by many clones of B1

B cells. All the antibodies that contain the same idio*tope* are said to be of the same idio*type*. Allotopes are different determinants encoded by allelic differences in conserved regions of antibodies, and isotypes are encoded by distinct heavy chain genes. Production of both anti-allotope and anti-isotype antibodies can be stimulated by Ig immunization. Rheumatoid factors are anti-IgG antibodies found in the setting of some autoimmune diseases. Conformational determinants, which are dependent on the three-dimensional folding of protein antigens, are not unique to Ig molecules.
CMI5 54, 150-151; BI2 67

24. (C) The Fc region corresponds to the Fc fragment derived by proteolytic cleavage of an IgG molecule and includes the heavy chain constant region domains. The Fc region contains the sites that bind to membrane Ig Fc receptors on other cells and the complement protein C1q.
CMI5 48; BI2 6

25. (B) The Fab region corresponds to the Fab fragment derived by proteolytic cleavage of an IgG molecule and includes one intact light chain paired with the N-terminal two Ig domains of the one heavy chain.
CMI5 48; BI2 6

26. (D) The hinge region is a part of the heavy chain of Ig molecules and is generally found between the C_H1 and C_H2 domains. The amino acid composition of the hinge region confers a flexibility to the conformation of the heavy chain, allowing the two antigen-binding sites to be at varying distances from one another.
CMI5 48; BI2 6

27. (A) The antigen-binding site is composed of the paired N-terminal Ig variable domains of the heavy and light chains. There are two identical antigen-binding sites in each IgG molecule.
CMI5 48; BI2 6

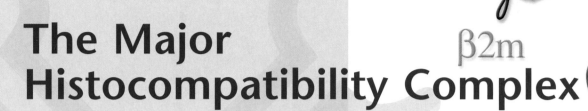

Chapter 4

The Major Histocompatibility Complex

Cellular and Molecular Immunology, 5/E: Chapter 4—The Major Histocompatibility Complex

Basic Immunology, 2/E: Chapter 3—Antigen Capture and Presentation to Lymphocytes

1. The major histocompatibility complex (MHC) was originally discovered by which of the following types of studies?

   A. Analysis of the human genome sequence
   B. Polymerase chain reaction (PCR) amplification of genes expressed in lymphocytes
   C. Genetic studies of transplant rejection and transfusion reactions
   D. Purification and sequencing of dendritic cell membrane proteins
   E. Studies of the pattern of inheritance of immune responsiveness to certain proteins

2. Which one of the following descriptions of class I MHC molecules is NOT true?

   A. The principal function of class I MHC molecules is to display peptides derived from cytosolic proteins on the cell surface.
   B. Class I MHC molecules bind to CD8 molecules on T cells.
   C. Human class I MHC molecules include HLA-A, HLA-B, and HLA-C.
   D. Class I MHC molecules are normally expressed only on dendritic cells and other professional antigen-presenting cells.
   E. A cell expresses class I MHC molecules encoded by genes inherited from both parents.

3. Which of the following statements about class II MHC molecules is NOT true?

   A. Class II MHC molecules bind peptides derived from extracellular proteins.
   B. Class II MHC molecules bind to CD4 molecules on T cells.
   C. Class II MHC molecules are expressed on a limited number of cell types, including dendritic cells.
   D. HLA-DR and HLA-DQ are human class II MHC molecules.
   E. Class II MHC molecules are not expressed on cells that express class I MHC molecules.

4. Which one of the following statements about polymorphism of MHC genes is NOT true?

   A. There are many allelic variants of MHC genes in outbred populations.
   B. MHC polymorphism is generated by somatic recombination of gene segments encoding different exons of MHC molecules.
   C. MHC polymorphism is the major barrier to acceptance of allogeneic organ grafts.
   D. Two allelic variants of an MHC molecule are most likely to differ in amino acid sequences around their peptide-binding clefts.
   E. Both class I and class II MHC genes are polymorphic.

5. A patient with chronic renal failure undergoes transplantation of a kidney donated by his older brother. During the first month after transplantation, there is clinical evidence of immunologic rejection of the graft. Which one of the following statements about the patient is true?

   A. Graft rejection was most likely due to the patient's immune response to allelic forms of MHC molecules found in both the patient and his brother.
   B. Future attempts at transplantation in this patient may be complicated by the presence of preformed antibodies specific for his brother's MHC alleles.
   C. CD4⁺ T cells in the patient recognized allogeneic class I MHC molecules expressed by cells in the kidney graft.
   D. The patient and his brother cannot share any class II MHC alleles.
   E. The kidney graft was syngeneic to the patient.

6. Which of the following is NOT a feature of class I MHC molecules?

   A. Class I MHC molecules bind peptides of 8-11 amino residues.
   B. Class I MHC molecules bind to CD8 molecules.
   C. The peptide-binding region of class I MHC molecules is composed of parts of both α and β chains.
   D. The nonpolymorphic polypeptide β_2-microglobulin is a part of class I MHC molecules.
   E. Class I MHC molecules are members of the immunoglobulin superfamily.

7. Which of the following is NOT a feature of class II MHC molecules?

   A. Class II MHC molecules bind to T cell receptors on CD8⁺ T cells.
   B. Stable cell surface expression of class II MHC molecules requires the presence of peptide in the peptide-binding cleft.
   C. Class II MHC molecules are composed of a heterodimer of two transmembrane polypeptide chains, both of which contain extracellular Ig-like domains.
   D. The peptide-binding cleft of class II MHC molecules accommodates peptides of up to 30 amino acid residues in size.
   E. Polymorphic residues of class II MHC molecules are mostly located in the N-terminal region of the β chain.

8. Which one of the following statements about peptide binding to MHC molecules is true?

   A. MHC molecules preferentially bind peptides derived from foreign (e.g., microbial) proteins and not peptides derived from self proteins.
   B. Each type of MHC molecule and each allelic variant of each type have a narrow specificity for a single peptide with a particular amino acid sequence.
   C. The affinity of peptide binding to MHC molecules is higher, on average, after chemokine stimulation of a cell.
   D. An MHC molecule has only one peptide-binding site, which accommodates only a single peptide at a time.
   E. Peptide binding to class I MHC molecules involves noncovalent interactions, whereas peptide binding to class II MHC molecules is covalent.

9. Which of the following statements about the human MHC is NOT true?

   A. It is located on chromosome 6.
   B. It includes genes encoding cytokines of the innate immune system.
   C. It includes genes encoding the transporter associated with antigen processing (TAP) and proteasome proteins required for antigen processing.
   D. It includes genes encoding both chains of class I MHC molecules.
   E. It is larger than the entire genome of many bacteria.

10. A 2-year-old child suffers from recurrent bacterial and viral infections. Immunologic workup of the patient reveals very low or absent class II MHC expression on any cells examined, including dendritic cells and B cells. Which of the following mutations is a likely cause of impaired class II MHC expression in this patient?

    A. Mutation of the *CIITA* gene
    B. Mutation of the interferon-α gene
    C. Mutations in the Ig ε heavy chain gene

D. Mutation of an HLA-A β chain gene

E. Mutation of the gene encoding one of the chains of the transporter associated with antigen processing (TAP)

Questions 11-15

Match each of the definitions in questions 11-15 with the MHC nomenclature (A-F).

A. HLA-A1, -B7, -Cw4, -DPw5, -DQw10, -DR8
B. H-2
C. HLA-DQ7
D. I-A^d
E. HLA-B5
F. H-2K^{d}I-A^{d}I-E^{d}D^{d}L^d

11. Human class I MHC allele (   )

12. Mouse class II MHC allele (   )

13. Mouse major histocompatibility complex (   )

14. Human MHC haplotype (   )

15. Inbred mouse strain MHC haplotype (   )

Questions 16-19

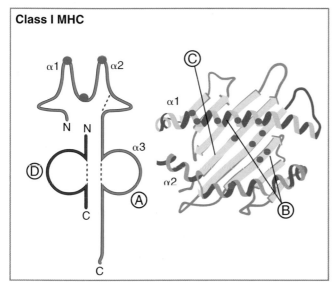

Class I MHC

For each region of a class I MHC molecule listed in questions 16-19, match the lettered label (A-D) from the diagram shown above.

16. Peptide-binding groove (   )

17. CD8-binding site (   )

18. β$_2$-Microglobulin (   )

19. Polymorphic region (   )

20. What is the name of a nonpolymorphic molecule that is structurally homologous to the class I MHC α chain, associates with β$_2$-microglobulin, and displays nonpeptide antigens for recognition by subsets of T cells with limited T cell receptor diversity?

A. CD1
B. CD2
C. CD3
D. CD4
E. CD8

Answers

1. (C) The existence of the major histocompatibility complex (MHC) was first discovered in mouse studies involving transplantation of tumors and then normal tissues between inbred mouse strains. The human MHC was discovered by studies of the presence of antibodies in transfusion and transplant, recipients that recognized antigens on leukocyte cell surfaces. The development of the polymerase chain reaction (PCR) technique and large-scale human genome sequencing occurred decades after the MHC was discovered. The MHC was not discovered by reverse genetics after protein purification and sequencing. Although the discovery of the role of MHC genes controlling immune responsiveness to nonallogeneic antigens was a fundamental advance in understanding the physiologic role of MHC molecules, this advance occurred many years after the MHC was defined as a locus controlling alloantigen responses.
CMI5 66-69; BI2 47

2. (D) Class I MHC molecules are expressed by almost all nucleated cells.   The principal function of both class I and class II MHC molecules is peptide display for T cell immunosurveillance. Class I MHC molecules display peptides derived from cytosolic proteins for recognition by CD8$^+$ T cells. CD8 binds to nonpolymorphic parts of the class I MHC α chain. The MHC genes inherited from both parents are codominantly expressed on cells.
CMI5 65-68; BI2 47-53

3. (E) Class I MHC molecules are ubiquitously expressed on all nucleated cells, including the more limited subset of cells that also express class II MHC molecules, such as dendritic cells. CD4 binds to the nonpolymorphic β$_2$ domain of class II MHC molecules. HLA-DP, HLA-DQ, and HLA-DR are the three types of human class II MHC molecules. The function of class II MHC molecules is to bind and display peptides derived from proteins in the extracellular environment.
CMI5 69-70; BI2 47-53

4. (B) MHC polymorphisms have been generated as an evolutionary process by mechanisms such as gene conversion and not by somatic events in one individual. Somatic recombination is the mechanism of generating antigen receptor diversity in each individual. MHC polymorphism refers to the presence of many different allelic variants of MHC genes in the population, but each individual inherits no more than two different alleles of each MHC gene. Both class I and class II MHC genes are polymorphic, although class I MHC genes are more polymorphic than class II MHC genes. The location of polymorphic amino acid residues in MHC molecules is concentrated in the peptide-binding grooves. Allelic differences in MHC genes are recognized by the adaptive immune system, and this is

the strongest immunologic barrier to successful grafting between individuals.
CMI5 66-72; BI2 48

5. (B) Exposure to another individual's MHC molecules, because of prior blood transfusions, organ transplants, or pregnancies, induces the production of MHC-specific alloantibodies. These antibodies can mediate rejection of grafts expressing the MHC molecules for which the antibodies are specific. The patient will not react to the MHC proteins encoded by shared MHC alleles because of self tolerance. Alloreactive CD4+ T cells recognize class II MHC molecules, not class I MHC molecules. The patient and his brother will share some class II MHC alleles that they both inherited from the same parent, but they are not genetically identical; therefore, the graft is not syngeneic to the patient.
CMI5 66-69; BI2 47-53

6. (C) The peptide-binding cleft of a class I MHC molecule is formed exclusively from the N-terminal end of a single α chain, in contrast to the peptide-binding cleft of class II MHC molecules, which is formed by the N-terminal ends of both α and β chains. The class I MHC binding cleft has closed ends and accommodates peptides of 8 to 11 amino acids, compared with the open-ended cleft of class II MHC molecules, which can bind peptides up to 30 amino acids long. Both the class I MHC α chain and the noncovalently associated β_2-microglobulin contain Ig-like domains, and therefore class I MHC molecules are members of the Ig superfamily. The Ig domain of the α chain binds to CD8.
CMI5 70-71; BI2 47-53

7. (A) Class II MHC molecules on the surface of antigen-presenting cells bind T cell receptors on CD4+ T cells and simultaneously bind the CD4 molecules. Stable surface expression of both class II and class I MHC molecules requires peptides to be bound within the peptide-binding grooves. Class II MHC molecules are composed of heterodimers of α and β chains, both of which have Ig-like domains. The peptide-binding cleft of class II MHC molecules is open ended and binds polypeptides of 10 to 30 amino acid residues. Most of the polymorphism of class II MHC molecules is limited to the N-terminal β chain, even though the N termini of both α and β chains contribute to the formation of the peptide-binding cleft.
CMI5 71-73; BI2 47-53

8. (D) There is only one peptide-binding site in both class I and class II MHC molecules that can fit only a single peptide at one time. MHC molecules do not distinguish foreign from self proteins; self-nonself discrimination is achieved by T cells. Each MHC molecule has a broad specificity for large numbers of peptides with varying sequences, although there are some structural constraints that result in each type of MHC molecule binding a different subset of peptides. The affinity of peptide-MHC interactions is not altered by chemokines. Peptide binding to both class I and class II MHC molecules involves only noncovalent interactions.
CMI5 73-77; BI2 49-53

9. (D) Only the polymorphic α chain of class I MHC molecules is encoded by a gene in the MHC, which is located on chromosome 6. The smaller, nonpolymorphic β_2-microglobulin is encoded by a gene outside the MHC, on chromosome 15. In addition to the polymorphic genes encoding class I and II MHC polypeptides, the MHC includes genes encoding tumor necrosis factor-α, lymphotoxin, and lymphotoxin β, which are cytokines of innate immunity. Also within the MHC are genes encoding the transporter in antigen processing (TAP), proteasomal subunits, and HLA-DM, which are all involved in antigen processing and presentation. The MHC is about 3500 kilobases long, which is larger than many bacterial genomes.
CMI5 76-78; BI2 47-48

10. (A) CIITA (class II transcription activator) is a protein required for the transcriptional activation of class II MHC genes, and mutations of the *CIITA* gene are a cause of severe immunodeficiency diseases in children. Interferon-α induces class I MHC expression but is not required for class II MHC expression. Ig ε heavy chain, a part of IgE molecules, has no direct effect on class II MHC expression. HLA-A is a class I MHC molecule, and TAP is involved in peptide loading of class I MHC, not class II MHC.
CMI5 78-80

11. (E) There are three human class I genes, *HLA-A*, *HLA-B*, and *HLA-C*, and each gene has many allelic forms, designated by numbers following A, B, or C.
CMI5 68-69; BI2 47

12. (D) The mouse class II MHC genes include *I-A* and *I-E*, and the allelic forms of each are designated by superscripted letters.
CMI5 68-69; BI2 47

13. (B) The mouse MHC is called the *H-2* complex.
CMI5 68-69; BI2 47

14. (A) An MHC haplotype is a complement of MHC genes on one chromosome, inherited from one parent. A human MHC haplotype (or HLA haplotype) includes single alleles of *HLA-A*, *HLA-B*, and *HLA-C* genes encoding class I MHC molecules, and *HLA-DP*, *HLA-DQ*, and *HLA-DR* genes, encoding class II MHC molecules.
CMI5 68-69

15. (F) A mouse MHC *(H-2)* haplotype from an inbred mouse strain will include one allele each of K, D, and L class I MHC genes and one allele each of *I-A* and *I-E* class II MHC genes. In an inbred strain, all the alleles have the same letter designation and the mice are homozygous for these alleles.
CMI5 68-69

16. (C) The peptide-binding groove of class I MHC molecules is formed by approximately 90 amino acids of the N-terminal α heavy chain, which includes the α1 and α2 domains. This groove is composed of a floor of β-pleated sheet and two parallel strands of α helix.
CMI5 71, 73; BI2 49

17. (A) Class I MHC molecules bind to CD8 on T cells via the α3 Ig domain of the α heavy chain.
CMI5 73; BI2 49

18. (D) β_2-Microglobulin is a separate polypeptide containing a single Ig domain, which is noncovalently associated with the extracellular region of the α heavy chain of class I MHC molecules.
CMI5 73; BI2 49

19. (B) All the polymorphic residues of class I MHC molecules are in the walls or floor of the peptide-binding groove.
CMI5 73; BI2 49

20. (A) CD1 is encoded outside the MHC, but is structurally homologous to class I MHC molecules. Some subsets of T cells, all with invariant T cell receptors, recognize lipid or glycolipid antigens bound to CD1 on antigen-presenting cells. CD2, CD3, CD4, and CD8 are all present on these T cells. Although they are members of the Ig superfamily, like class I MHC, they are not otherwise homologous to class I MHC and do not bind and display antigens for T cell recognition.
CMI5 77

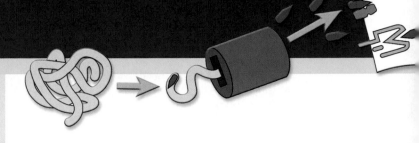

Chapter 5

Antigen Processing and Presentation to T Lymphocytes

Cellular and Molecular Immunology, 5/E: Chapter 5—Antigen Processing and Presentation to T Lymphocytes

Basic Immunology, 2/E: Chapter 3—Antigen Capture and Presentation of Lymphocytes

1. Antigen-presenting cells (APCs) perform which of the following functions in adaptive immune responses?

   A. Display major histocompatibility complex (MHC)-associated peptides on their cell surfaces for surveillance by B lymphocytes
   B. Initiate T cell responses by specifically recognizing and responding to foreign protein antigens
   C. Display MHC-associated peptides on their cell surfaces for surveillance by T lymphocytes
   D. Display polysaccharide antigens on their cell surfaces for surveillance by B lymphocytes
   E. Secrete peptides derived from protein antigens for binding to T cell antigen receptors

2. A child who suffers from a persistent viral infection is found to have a deficiency in lymphocyte production and very few T and B cells. Other bone marrow–derived cells are produced in normal numbers, and MHC molecule expression on cells appears normal. Transfusion of mature T cells from an unrelated donor who had recovered from a previous infection by the same virus would not be expected to help the child clear his infection. Which one of the following is a reasonable explanation for why this therapeutic approach would fail?

A. Viral infections are cleared by antibodies, not T cells.
B. The patient's own immune system would destroy the transfused T cells before they could respond to the viral infection.
C. T cells recognize peptides, not viral particles.
D. Donor T cell viral antigen recognition is restricted by MHC molecules not expressed in the patient.
E. In responding to the previous infection, the donor would have used up all his T cells specific for that virus.

3. Many vaccines now in development will include highly purified, recombinant, or synthetic peptide antigens. These vaccine antigens are expected to stimulate highly specific immune responses, but they are less immunogenic than vaccines containing intact killed or live microbes. Adjuvants are substances added to such vaccines to enhance their ability to elicit T cell immune responses. Which of the following statements about adjuvants is NOT correct?

A. Adjuvants induce local inflammation, thereby increasing the number of antigen-presenting cells (APCs) at the site of immunization.
B. Adjuvants stimulate the expression of costimulators on local APCs.
C. Adjuvants enhance local production of cytokines that promote T cell activation.
D. Adjuvants prolong the expression of peptide-MHC complexes on the surface of APCs.
E. Adjuvants bind to T cell antigen receptors and promote their proliferation.

4. A helper T cell response to a protein antigen requires the participation of antigen-presenting cells that express which of the following types of molecules?

A. Class II MHC and costimulators
B. Class I MHC and CD4
C. Class II MHC and CD8
D. CD4 and costimulators
E. Class II MHC and CD4

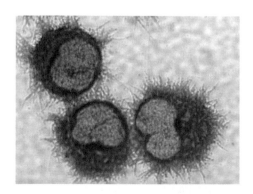

5. The cell type shown above is found between follicles in lymph nodes and expresses B7-1, B7-2, and class II MHC. What type of cell is this?

A. B cell
B. Follicular dendritic cell
C. Thymic epithelial cell
D. Dendritic cell
E. Plasma cell

6. Which type of antigen-presenting cell is most important for activating naive T cells?

A. Macrophage
B. Dendritic cell
C. Endothelial cell
D. B lymphocyte
E. Epithelial cell

7. Which of the following statements about the antigen-presenting function of macrophages is NOT correct?

A. Macrophages are particularly important at presenting peptides derived from particulate or opsonized antigens that are internalized by phagocytosis.
B. Macrophages become activated by the helper T cells to which they present microbial peptides, and as a result of this activation they become efficient at killing the microbes.
C. Resting macrophages express low levels of class II MHC molecules, but higher class II MHC expression is induced on activation by the T cells to which they present antigen.
D. Macrophages express highly variable, high-affinity receptors for many different antigens, and these receptors facilitate the internalization of the antigens for processing and presentation.
E. Macrophages present antigen to T cells in lymphoid organs and many nonlymphoid organs.

8. Which one of the following statements about dendritic cells is true?

A. Immature dendritic cells are ubiquitously present in skin and mucosal tissues.
B. Dendritic cell maturation occurs after migration to lymph nodes in response to signals derived from activated T cells.
C. Class II MHC and T cell costimulators are highly expressed on immature dendritic cells and are down-regulated during maturation.
D. Dendritic cells that enter lymph nodes through draining lymphatics migrate to the B cell-rich follicles in response to chemokines.
E. The principal function of mature dendritic cells is antigen capture.

9. Maturing dendritic cells that migrate to a lymph node from peripheral tissues end up mainly in:

A. Follicles
B. High endothelial venules
C. The medullary sinus
D. T cell zones
E. Efferent arterioles

10. A young adult is exposed to a virus that infects and replicates in mucosal epithelial cells of the upper respiratory tract. One component of the protective immune response to this viral infection is mediated by CD8$^+$ cytolytic T lymphocytes (CTLs), which recognize and kill virus-infected cells. The CTLs can recognize and kill the infected cells because:

    A. In response to interferon-γ secreted during the innate immune response to the virus, the mucosal epithelial cells express class II MHC, with bound viral peptides, on their cell surfaces.
    B. Mucosal epithelial cells, like all nucleated cells, express class I MHC molecules and are able to process cytoplasmic viral proteins and display complexes of class I MHC and bound viral peptides on their cell surfaces.
    C. Antibodies specific for viral antigens bind to these antigens on infected cell surfaces and engage Ig Fc receptors on the CTL, thereby targeting the CTL to the infected cells.
    D. Virus-infected mucosal epithelial cells migrate to draining lymphoid tissues, where they present viral peptide antigens to naive CD8$^+$ T cells.
    E. Viral infection of the mucosal epithelial cells stimulates them to express E-selectin, which promotes CD8$^+$ T cell adhesion.

11. Naive CD8$^+$ T cells require signals in addition to T cell receptor recognition of peptide-MHC to become activated and differentiate into cytolytic T cells. These signals are called costimulatory signals and are provided by professional antigen-presenting cells (APCs), such as dendritic cells. If a virus infects epithelial cells in the respiratory tract but does not infect professional APCs, what process ensures that naive T cells specific for viral antigens will become activated?

    A. Cross-reactivity, whereby the naive CD8$^+$ T cell recognizes a self antigen that is structurally similar to a viral antigen presented by dendritic cells
    B. Crossover, whereby part of the viral genome is exchanged with part of one chromosome of the host
    C. Crosstalk, whereby signals generated by the virus binding to class I MHC molecules intersect with T cell receptor signaling pathways
    D. Cross-presentation, whereby infected epithelial cells are captured by dendritic cells, and the viral proteins originally synthesized in the epithelial cells are processed and presented in association with class I MHC molecules on the dendritic cell
    E. Cross-dressing, whereby viral infection of the epithelial cell stimulates the expression of surface molecules that are typically found only on dendritic cells

12. Which of the following is the main criterion that determines whether a protein is processed and presented via the class I MHC pathway in an antigen-presenting cell (APC)?

    A. Encoded by a viral gene
    B. Present in an acidic vesicular compartment of the APC
    C. Present in the cytosol of the APC
    D. Internalized into the cell from the extracellular space
    E. Small in size

13. Which one of the following molecules does NOT play an important role in the class II MHC pathway of antigen presentation?

    A. β_2-Microglobulin
    B. Cathepsin
    C. Invariant chain
    D. HLA-DM
    E. Calnexin

14. In the class I MHC pathway of antigen presentation, peptides generated in the cytosol are translocated into the endoplasmic reticulum in which of the following ways?

    A. By ATP-dependent transport via the transporter associated with antigen-processing (TAP) 1/2 pump
    B. By passive diffusion
    C. By receptor-mediated endocytosis
    D. Through membrane pores
    E. Via the proteasome

15. In the class I MHC pathway of antigen presentation, cytoplasmic proteins are tagged for proteolytic degradation by covalent linkage with which of the following molecules?

    A. Calreticulin
    B. Nuclear factor (NF)-κB
    C. Tapasin
    D. Ubiquitin
    E. Calnexin

Questions 16-20

Match the description in questions 16-20 with the lettered item (A-I) related to antigen-presentation pathways.

    A. T cell receptor on CD4$^+$ T cells
    B. Endosomes
    C. Endoplasmic reticulum
    D. MHC class II compartment/class II vesicle (MIIC/CIIV)
    E. Class II-associated invariant chain peptide (CLIP)
    F. LMP-2 and LMP-7
    G. Acidic proteases
    H. T cell receptor on CD8$^+$ T cells
    I. HLA-DM

16. Site of proteolysis of antigens in the class II MHC pathway (   )

17. Site of peptide loading of class II MHC molecules ( )

18. The molecule that binds to the final product of the class II antigen-presenting pathway ( )

19. Required for proteolytic generation of class I MHC-binding peptides ( )

20. Site of peptide loading of class I MHC molecules ( )

21. Which one of the following statements about T cell tolerance to self proteins is accurate?

    A. Self proteins are not presented by the class I pathway because only microbial proteins, and not self proteins, are ubiquinated in the cytosol.
    B. Peptides derived from self proteins are not presented by the class I or class II pathways because MHC molecules are expressed only in response to infections.
    C. Self proteins are not presented by the class II pathway because endosomal acidic proteases digest microbial proteins but not eukaryotic proteins.
    D. Self peptide/self MHC complexes are formed and displayed by antigen-presenting cells in both class I and class II MHC pathways, but T cells that recognize these complexes usually are not present or are functionally inactive.
    E. Peptides derived from self proteins are not displayed by MHC molecules because they usually are displaced by the more abundant microbial peptides.

22. In a clinical trial of a new antiviral vaccine composed of a recombinant viral peptide and adjuvant, 4% of the healthy recipients did not show evidence of response to the immunization. Further investigation revealed that all the nonresponders expressed the same, single allelic variant of HLA-DR but all the responders were heterozygous for HLA-DR alleles. Which of the following is the most likely explanation for this finding?

    A. Response to the vaccine requires T cell recognition of complexes of the viral peptide with HLA-DR, but the peptide cannot bind to the allelic variant of HLA-DR found in the nonresponders.
    B. The nonresponders could not express class II MHC proteins.
    C. The viral peptide is not an immunodominant epitope.
    D. The nonresponders underwent determinant selection of another viral epitope.
    E. Because of technical errors, the nonresponders had not received adequate doses of the vaccine.

23. The required number of complexes of a microbial peptide and a particular class II MHC allele on the surface of an antigen-presenting cell to initiate a T cell response specific for the viral peptide is:

    A. At least equal to the number of complexes of self peptides with class II MHC on the cell surface

B. Greater than 10^3
C. Less than or equal to 0.1% of the total number of class II MHC molecules on the cell surface
D. Greater than 10^6
E. Zero

Answers

1. (C) Antigen-presenting cells (APCs) degrade proteins derived from either the extracellular environment or the cytoplasm. They form complexes of peptide fragments of these proteins with major histocompatability complex (MHC) molecules and display these complexes on their cell surfaces, where T cells can "see" them. Neither processing nor MHC association of protein or polysaccharide antigens by B cells is required for recognition. APCs do not distinguish between self and foreign proteins and will display peptides derived from a sampling of all cytoplasmic and extracellular proteins. APCs do not secrete peptide antigens, and T cell antigen receptors do not bind free peptides.
CMI5 81-84; BI2 43-46

2. (D) T cells are "self MHC restricted," meaning they specifically recognize infected cells that display microbial peptides displayed by self MHC molecules. There may be no MHC molecules shared by donor and patient, and therefore the transfused T cells would not recognize virus-infected cells in the patient. Because the patient has very few B cells and T cells, his immune system is unlikely to be able to recognize and destroy (i.e., "reject") the transfused T cells. T cells do not recognize structures on intact viral particles but rather peptides derived from viral proteins bound to MHC molecules. Prior viral infection in the donor would be expected to generate memory T cells specific for the virus.
CMI5 81-84; BI2 42-43

3. (E) Adjuvants are not necessarily T cell antigens. Some adjuvants may be T cell antigens, but their adjuvant activity is unrelated to their ability to be recognized, in peptide form, by T cells. Adjuvants are surrogates of the innate immune response to a microbe, required along with antigen component of a vaccine for naive T cell activation. Adjuvants stimulate local inflammation, influx of antigen-presenting cells (APCs), and activation of APCs to secrete cytokines and express costimulatory molecules, and they prolong peptide-MHC expression on the APC membrane.
CMI5 85; BI2 37

4. (A) Helper T cells are almost always CD4+. The activation of naive CD4+ T cells requires T cell receptor recognition of class II MHC-peptide complexes and the binding of costimulators, both on the antigen-presenting cell (APC) surface. CD4+ helper T cells bind to class II MHC molecules on the APC, not to class I MHC molecules. CD4 or CD8

expression on the APC surface is of no known relevance to T cell activation.
CMI5 85; BI2 59

5. (D) Dendritic cells have delicate cytoplasmic extensions, which may serve to enhance interactions with T cells. They express molecules required for naive T cell activation, and they migrate from infected tissues into the parafollicular (T cell) areas of lymph nodes.
CMI5 87; BI2 43-44

6. (B) Dendritic cells are the key type of antigen-presenting cell (APC) for activation of naive T cells and initiation of T cell immune responses. Macrophages and B lymphocytes function as APCs for already differentiated effector T cells in cell-mediated and humoral immune responses, respectively. Epithelial cells usually do not function as APCs.
CMI5 86-87; BI2 43-44

7. (D) The description of high-affinity and highly variable receptors for antigen applies to B cells, which can present antigen to helper T cells, but does not apply to macrophages. Macrophages express receptors for the Fc region of Ig molecules, and these receptors do facilitate internalization of antibody-opsonized antigens. These Fc receptors are not highly variable and do not recognize the antigen. Macrophages are also highly competent at internalizing intact microbes and other large particulate antigens through phagocytosis. Macrophage class II MHC expression and microbicidal activity are enhanced by signals from the T cells to which they present antigen, including cytokines and CD40 ligand. Macrophages are abundant in spleen, lymph nodes, and most nonlymphoid tissues. They may perform antigen-presenting functions in all these locations.
CMI5 86-87; BI2 59, 95-96

8. (A) Tissues that are barriers between the external environment and the inside of the body, such as skin and mucosa, are rich in resting dendritic cells. In this location, the dendritic cells are well positioned to internalize samples of the environment and respond to innate immune system signals, which will drive their maturation into competent antigen-presenting cells. Dendritic cell maturation occurs during migration from infected tissues via lymphatics to the T cell zones of draining lymph nodes. Maturation must occur before, and is required for, activation of T cells, not vice versa. Class II MHC molecule up-regulation occurs during dendritic cell maturation and is one of the changes that make mature dendritic cells better able to present antigen to CD4+ T.
CMI5 86, 88-90; BI2 43-47

9. (D) Migrating dendritic cells express the chemokine receptor CCR7 and move into the T cell zones, where SLC and ELC, the chemokines that bind CCR7, are expressed. In this location, the dendritic cells they are most likely to interact with are naive T cells that also migrate to the same area.
CMI5 88-89; BI2 43-47

10. (B) Differentiated CD8+ cytolytic T lymphocytes (CTLs) can recognize class I–associated viral peptides on epithelial cells, as well as most other cell types, and become activated to kill those cells. Interferon-γ may be secreted during the innate immune response to a virus, and this cytokine can up-regulate both class I and class II MHC expression of various cell types, but CD8+ T cells do not recognize class II–associated peptides. Antibodies may form a bridge between Fc receptor-bearing natural killer cells and infected cells expressing viral antigens on their surface, but this phenomenon does not apply to CD8+ CTLs. Mucosal epithelial cells do not migrate to draining lymph nodes in response to viral infection, nor do they express E-selectin, which is an endothelium-specific adhesion molecule.
CMI5 90; BI2 55-58

11. (D) Cross-presentation (or cross-priming) is the phenomenon by which a protein antigen made within one cell is processed and presented by the class I MHC pathway of a separate professional antigen-presenting cell (APC). Cross-presentation requires that the protein antigen from one cell be internalized from the extracellular milieu into the APC to gain access to the cytoplasm of the APC. *Crossover* and *crosstalk* are terms referring to genetic and signaling phenomena, which are not accurately described in the question. *Cross-dressing* is not a term used in immunology.
CMI5 90-91; BI2 92

12. (C) Regardless of the source of the protein, its presence in the cytosol makes it accessible to the tagging and proteolytic processing mechanisms that initiate the class I MHC antigen presentation pathway. Microbial proteins and self proteins have equal access to this pathway if they are present in the cytosol. Presence in acidic vesicles is the comparable major criterion for inclusion in the class II MHC pathway; such proteins are usually, but not always, internalized from the extracellular space. The size of an intact protein is not relevant to which processing and presentation pathway it will enter.
CMI5 92; BI2 53-58

13. (A) β2-Microglobulin is one of the polypeptide chains of a class I MHC molecule and is required for assembly of the peptide-class I MHC complex. All the other molecules listed are involved in the class II MHC of antigen presentation. Cathepsins are acid proteases that degrade proteins in acidic vesicles in the class II MHC pathway. The invariant chain directs appropriate sorting of new class II MHC molecules from the Golgi to endosomes, and it protects the class II MHC peptide binding groove from occupancy by peptides until the class II MHC molecules are delivered to the endosome. Calnexin

is an endoplasmic reticulum chaperone involved in the assembly of both class I and class II molecules.
CMI5 93-100; BI2 53-55

14. (A) The TAP1/TAP2 heterodimer is an ATP-dependent pump that delivers peptides generated by the proteasome into the endoplasmic reticulum.
CMI5 99; BI2 55-58

15. (D) In the class I pathway, proteins are tagged for proteasomal degradation by covalent addition of several copies of the polypeptide ubiquitin. Ubiquitin-dependent proteasomal degradation is also important in many other cellular processes besides antigen presentation. For example, NF-κB is a transcription factor whose activation is dependent on ubiquitination and proteasomal degradation of an inhibitor (called IκB). Calreticulin, tapasin, and calnexin regulate the assembly of class I MHC proteins within the endoplasmic reticulum.
CMI5 94-100; BI2 55-58

16. (B) Endosomes are membrane-bound acidic vesicles in which internalized proteins are proteolytically degraded in the class II MHC pathway.
CMI5 94-95; BI2 53-55

17. (D) The MIIC or CIIV compartment is a specialized organelle with class II MHC molecules and HLA-DM in its limiting membrane. This is the site where peptides derived from endosomal proteolytic cleavage of internalized proteins bind to class II MHC molecules.
CMI5 96-97; BI2 53-55

18. (A) The final product of the class II MHC pathway of antigen presentation is a peptide-class II MHC complex. This is displayed on the antigen-presenting cell surface, where it can be recognized by the T cell receptor on $CD4^+$ T cells.
CMI5 94, 97; BI2 53-55

19. (F) LMP-2 and LMP-7 are subunits of the proteasome that are needed to efficiently generate peptides of the correct length and composition for optimal binding to class I MHC molecules. The expression of these proteasomal subunits is induced by innate immune responses.
CMI5 98

20. (C) Peptides generated in the cytoplasm are pumped into the endoplasmic reticulum, via the transporter associated with antigen-processing (TAP) 1/2 pump, and bind to newly formed class I MHC molecules in the lumen of the endoplasmic reticulum.
CMI5 98-99; BI2 55-58

21. (D) T cell tolerance is a result of deletion or inactivation of self-reactive T cells. The various steps in both the class I and the class II MHC antigen-presenting pathways do not discriminate between self and microbial proteins. Although expression of MHC molecules is up-regulated as a result of the innate immune responses to infections, there is some degree of constitutive expression of class II MHC on professional antigen-presenting cells, and class I MHC is constitutively expressed on most cells in the body. Only a small fraction of the surface MHC molecules of an infected cell will express peptides derived from microbial peptides.
CMI5 100-101; BI2 53

22. (A) The response to a viral protein (or peptide) requires T cell recognition of the peptide bound to an MHC molecule. Although the viral peptide in the vaccine may bind to many different MHC alleles, it likely will not bind to all. The nonresponders express an allelic variant of HLA-DR, which is a class II MHC molecule. Because the peptide evoked a response in 96% of the people in the trial, it can be considered a dominant epitope. Formally, this can be concluded only when the whole protein is the immunogen and the specificities of the responses for different epitopes are compared. *Determinant selection* is an older term that predates our knowledge of peptide-MHC binding, but it does not mean active selection for one versus another epitope. It is highly unlikely that the only people in the trial who were not adequately immunized for technical reasons happen to be the only ones homozygous for a particular MHC allele.
CMI5 102-103

23. (C) As few as 100 complexes of a particular peptide and a particular class II MHC molecule are needed to activate naive T cells specific for that complex and thereby initiate a detectable T cell response. This represents less than 0.1% of the total class II MHC molecules on a typical antigen-presenting cell surface.
CMI5 97; BI2 53

Chapter 6

Antigen Receptors and Accessory Molecules of T Lymphocytes

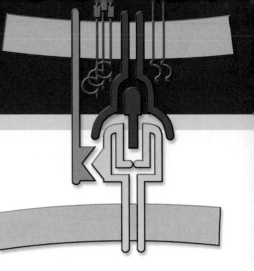

Cellular and Molecular Immunology, 5/E: Chapter 6—Antigen Receptors and Accessory Molecules of T Lymphocytes

Basic Immunology, 2/E: Chapter 4—Antigen Recognition in the Adaptive Immune System, Chapter 5—Cell-Mediated Immune Responses, and Chapter 6—Effector Mechanisms of Cell-Mediated Immunity

1. Most T lymphocytes have a dual specificity for which one of the following pairs of molecules?

   A. A particular allelic form of a major histocompatibility complex (MHC) molecule and a peptide bound to the MHC molecule
   B. Both MHC class I and class II molecules
   C. Both peptide and glycolipid antigens
   D. Both soluble peptides and peptide-MHC complexes
   E. MHC molecules and CD4 or CD8

2. The T cell receptor (TCR) complex contains:

   A. A highly variable antigen coreceptor
   B. CD28
   C. Three homologous CD3 chains, each covalently linked to the TCR αβ heterodimer
   D. Invariable ζ chains noncovalently linked to the TCR αβ heterodimer
   E. Igβ

Questions 3-5

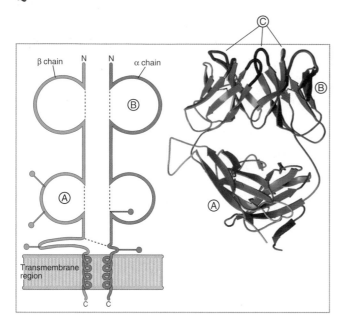

For each component of a T cell receptor listed in questions 3-5, match the lettered region (A-C) shown in the figure above.

3. Variable Ig domain (   )

4. Constant Ig domain (   )

5. Complementarity-determining regions (   )

Questions 6-9

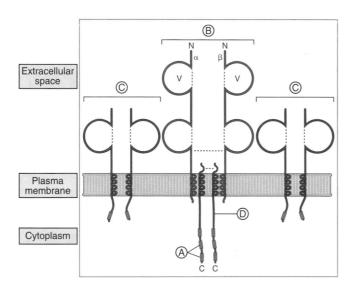

For each component of a T cell receptor complex listed in questions 6-9, match the lettered item (A-D) shown in the figure above.

6. Antigen-binding region (   )

7. CD3 protein (   )

8. ζ protein (   )

9. Immunoreceptor tyrosine-based activation motif (ITAM) (   )

10. A 4-year-old boy suffers from an immunodeficiency disease characterized by impaired T cell activation. The disease is caused by genetic deficiency of a membrane protein whose cytoplasmic tail is involved in intracellular signaling in response to T cell receptor (TCR) recognition of antigen. Which one of the following proteins does NOT fit this description?

   A. TCRα
   B. CD3γ
   C. ζ
   D. CD4
   E. CD3ε

11. A healthy 45-year-old child-care worker becomes infected with a virus and develops a sore throat, cough, and fever. Infected cells in the bronchial mucosa of this patient process virus-encoded proteins through an intracellular pathway and display peptides derived from the protein on the cell surface bound to class I MHC molecules. CD8⁺ T cells migrate to the mucosa and recognize these peptide-MHC complexes. Which of the following components of the TCR actually bind to the viral peptide-MHC complex?

   A. Hypermutated regions: 1 in the α chain, 2 in the β chain
   B. Complementarity-determining regions: 3 in the α chain, 3 in the β chain
   C. Hypervariable regions: 2 in the α chain, 2 in the β chain
   D. Congenic regions: 1 in the α chain, 1 in the β chain
   E. One peptide-binding groove formed by the α chain and the β_2-microglobulin chain

12. The T cell receptor (TCR) complex differs from an immunoglobulin molecule in which one of the following ways?

   A. On average, a TCR binds antigen with much lower affinity than does an Ig molecule.
   B. The TCR can serve as a lymphocyte antigen receptor, but an Ig molecule cannot.
   C. Only the TCR can bind soluble antigen directly.
   D. The TCRs expressed by one clone of T cells can undergo changes in constant region structure after cellular activation, whereas Ig molecules expressed by one clone of B cells do not.
   E. The TCR polypeptide chains have short cytoplasmic tails and rely on associated proteins for signaling functions, whereas membrane Ig receptors are competent signaling molecules on their own.

13. CD1-restricted T cells differ from other T cells restricted to class I or class II MHC molecules in which one of the following ways?

   A. CD-1 restricted T cells cannot rapidly secrete cytokines.

B. CD-1 restricted T cells recognize non-peptide antigens, such as lipids.

C. CD-1 restricted T cells bind both cell-associated and soluble antigens.

D. CD-1 restricted T cells express both CD4 and CD8 coreceptors.

E. CD-1 restricted T cells are actually natural killer (NK) cells.

14. γδ T cells may be important for recognition of common antigens at epithelial boundaries between the host and the external environment. The γδ T cells differ from the αβ T cells in which one of the following ways?

A. γδ T cells recognize only nonprotein antigens.

B. γδ T cells are not MHC-restricted and do not recognize MHC-associated antigens.

C. The γδ TCR complex contains CD3γ or CD3δ but not CD3ε.

D. Most mature γδ T cells express either CD4 or CD8 but not both.

E. γδ T cells lack key biologic activities, including the ability to lyse target cells.

15. CD8 is a protein that functions as a coreceptor for a subset of T cells and plays a significant role in all of the following EXCEPT:

A. Recognition of peptide antigen bound to class I MHC molecules

B. Maturation of MHC class I–restricted T cells

C. Infection of T cells by human immunodeficiency virus (HIV)

D. Signaling via Lck tyrosine kinase to initiate T cell activation

E. Strengthening the binding of T cells to antigen-presenting cells, albeit with low affinity

16. After 2 years of hard work, a graduate student finally succeeds in creating a gene knockout mouse lacking CD4. The student is particularly careful to keep this mouse line in a microbe-free animal facility because these mice are expected to show:

A. No ability to produce IgM antibodies

B. Impaired ability to produce antibodies and activate macrophages

C. No ability to activate naive class I–restricted T cells

D. Complete absence of cytotoxic T lymphocyte (CTL) responses to viral infections

E. Failure to produce neutrophils

17. Which of the following is NOT a property shared by both CD4 and CD8?

A. Binds to nonpolymorphic regions of MHC molecules

B. Cytoplasmic tail associates with the Src family kinase Lck

C. Is a member of the Ig superfamily

D. Functions as a coreceptor for αβ TCRs

E. Is expressed on the majority of mature blood T cells

Questions 18 and 19

A 15-year-old girl develops malaise, headache, and low-grade fever, followed by pharyngitis and cervical lymph node enlargement as a result of infectious mononucleosis caused by Epstein-Barr virus (EBV). Her acute symptoms resolve within 2 weeks, and the fatigue improves within 3 months.

18. All of the following are required for CD8⁺ cytotoxic T lymphocyte (CTL) recognition and killing of EBV-infected cells EXCEPT:

A. β_2-Microglobulin

B. HLA-A, -B or -C

C. CD28

D. LFA-1 (leukocyte function-associated antigen-1)

E. TAP (transporter associated with antigen processing)

19. Following the primary infection described in this patient, the patient's subsequent exposure to Epstein-Barr virus (EBV) will trigger clonal expansion of EBV-specific T cells expressing which one of the following surface molecules?

A. CD62L^{high}

B. CD44^{low}

C. CD45RA^{high}

D. CD45RO^{high}

E. CD21^{high}

20. Both CD28 and CTLA-4 are receptors on T cells that are critical for regulating T cell activation. In which one of the following ways does CD28 differ from CTLA-4?

A. Only CD28 binds the costimulatory ligands B7-1 and B7-2 expressed on professional antigen-presenting cells.

B. CD28 counteracts positive, pro-proliferative T cell signals delivered by CTLA-4.

C. CD28 is constitutively expressed on naive T cells, whereas CTLA-4 is expressed on activated T cells.

D. CD28 binds its ligand with 10-fold greater affinity than does CTLA-4.

E. CD28 is important for delivering "signal 1" for T cell activation, whereas CTLA-4 is important for delivering "signal 2."

21. LFA-1 is an integrin that promotes T cell activation by which one of the following mechanisms?

A. Binds to the α3 domain of class I MHC molecules, mediating high avidity between T cells and antigen-presenting cells (APCs)

B. Binds to B7-1 or B7-2 on the surface of APCs, mediating "signal 2"

C. Binds to GlyCAM-1 on high endothelial venules of lymph nodes, mediating rolling of T cells on endothelium

D. Binds to ICAM-1 on the surface of a variety of cells, mediating firm adhesion between T cells and APCs or endothelial cells

E. Binds to VCAM-1 on the surface of cytokine-activated endothelial cells, mediating homing of T cells to peripheral sites of inflammation

22. Selectins differ from integrins in which one of the following ways?

    A. Selectins are expressed only on endothelial cells and integrins are expressed only on leukocytes.
    B. Selectins are important mediators of leukocyte adhesion to endothelium, but integrins are not.
    C. Selectins bind carbohydrate ligands, but integrins do not.
    D. Selectins mediate rolling of leukocytes on endothelium, but integrins do not.
    E. Selectins are a family of homologous molecules, but integrins are not.

23. A 2-year-old boy suffers from recurrent bacterial infection of his ears, sinuses, lungs, and skin; laboratory studies indicate absence of sialylated Lewis X on his leukocytes. He is diagnosed with leukocyte adhesion deficiency type 2 (LAD-2). Which type of adhesive interaction required for leukocyte migration is defective in this boy?

    A. E-selectin ligand binding to E-selectin
    B. CD4 binding to class II MHC
    C. VLA-4 binding to VCAM-1
    D. Ig Fc receptor binding to Ig-coated cells
    E. LFA-1 binding to ICAM-1

24. CD44 expressed on the surface of T cells is critical for the binding of activated T cells to endothelium at sites of inflammation, and for the retention of T cells in extravascular tissues at sites of infection. CD44 does this by binding to which one of the following molecules?

    A. VCAM-1
    B. Hyaluronate
    C. ICAM-1
    D. Fibronectin
    E. E-selectin

25. Neonates, elderly persons, and otherwise immunocompromised patients are particularly susceptible to infections with *Listeria monocytogenes*. These patients typically have fever and chills, often progressing to hypotension and septic shock. In healthy individuals, however, such intracellular microbes are usually effectively phagocytosed and killed by macrophages, which become activated via:

    A. CD40L-CD40 interactions between activated T helper cells and macrophages
    B. CD28-B7 interactions between activated T cells and macrophages
    C. Fas ligand–Fas interactions between activated cytotoxic T lymphocytes and macrophages
    D. TCR-MHC class II interactions between activated T helper cells and macrophages
    E. LFA-1–ICAM-1 interactions between activated T cells and macrophages

Questions 26-32

Match each receptor listed in questions 26-32 with the lettered ligand (A-E) that binds to the receptor. (Answers may be used more than once.)

A. B7-1, B7-2
B. Class II MHC
C. LFA-3
D. VCAM-1
E. Sialylated Lewis X

26. VLA-4 (   )
27. P-selectin (   )
28. CTLA-4 (   )
29. CD28 (   )
30. CD2 (   )
31. E-selectin (   )
32. CD4 (   )

33. The strength of integrin-dependent binding of T cells to antigen-presenting cells (APCs) may be rapidly increased by which one of the following mechanisms?

    A. Integrin clustering and increased integrin affinity are induced by chemokines and antigen recognition.
    B. Integrins stored in cytoplasmic organelles are mobilized to the T cell surface in response to TCR-mediated signals.
    C. Integrin gene transcription is enhanced by chemokine-generated signals.
    D. The affinity of integrin ligands on APCs is increased in response to chemokines.
    E. Integrin ligands stored in cytoplasmic granules in the APCs are mobilized to the cell surface in response to CD40-CD40 ligand interaction.

Answers

1. (A) Most T cells are specific for polymorphic residues of a self major histocompatibility complex (MHC) molecule, which accounts for their MHC restriction, and for residues of a peptide antigen displayed by the MHC molecule, which accounts for antigen specificity. The receptor that recognizes peptide-MHC complexes is called the T cell receptor (TCR). Mature αβ T cells (the predominant type) express either CD4 or CD8, but not both. As such, each αβ T cell is restricted to bind either MHC class II or class I molecules, but not both. Although a small subset of T cells may recognize glycolipid antigens bound to class I MHC-like molecules called CD1, these T cells do not also recognize peptide antigens. Unlike the B cell receptor (immunoglobulins), the TCR can recognize only peptides displayed on MHC molecules, not soluble peptides alone. T cells express CD4 or CD8 and do not recognize CD4 or CD8 on other cells.
CMI5 105; BI2 42-43

2. (D) The T cell receptor (TCR) complex contains a highly variable antigen receptor, usually composed of a heterodimer of α and β chains, called the TCR, which is responsible for antigen recognition, as well as invariant signaling proteins, CD3δ,

CD3ε, and CD3λ, and the ζ protein. These signaling molecules are all noncovalently associated with the TCR. Coreceptors for T cells include CD4 and CD8; these are invariant proteins and are not part of the TCR complex itself. CD28 is involved in T cell costimulation, but it is not a member of the TCR complex. Igβ is a component of the B lymphocyte antigen receptor complex.
CMI5 105, 108, 110-111; BI2 87-88

3. (B) The variable regions of TCR molecules are composed of Ig V-like domains at the N termini of both the α and the β chains.
CMI5 108; BI2 71-72

4. (A) The constant regions of TCR molecules are composed of membrane-proximal Ig C-like domains of both the α and the β chains.
CMI5 108; BI2 71-72

5. (C) Complementarity-determining regions (or hypervariable regions) are composed of three loops each of the α- and β-chain V domains. They form the antigen-binding surface of the TCR.
CMI5 108; BI2 71-72

6. (B) The antigen-binding region of the TCR complex is made up of the N-terminal V regions of the α and the β chains.
CMI5 108; BI2 88

7. (C) The CD3 proteins are three highly homologous Ig family members, γ, δ, and ε, which are noncovalently associated with the T cell αβ heterodimer.
CMI5 111; BI2 88

8. (D) The ζ (zeta) protein, which is noncovalently associated with the αβ heterodimer, has a short extracellular domain and a long cytoplasmic domain. It is present in the TCR complex as a homodimer.
CMI5 111; BI2 88

9. (A) Immunoreceptor tyrosine-based activation motifs (ITAMs) are signaling motifs present in the cytoplasmic tails of the CD3 and ζ proteins. Tyrosine residues within ITAMs become phosphorylated after antigen binding to the TCR and serve as docking sites for ZAP-70 (ζ-associated protein of 70 kD).
CMI5 111; BI2 88

10. (A) Although the T cell receptor (TCR) α and β chains are responsible for antigen recognition, they are not directly involved in signaling. Rather, the αβ heterodimer is noncovalently associated with signaling molecules CD3γ, CD3δ, CD3ε, and ζ, all of which have ITAMs in their cytoplasmic tails. Although CD4 is not part of the TCR complex, it does play a critical role in initiating signaling during TCR recognition of antigen by binding Lck to its cytoplasmic tail and bringing this tyrosine kinase near the ITAMs of CD3 and ζ.
CMI5 105-107, 110-113; BI2 88

11. (B) Each α and β chain of the T cell receptor (TCR) contains both a constant and a variable domain. The variable domain contains short stretches of amino acids where the variability between different TCRs is concentrated, and these form the hypervariable or complementarity-determining regions (CDRs). Three CDRs in the α chain are juxtaposed to three similar regions in the β chain to form the part of the TCR that specifically recognizes peptide-MHC complexes. The variable regions of Ig molecules may undergo hypermutation during humoral immune responses, but this does not happen in TCRs. Congenic does not refer to a part of a protein, but rather to an inbred strain of animal. Peptide-binding grooves are part of MHC molecules, not TCRs.
CMI5 108; BI2 71-72

12. (A) TCRs bind antigen with much lower affinity than immunoglobulins (the dissociation constant for the TCR is 10^{-5} to 10^{-7} versus 10^{-7} to 10^{-11} for secreted Ig). Both T cell receptors (TCRs) and membrane Ig serve as lymphocyte antigen receptors on T cells and B cells, respectively. TCRs do not bind soluble antigens, but rather cell surface–associated peptide-MHC molecule complexes. Only immunoglobulins undergo constant region changes, called heavy chain isotype switching. Both TCRs and Ig have short cytoplasmic tails and rely on associated signaling molecules (CD3 and ζ for TCR, Igα and Igβ for membrane Ig).
CMI5 109; BI2 73

13. (B) A small population of T cells express T cell receptors that recognize lipids bound to class I MHC–like molecules called CD1 molecules. These lipid antigen specific T cells include CD4⁺CD8⁺, or CD4⁻CD8⁻ αβ T cells. Many of these T cells also express markers found on natural killer (NK) cells and are therefore called NK T cells, although they are not actually NK cells. CD1-restricted T cells are still capable of rapidly producing cytokines such as IL-4 and IFN-γ, but their physiologic function is unknown.
CMI5 110

14. (B) T cells expressing the γδ TCR are a lineage distinct from the much more numerous αβ-expressing T lymphocytes. The γδ T cells do not recognize MHC-associated peptide antigens and are not MHC restricted. Some γδ T cells recognize protein or nonprotein antigens that do not require processing or particular types of antigen-presenting cells for their presentation. The γδ heterodimer associates with the same CD3 and ζ proteins as do αβ receptors. Most γδ cells do not express CD4 or CD8. The γδ cells are capable of several biologic activities, including secretion of cytokines and lysis of target cells.
CMI5 113; BI2 71

15. (C) CD4, but not CD8, serves as a receptor for the human immunodeficiency virus (HIV). CD8 is a coreceptor that binds to class I MHC molecules.

It is expressed on T cells whose T cell receptors (TCRs) recognize complexes of peptide and class I MHC molecules. CD8 plays a critical role in the maturation of class I MHC–restricted T cells in the thymus because this process requires the maturing T cells to recognize class I MHC on thymic antigen-presenting cells (APCs). Both CD8 and CD4 associate with the Src family tyrosine kinase, called Lck, and thus they participate in the early signal transduction events that occur after T cell recognition of peptide-MHC complexes on APCs. The affinities of CD8 and CD4 for MHC molecules are very low, but they are still thought to play some role in mediating adhesion between T cells and APCs.
CMI5 117-118; BI2 86-88

16. (B) Knockout mice lacking CD4 do not contain mature class II–restricted T cells because the CD4 coreceptor plays an essential role in the maturation of T cells in the thymus. Most CD4+ class II–restricted T cells are cytokine-producing helper cells that function in host defense against intracellular microbes. These helper T cells are critical for activating B cells to produce antibodies, and for activating macrophages to efficiently kill phagocytosed microbes. Knockout mice lacking CD4 therefore do not have any helper T cells. IgM antibody production is generally not dependent on help from CD4+ T cells. Because CD8 is still expressed, naive class I–restricted T cells are still present and able to respond to intracellular infections, although this ability may be impaired by lack of T cell help. Neutrophil production by the bone marrow should be relatively normal.
CMI5 116-117; BI2 80-82, 88

17. (E) CD4 is expressed on the majority (~65%) of mature blood T cells, whereas CD8 is expressed on a minority (~35%). Both CD4 and CD8 are transmembrane glycoprotein members of the Ig superfamily, both serve as MHC-binding coreceptors for the T cell receptor, and both participate in early signal transduction events via cytoplasmic tail binding of the Src family tyrosine kinase Lck.
CMI5 115, 117; BI2 86-89

18. (C) CD28 is not involved in antigen recognition by T cells, but rather, in costimulation. Cell-mediated immunity against intracellular organisms, such as viruses, is largely mediated by class I–restricted T cells, such as cytotoxic T lymphocytes (CTLs). The class I MHC molecules are HLA-A, HLA-B, and HLA-C. CTLs recognize complexes of viral peptides with class I MHC molecules. β_2-Microglobulin is the nonpolymorphic, noncovalently associated polypeptide chain of MHC class I molecules. TAP is a critical protein involved in the processing and presentation of antigen by class I MHC. LFA-1 is an important integrin mediating adhesion of the CD8+ T cells to virus-infected target cells.
CMI5 69, 99, 116; BI2 117-118

19. (D) After primary infection, subsequent exposure to Epstein-Barr virus (EBV) (i.e., secondary infection) will trigger clonal expansion of EBV-specific memory T cells. Memory T cells express CD45RO. CD45RA is expressed on naive human T cells. CD62L, or L-selectin, is a peripheral lymph node homing receptor that is expressed at high levels on naive T lymphocytes but not on activated or memory T lymphocytes. CD44 is an adhesion molecule that is expressed at low levels on naive T lymphocytes and at high levels on activated and memory T lymphocytes. CD21 is actually the EBV receptor, but it is expressed on B cells (and follicular dendritic cells). It normally functions as a coreceptor to deliver activating signals in B cells.
CMI5 10, 24, 508

20. (C) CD28 is constitutively expressed on more than 90% of CD4+ T cells and 50% of CD8+ T cells, whereas CTLA-4 is expressed only on activated T cells. Both B7-1 and B7-2, expressed on professional antigen-presenting cells (APCs), bind to both CD28 and CTLA-4 receptors on T cells. Binding of B7 molecules on APCs to CD28 delivers "positive" signals to the T cells that stimulate production of growth factors, promote T cell proliferation and differentiation, and induce expression of anti-apoptotic proteins. CTLA-4, however, functions to inhibit T cell activation by counteracting signals delivered by CD28. CTLA-4 also binds B7-1 with 10-fold greater affinity than CD28 binds B7-1; this difference may play an important role in the temporal sequence of T cell activation.
CMI5 118; BI2 89-92

21. (D) LFA-1 is an integrin expressed on the surface of leukocytes, which binds ICAM-1 to mediate specific, firm adhesion between T cells and antigen-presenting cells, as well as leukocytes and endothelial cells. As such, it plays an important role in the activation of T lymphocytes and in their migration to sites of infection and inflammation. In contrast, CD8 binds the $\alpha3$ domain of class I MHC molecules, CD28 and CTLA-4 bind B7 proteins, L-selectin is the receptor for GlyCAM-1, and VLA-4 is the receptor for VCAM-1.
CMI5 119-120; BI2 89-90

22. (C) Selectins specifically bind carbohydrate groups on cell surface glycoproteins, whereas integrins do not bind carbohydrate groups on Ig superfamily molecules. L-selectin and several integrins are both expressed on some lymphocytes. Both selectins and integrins are important mediators of leukocyte adhesion to endothelium. Both selectins and integrins (especially VLA-4) can mediate rolling interactions; selectins are more specialized in this regard. There are three members of the selectin family (E-, P-, and L-) and more than 30 different members of the integrin family.
CMI5 119, 122-123; BI2 108-111

23. (A) Leukocyte adhesion deficiency type 2 (LAD-2) is a rare genetic disorder characterized by severely impaired neutrophil rolling and adhesion to acti-

vated endothelium. The cause is a defect in the synthesis of sialylated Lewis X, the carbohydrate ligand on neutrophils and other leukocytes that is required for binding to E-selectin and P-selectin on cytokine-activated endothelium. In a clinically similar disorder called LAD-1, there is absent or deficient expression of the CD11CD18 family of integrins (of which LFA-1 is a member). Adhesion interactions mediated by CD4, Fc receptor, and VLA-4 are normal in patients with LAD-2.
CMI5 120, 123

24. (B) CD44 is a glycoprotein expressed on a variety of cells, particularly on recently activated and memory T cells. CD44 binds to hyaluronate, which allows for the retention of T cells in extravascular tissues at sites of infection and for the binding of activated and memory T cells to endothelium at sites of inflammation.
CMI5 123-124

25. (A) Activated CD4+ T cells express CD40 ligand (CD40L), which binds to CD40 on B lymphocytes, macrophages, dendritic cells, and endothelial cells thereby activating these cells. Only activated macrophages can effectively phagocytose and kill intracellular microbes such as *Listeria*. CD28-B7 and TCR-MHC class II interactions provide signals 2 and 1, respectively, in the activation of T cells by antigen-presenting cells (not the activation of macrophages by T cells). Engagement of Fas by Fas ligand (FasL) on T cells results in apoptosis and provides one of the mechanisms by which CTLs kill their targets. LFA-1–ICAM-1 mediates cell adhesion interactions important in T cell activation and homing.
CMI5 124; BI2 112-115

26. (D) VLA-4, an integrin expressed on T cells, binds to VCAM-1, an Ig superfamily member expressed on activated endothelium. VLA-4–VCAM-1 interactions promote T cell recruitment into inflammatory sites.
CMI5 120; BI2 87

27. (E) Sialylated Lewis X is a carbohydrate structure on glycoprotein ligands of E-selectin expressed by leukocytes. E-selectin binding to sialylated Lewis

X mediates leukocyte rolling interactions with activated endothelium. The same is true of P-selectin.
CMI5 123; BI2 109

28. (A) B7-1 and B7-2 on antigen-presenting cells bind to CTLA-4 on activated T cells, stimulating negative signals in the T cells.
CMI5 115; BI2 87

29. (A) B7-1 and B7-2 on antigen-presenting cells bind to CD28 on naive T cells, stimulating positive signals in the T cells.
CMI5 115; BI2 87

30. (C) LFA-3 on antigen-presenting cells binds to CD2 on T cells, and this interaction provides both adhesive and signaling functions that promote T cell activation.
CMI5 115

31. (E) Sialylated Lewis X is a carbohydrate structure on glycoprotein ligands of E-selectin expressed by leukocytes. E-selectin binding to sialylated Lewis X mediates leukocyte rolling interactions with activated endothelium. The same is true of P-selectin.
CMI5 123; BI2 109

32. (B) CD4 on T cells binds to a nonpolymorphic region of class II MHC during T cell recognition of antigen. This molecular interaction promotes signaling events required for T cell activation.
CMI5 115; BI2 87

33. (A) T cell integrin affinity is enhanced by "inside-out signaling" in response to antigen binding to the T cell receptor (TCR) and chemokine binding to chemokine receptors. In addition, antigen and chemokines can induce clustering of integrins in the region of the T cell membrane in contact with the antigen-presenting cell (APC). These changes cause stronger T cell binding to APCs displaying the peptide-MHC complex that the T cell recognizes, thus ensuring prolonged T cell/APC contact and T cell activation. Integrins are not stored in cytoplasmic granules, and transcriptional activity cannot account for rapid changes in integrin-mediated binding. Integrin ligands (such as ICAM-1) do not undergo changes in affinity, nor are they stored in cytoplasmic granules.
CMI5 121-122; BI2 90

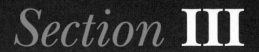
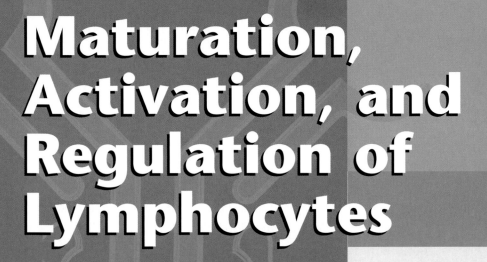

Maturation, Activation, and Regulation of Lymphocytes

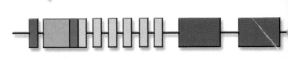

Chapter 7

Lymphocyte Maturation and Expression of Antigen Receptor Genes

Cellular and Molecular Immunology, 5/E: Chapter 7—Lymphocyte Maturation and Expression of Antigen Receptor Genes

Basic Immunology, 2/E: Chapter 4—Antigen Recognition in the Adaptive Immune System

1. Which of the following is NOT a required step in B and T lymphocyte maturation?

   A. Proliferative expansion of precursor cells
   B. Cell surface expression of complete antigen receptor complexes
   C. Positive selection
   D. Activation of precursors by foreign antigens
   E. Pre-antigen receptor expression

2. A 3-month-old boy begins to suffer recurrent severe infections, chronic diarrhea, and failure to thrive. A blood cell count reveals a complete absence of T cells, normal numbers of B cells, and abnormally low IgG titers. A mutation in the gene encoding which of the following proteins is the most likely explanation for this child's disease?

   A. γ_c chain
   B. Jak3
   C. RAG-1
   D. DRα chain
   E. CD4

3. Which of the following is NOT an example of a checkpoint in lymphocyte maturation that contributes to the selective maturation of cells with useful antigen receptors?

   A. B cell precursors that cannot express Ig γ heavy chains die by apoptosis.

23. Which of the following is the most accurate description of B1 B cells?

    A. A subset of B cells that respond first to newly encountered antigens
    B. A subset of B cells with limited receptor diversity that produce IgM specific for microbial polysaccharides and blood group antigens
    C. Cells that express both membrane IgM and γδ TCR antigen receptors and function in defense against peritoneal infections
    D. The most immature cells identifiable as committed B cell precursors in the bone marrow
    E. The subset of B cells responsible for production of IgB

24. The order of stages of T cell maturation is most accurately indicated by which of the following sequences?

    A. Stem cell → pre-T cell → pro-T cell → single positive thymocyte → double positive thymocyte → naive mature T lymphocyte
    B. Stem cell → pre-T cell → pro-T cell → double positive thymocyte → single positive thymocyte → naive mature T lymphocyte
    C. Stem cell → pro-T cell → pre-T cell → double positive thymocyte → single positive thymocyte → naive mature T lymphocyte
    D. Stem cell → pro-T cell → pre-T cell → single positive thymocyte → double positive thymocyte → naive mature T lymphocyte
    E. Pre-T cell → pro-T cell → double positive thymocyte → single positive thymocyte → naive mature T lymphocyte → stem cell

25. Which one of the following statements is an accurate description of the ways in which major histocompatibility complex (MHC) molecules are involved in thymic selection processes that shape the T cell repertoire?

    A. Class I MHC molecules are involved in positive selection only, and class II MHC molecules are involved in negative selection only.
    B. Class I and class II MHC molecules are required for positive selection of self-MHC–restricted T cells and negative selection of strongly autoreactive T cells.
    C. Class I and class II MHC molecules are required for negative selection of self-MHC–restricted T cells and positive selection of strongly autoreactive T cells.
    D. Class I and class II MHC molecules are required for positive selection of self-MHC–restricted T cells but not negative selection of strongly autoreactive T cells.
    E. MHC molecules are not required for either positive or negative selection of T cells, and are only required for activation of mature T cells outside the thymus.

26. A 1-year-old boy is treated for X-linked severe combined immunodeficiency disease (SCID) by bone marrow transplantation. The bone marrow donor is the patient's mother. The transplantation is successful, and the patient is cured of SCID. Within 2 years after the transplantation, he has normal levels of serum Ig and normal numbers of circulating lymphocytes. MHC typing of blood cells 1 year later, when the patient is 2 years of age, indicates that the patient's bone marrow contains a mixture of his own stem cells and stem cells of maternal origin. When the patient is 5 years of age, all hematopoiesis is from stem cells of maternal origin. The patient is given a series of routine childhood immunizations, including tetanus toxoid, between the ages of 3 and 11. At age 12, immunology researchers obtain permission from the family to test the MHC restriction of the patient's blood T cells using in vitro antigen-presenting assays. The researchers find that some of the patient's T cells recognize tetanus toxoid presented by antigen-presenting cells (APCs) from the mother but not the father and that other of the patient's T cells recognize tetanus toxoid presented by APCs from the father but not from the mother. Which of the following most likely explains these findings?

    A. Some T cell precursors were positively selected in the thymus by maternal MHC molecules on bone marrow–derived APCs and others by paternally derived MHC molecules on thymic epithelial cells.
    B. Memory T cells restricted by paternal MHC molecules were generated before transplantation and are still detectable at age 12.
    C. Some of the T cells use TCR genes that were inherited from the mother, and other T cells use TCR genes inherited from the father.
    D. The patient's CD8+ T cells recognize peptide antigens presented by paternally inherited class I MHC molecules, and his CD4+ T cells recognize antigens presented by maternally inherited class II MHC molecules.
    E. T cells derived from maternal stem cells will be restricted to recognize only peptide antigen in the context of maternal MHC molecules, and T cells derived from the patient's own stem cells may be restricted by maternal or paternal MHC alleles.

27. Which one of the following statements about γδ T cell development is NOT true?

    A. γδ T cells are derived from a bone marrow stem cell precursor.
    B. γδ T cells theoretically could have greater diversity than αβ T cells, but in reality they show very limited diversity.
    C. γδ T cells are derived from αβ T cells.
    D. γδ T cells mature in the thymus.
    E. γδ T cells are not MHC-restricted.

Answers

1. (D) Foreign antigens are not likely to be present in the generative lymphoid organs where lymphocytes mature and thus are not involved in the process. Both B cell and T cell maturation include sequential steps, including cytokine-induced proliferation and expansion of immature precursors, somatic recombination of Ig heavy chain or T cell receptor (TCR) β chain genes, expression of μ heavy chain or TCR β chain with a surrogate nonvariable partner to form a pre-Ig or pre-TCR, somatic recombination of Ig light chain or TCR α chain genes, expression of complete antigen receptors and associated signaling molecules, and positive selection by recognition of self antigens.
CMI5 129; BI2 74

2. (A) The γ_c chain (common cytokine receptor γ chain) is required for signaling by several cytokines including interleukin (IL)-7, and IL-7 is essential for proliferation of early T cell precursors in the thymus. Mutations of γ_c are the main cause of X-linked severe combined immunodeficiency disease (SCID) and account for about 50% of cases of SCID. JAK3 is a kinase required for IL-7 signaling, and patients with JAK3 kinase deficiencies have a very similar disease to patients with γ_c deficiency. However, JAK3 deficiency is due to homozygous recessive mutations and is very rare. RAG-1 deficiency would prevent somatic recombination of both TCR and Ig genes, resulting in an absence of both B cells and T cells. Mutations in CD4 or a DR2 α (a chain of class II MHC molecules) would be expected to have selective defects in T cell maturation but not a complete absence of T cells.
CMI5 130; BI2 72-73, 211

3. (A) B cell precursors must express Ig μ heavy chains (not Ig γ heavy chains) to survive. The μ chains associate with surrogate light chains in pre-B cells, which allows for the generation of survival signals. Otherwise, the cells die by a default apoptotic pathway. A similar checkpoint exists in T cell precursors, which must express TCR β chains that associate with pre-Tα chains to avoid apoptotic death. Developing T cells must progress to express TCR α chains and form αβ TCRs to be positively selected and continue to survive. Both immature B cells and developing T cells will undergo apoptosis if they express high-affinity receptors that bind to self antigens. In the case of developing T cells, high-affinity binding to self MHC will lead to apoptotic death.
CMI5 131-133; BI2 74, 76-82

4. (B) Negative selection is a mechanism that promotes a self-tolerant lymphocyte repertoire for both B and T cells. It occurs in the generative lymphoid organs (bone marrow and thymus) when developing lymphocytes express antigen receptors that bind strongly to self antigens. The major mechanism is actively induced apoptosis; immature lymphocytes that receive strong antigen receptor–mediated signals are particularly susceptible to death by apoptosis. Positive selection in the thymus promotes a self-MHC–restricted T cell repertoire.
CMI5 133-134,160; BI2 74, 80-81

5. (B) Ikaros is a transcription factor required for transition of a pluripotential stem cell to a cell committed to either B or T lymphocyte lineages.
CMI5 131

6. (A) Pro-B to pre-B transition requires expression of Ig μ heavy chains. Functional μ heavy chain genes are formed by RAG-1– and RAG-2–dependent VDJ recombination.
CMI5 132; BI2 74, 76-80

7. (E) Maturation to a single positive CD8⁺ thymocyte requires positive selection of cells whose TCRs recognize self class I MHC-peptide complexes on other cells in the thymus. TAP-1 and TAP-2 are needed to deliver peptides that participate in the assembly of class I-peptide complexes into the endoplasmic reticulum. Mutations in *RAG-2, Ikaros, CD3e,* or *JAK3* would block development before the double positive thymocyte stage.
CMI5 132; BI2 80-82

8. (E) Natural killer (NK) cells do not express clonally distributed antigen receptors encoded by genes formed by RAG-1– and RAG-2–dependent VDJ recombination (i.e., they do not express Ig or TCRs). Therefore, NK cells are expected to be present in normal or even increased numbers in patients with B and T lymphocyte deficiencies. Double positive thymocytes mature from pre-T cells in response to signals generated by a functional pre-TCR, which includes a TCR β chain. RAG-1 and RAG-2 are needed to form a functional β chain gene. Plasma cells, IgA-secreting B cells, and cytolytic T lymphocytes are all differentiated effector lymphocytes. The development and differentiation of these lymphocytes require expression of functional antigen receptors encoded by genes formed by RAG-1– and RAG-2–dependent VDJ recombination.
CMI5 130, 141; BI2 750

9. (C) Naive T cells leave the thymus to recirculate and populate peripheral lymphoid tissues. Both effector T cells and memory T cells differentiate from naive T cells after an encounter with antigens in the periphery. Immature T cells normally do not exit the thymus, and B cell maturation occurs in the bone marrow, not in the thymus.
CMI5 134-135; BI2 80-83

10. (D) Naive B cells produce IgM and IgD antibody isotypes. The IgM isotype is a characteristic of the heavy chain constant region, encoded by the C_μ gene segment.
CMI5 135-137; BI2 76

11. (A) One variable (V) gene segment, from as many as 45 possible V gene segments, is used in each functional Ig heavy chain gene. This V gene segment encodes an Ig domain that includes complemen-

tarity-determining regions (CDRs) 1 and 2 of the antigen-binding region of the heavy chain.
CMI5 135-137; BI2 76

12. (B) Diversity (D) segments are found in the Ig heavy chain and TCR β chain loci, but not in the Ig light chain or the TCR α chain loci. D segments are joined to V and J segments through somatic recombination and encode part of CDR3.
CMI5 135-137, 146-147, 153-155; BI2 76

13. (C) Joining (J) segments are found in all antigen receptor loci. In the first somatic recombination event in Ig heavy chain and TCR β chain loci, J segments are joined to D segments. In the only somatic recombination event in the Ig light chain and the TCR α chain loci, J segments are joined to V segments.
CMI5 135-137, 146-147, 153-155; BI2 76

14. (E) The V(D)J recombinase is an enzyme complex that includes the lymphocyte-specific RAG-1 and RAG-2 proteins, as well as other more widely expressed DNA repair enzymes. This recombinase acts on DNA in the antigen receptor gene loci but does not mediate RNA splicing. The RAG-1 protein binds to recombination signal sequences (RSSs), cleaves the adjacent DNA, and promotes alignment of the different segments to be joined. Other enzymes in the complex ligate the cleaved DNA ends to form the functional gene, encoding a chain of the antigen receptor.
CMI5 138-141; BI2 75

15. (D) Heptamers and nonamers are identical in the Ig and TCR loci, which is why RAG-1 can recognize recombination sites in all these loci. Gene segment joining in all Ig and TCR loci obeys the 12/23 rule, which allows joining only of segments with different spacers. Direct V-to-J joining cannot occur in the Ig heavy chain locus because of the 12/23 rule, but D segments can join to both V and J segments. During recombination, RAG-1 cleaves the DNA between the heptamer and the coding sequence, and a piece of DNA that includes the RSSs with heptamers joined together is removed.
CMI5 139-141

16. (D) Burkitt's lymphoma, a neoplasm of the B lymphocyte lineage, always carries a *myc* gene (t8) translocation to one of the Ig gene loci, usually the heavy chain locus (t14). Many other lymphoid malignancies carry chromosomal translocations that involve antigen receptor loci. These include t(14;18) (q32.3;q21.3) involving *bcl-2* and *IgH* in follicular lymphomas; t(9;22) (q34;q11.2) involving *bcr* and *Igγ* in pre-B cell acute leukemias; t(1;14) (p32p;q11.2) involving *TAL1* and *TCRa* in pre-T cell acute leukemias; and t(3;14) (q27;q32.3) involving *cyclin D1* and *IgH* in mantle cell lymphomas.
CMI5 142-143

17. (B) Junctional diversity is caused by deletions and additions of base pairs between V, D, and J segments during somatic recombination, resulting in new junctional sequences not present in the germline. This accounts for the majority of Ig and TCR diversity. Combinatorial diversity is the second major mechanism for diversity, based on the large number of different V, D, and J segments inserted in the germline that can be used during somatic recombination. Isotype switching (of Ig molecules only) changes the non–antigen-binding region and does not contribute to diversity of antigen receptor specificity. Polymorphism refers to the presence of different alleles of a gene in the population, not in an individual, and is not a mechanism of diversity of the antigen receptor repertoires.
CMI5 143-146; BI2 75-76

18. (A) Terminal deoxyribonucleotidyl transferase (TdT) is the enzyme that adds random nontemplate nucleotides (called N nucleotides) at the junctions between V, D and J segments, mainly in the recombined Ig heavy chain and TCRβ chain genes. The enzyme is expressed mainly during the time in B cell and T cell development when the IgH and TCRβ chain genes are undergoing recombination. Activation-induced deaminase is an enzyme involved in somatic mutation and isotype switching of Ig genes. Recombinase activating gene-1 *(RAG-1)* and DNA-dependent protein kinase are components of the V(D)J recombinase that mediates the joining of the discrete gene segments, but these enzymes do not contribute on their own to junctional diversity.
CMI5 141, 144, 206; BI2 75

19. (C) The μ heavy chain gene is the first to undergo somatic recombination and expression as a protein during B cell maturation. In fact, μ expression is required for signals to be generated that stimulate recombination and expression of light chain genes. Although the δ heavy chain and IgD molecules are expressed simultaneously with IgM in immature B cells, this is a result of alternative spicing of a primary RNA transcript containing both μ and δ coding sequences. Other Ig heavy chains, such as α, are expressed only after mature B cells are activated and undergo isotype switching.
CMI5 146-148; BI2 79

20. (C) The surrogate light chain, which is composed of the λ5/14.1 and the variable (V) pre-B proteins, associates with μ heavy chains in pre-B cells to form the pre-B cell receptor. The pre-B cell receptor is not required for somatic recombination and expression of μ heavy chain genes. The pre-B cell receptor does deliver signals that are required for proliferation of B cell precursors and heavy chain allelic exclusion. Light chain gene recombination is also largely dependent on pre-B cell receptor signals. This boy's mutations in both λ5/14.1 alleles have caused a failure to produce pre-B cell receptors and therefore a failure to produce mature B cells. Little or no antibody will be produced, regardless of specificity.
CMI5 148-149; BI2 79

21. (E) The *RAG-1* gene is only transiently expressed during short periods in development of a B cell and is then permanently shut off once the mature B cell stage is reached. This ensures that after a functional Ig antigen receptor is produced, V gene usage cannot be changed. *RAG-1* expression can occur in the immature B cell stage in response to recognition of self antigens, allowing for changes in light chain V gene usage (receptor editing), thereby maintaining self tolerance. Mature naive B cells express membrane forms of both IgM and IgD, and these antibodies may use the κ or λ light chains. These membrane Ig molecules are noncovalently associated with the Igα and Igβ signaling molecules.
    CMI5 146, 149-150; BI2 75, 79

22. (D) In TCR allelic exclusion, expression of the β chain gene encoded by a successfully recombined gene on one chromosome inhibits recombination of the β chain gene on the other chromosome. The inhibitory signals are generated by the pre-TCR. This ensures that the T cell will not produce receptors with two different β chains. However, allelic exclusion does not occur for TCR α chain genes, and many T cells may express TCRs with two different α chains. Positive selection requires that only one of the receptors be self-MHC–restricted, and the chance that both TCRs can recognize peptide-self MHC complexes is minimal. Heavy chain allelic exclusion occurs by a similar mechanism in B cell development.
    CMI5 149, 153, 155; BI2 80

23. (B) B1 B cells residing in the peritoneum produce most of the IgM antibody in the body. These antibodies have no junctional diversity and limited use of V, D, and J gene segments. B1 B cells are thought to provide an antibody-mediated innate response to commonly encountered microbial antigens. The "natural" antibodies against blood group antigens are also produced by B1 B cells, and almost all chronic lymphocytic leukemias are derived from this subset. B1 B cells do not necessarily respond earlier than other B cells to newly encountered antigens. γδ T cells also have limited receptor diversity and may play a similar role in protection against commonly encountered microbial antigens, but B1 B cells do not express γδ TCRs. B1 B cells

are not a stage in B cell maturation. There is no IgB isotype.
    CMI5 151; BI2 24-25

24. (C) In T cell maturation, stem cells in the bone marrow give rise to lymphocyte progenitors that migrate to the thymus, begin to undergo TCR gene locus recombination in the pro-T cell stage, express pre-TCRs in the pre-T cell stage, express TCRs and both CD4 and CD8 in the double positive thymocyte stage, and become single $CD4^+$ or $CD8^+$ T cells in the naive mature T cell stage.
    CMI5 151-155; BI2 74, 76-80, 81

25. (B) Both positive and negative selection requires that the T cell precursors recognize the selecting antigens in the thymus. Because antigen recognition is based on TCR binding to peptide-MHC complexes, as is the case for mature T cells, both class I and class II MHCs are required for both positive and negative selection.
    CMI5 155-160; BI2 80-82

26. (A) The antigen-presenting cells (APCs) that mediate positive selection in the thymus can be either thymic epithelial cells or bone marrow–derived cells (dendritic cells, macrophages). The patient's bone marrow–derived APCs will have both maternal and paternal MHC molecules at 3 years of age, but only maternal MHC molecules after age 3. His thymic epithelial cells will always have both maternal and paternal MHC molecules. Tetanus toxoid-specific memory T cells would not have been generated before bone marrow transplantation because he had few or no T cells and he had not been immunized. The origin of the stem cells has no relevance to the MHC restriction of the T cells that eventually develop, because essentially the same set of TCR genes will be inherited from either parent, and MHC restriction will result from selection processes superimposed on a randomly generated set of TCRs. There is no basis for predicting that $CD8^+$ and $CD4^+$ T cells will be restricted by MHC alleles inherited from different parents.
    CMI5 157-160; BI2 80-82

27. (C) γδ T cells are a separate lineage from αβ T cells. This is indicated because TCRαβ genes have not undergone somatic recombination in γδ T cells, and γδ T cells develop normally in mice with null mutations in TCR αβ genes.
    CMI5 160-161; BI2 24

Chapter 8

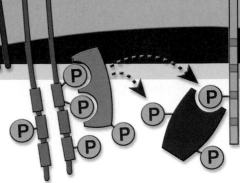

Activation of T Lymphocytes

Cellular and Molecular Immunology, 5/E: Chapter 8—Activation of T Lymphocytes

Basic Immunology, 2/E: Chapter 5— Cell-Mediated Immune Response

1. All of the following protein-protein interactions are involved in activation of naive helper T cells by antigen-presenting cells (APCs) EXCEPT:

   A. Binding of peptide-MHC complexes on the APC to the TCR on the T cell
   B. Binding of CD4 on the T cell to nonpolymorphic regions of class II MHC molecules on the APC
   C. Binding of integrins on the T cell with adhesion ligands on the APC
   D. Binding of B7-2 on the APC with CD28 on the T cell
   E. Binding of CD40L on the T cell with CD40 on the APC

2. Which one of the following statements about MHC-TCR interactions is NOT true?

   A. Antigen receptors on T cells bind to MHC molecules for only brief periods of time.
   B. The affinity of most TCRs for peptide-MHC complexes is similar to the affinity of antibodies for their antigens.
   C. Only 1% or less of the MHC molecules on any antigen-presenting cell (APC) display a peptide recognized by a particular T cell.
   D. T cells usually require multiple engagements with an APC before a threshold of activation is reached.
   E. A subthreshold number of MHC-TCR interactions can lead to T cell inactivation.

3. Which one of the following cell types would be most potent at activating naive T cells?

   A. Kupffer cells
   B. B cells

C. Follicular dendritic cells
D. Neutrophils
E. Langerhans cells

4. Which one of the following descriptions of cytokine interleukin-2 is NOT true?

   A. Expression of its gene requires multiple transcription factors, such as Fos, Jun, and NFAT.
   B. It acts as an autocrine growth factor for T cells.
   C. It binds to CD25 on the cell membrane of T cells.
   D. It is only involved in the proliferation of helper T cells and not CTLs.
   E. It promotes susceptibility of T cells to apoptosis.

5. Which one of the following statements about T cells involved in an immune response is NOT true?

   A. Activated T cells receive survival signals from antigen during an infection.
   B. Activated T cells contribute to the activation of antigen-presenting cells via CD40 ligand.
   C. Memory T cells generated during a primary immune response express high levels of interleukin-2 receptors and actively proliferate long after the primary response is completed.
   D. The major effector function of helper T cells is to activate macrophages and other cells by releasing cytokines.
   E. When an infection is eliminated, activated T cells die by apoptosis.

6. Which one of the following statements about the molecules B7-1 and B7-2 is NOT true?

   A. B7-1 and B7-2 expression on antigen-presenting cells (APCs) is upregulated by the presence of "danger" signals, such as lipopolysaccharide, as well as cytokines, such as interferon (IFN)-γ.
   B. B7-1 and B7-2 are expressed at low levels on some resting APCs.
   C. Induction of B7-1 usually occurs before the induction of B7-2 in an immune response.
   D. B7-1 and B7-2 bind to CD28 on T cells and provide "second signals" for naive T cell activation.
   E. Activated helper T cells can induce expression of B7-1 and B7-2 on APCs via CD40L binding to CD40.

7. In patients with hyper IgM syndrome, there is a genetically based deficiency in expression of CD40 ligand. In addition to defects in antibody isotype switching, these patients have defects in T cell–mediated immune responses and become infected with intracellular parasites. Which one of the following normal functions of CD40 ligand is important in T cell–mediated immunity?

   A. CD40-dependent isotype switching is required to produce antibody isotypes that activate T cells.

B. CD40 ligand is required for CTL killing of CD40-expressing infected cells.
C. CD40 ligand is required for maturation of CD4⁺ T cells in the thymus.
D. CD40 ligand on activated T cells binds to CD40 on antigen-presenting cells (APCs), and this enhances the expression of B7-1, B7-2, and cytokines by the APCs.
E. CD40 ligand on T cells binds to B7-1 and B7-2 on APCs, and this enhances the function of the APCs.

8. All of the following molecules act as transcription factors in T cell activation signaling EXCEPT:

   A. NF-κB
   B. Jun
   C. Fos
   D. NFAT
   E. Ras

9. Which one of the following statements about the molecule Lck is NOT true?

   A. It is a member of the Src family of kinases.
   B. It binds to the cytoplasmic tails of T cell coreceptors CD4 or CD8.
   C. It phosphorylates ITAM motifs on the CD3 complex.
   D. It phosphorylates tyrosine residues on Zap-70 and activates it.
   E. It phosphorylates PIP2 to PIP3 and leads to the activation of Itk.

10. A 7-month-old boy, the only child of second-degree cousins, saw a pediatrician for immunologic evaluation after developing *Pneumocystis carinii* pneumonia. Serum IgG, IgM, and IgA levels were normal. Blood cell count showed 10,600 leukocytes/mm³ and 80% lymphocytes; 90% of the lymphocytes were TCR αβ⁺ CD4⁺. In vitro lymphocyte-proliferative responses to PHA and anti-CD3 were absent, and the pattern of tyrosine-phosphorylated cytoplasmic proteins after anti-CD3 treatment of the T cells was distinctly abnormal. This boy most likely carries homozygous mutations in the gene encoding which one of the following proteins?

   A. Zap-70
   B. RAG-1
   C. CD3
   D. Pre-Tα
   E. TCRα

11. Which one of the following signaling molecules, if mutated, would affect B cell maturation and function primarily without affecting T cell function?

   A. Btk
   B. Itk
   C. Tec
   D. PI-3 kinase
   E. Zap-70

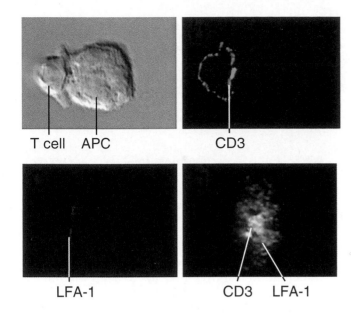

T cell   APC   CD3

LFA-1   CD3   LFA-1

12. The figure above shows the distribution of the TCR complex (as indicated by the localization of CD3) and the integrin LFA-1 on a T cell as it interacts with an antigen-presenting cell (APC) displaying the peptide-MHC complex recognized by the T cell. The focal concentration of these and several other molecules at the point of contact of the T cell and APC membranes is called the:

   A. Immune complex
   B. Supramolecular activation cluster
   C. Inferiority complex
   D. Excitatory synapse
   E. Lipid raft

13. All of the following are early T cell events that occur after antigen recognition by the TCR EXCEPT:

   A. Formation of the immunologic synapse
   B. Recruitment of signaling molecules, such as LAT, to glycolipid-enriched domains known as lipid rafts
   C. Enhanced adhesion between T cells and antigen-presenting cells (APCs) via T cell integrin LFA-1 and its ligand on the APC, ICAM-1, at the central zone of the immunologic synapse
   D. Clustering of the TCR and coreceptors leading to phosphorylation of ITAMs on CD3 by Lck
   E. Binding of CD28 with costimulators on APCs in the cSMAC, resulting in signal transduction activation

14. An experiment is performed in which a point mutation is introduced randomly into the *Zap-70* gene for a particular strain of mice. The mutant mice display a defect in T cell development. However, precursor T cells isolated from the thymus of these mice show normal expression levels of Zap-70 of the correct molecular weight. On further in vitro analysis, the mutant Zap-70 is found to bind to ITAM motifs in the cytoplasmic tail of the ζ chain, but only when the ζ chain is phosphorylated. No phosphorylated LAT is detected, however. Given these data, in which of the following protein domains is the mutation most likely to be present?

   A. Pleckstrin homology (PH) domain
   B. Proline-rich (PR) domain
   C. SH1 domain
   D. SH2 domain
   E. SH3 domain

15. Which one of the following accurately depicts the correct order of events in a TCR signal transduction pathway?

   A. TCR → Lck → Zap-70 → LAT → Grb-2 → SOS → Ras → Erk → Fos
   B. TCR → Lck → Zap-70 → LAT → SOS → Grb-2 → Ras → Erk → Fos
   C. TCR → Lck → ITK → LAT → Grb-2 → SOS → Ras → Erk → Fos
   D. TCR → Lck → Zap-70 → LAT → SOS → Grb-2 → Ras → Erk → Jun
   E. TCR → Lck → Zap-70 → LAT → PLCγ → DAG → calcium release

Questions 16-23

   For each of the descriptions in questions 16-23, choose the T cell signaling molecule that best matches it from the list below (A-O).

   A. CD3
   B. Lck
   C. Zap-70
   D. LAT
   E. Ras
   F. PLCγ
   G. PIP2
   H. PIP3
   I. IP3
   J. DAG
   K. Calcineurin
   L. NFAT
   M. Jun
   N. Fos
   O. NF-κB

16. This molecule becomes an active transcription factor on dephosphorylation. (   )

17. This protein is a well-characterized proto-oncogene product that on mutation to a constitutively active form has been associated with multiple neoplasms. (   )

18. Binding of this molecule to Jun is needed for transcriptional activation of the IL-2 gene. (   )

19. This is a transcription factor that exists in the phosphorylated form within the nucleus. (   )

20. Immunosuppressive therapy with the drugs cyclosporine and FK506 inhibits T cell activation by blocking the protein phosphatase activity of this molecule. (   )

21. This molecule binds to a receptor on the endoplasmic reticulum and stimulates release of calcium into the cytosol. (   )

22. This molecule has the same downstream effect as addition of the drug phorbol myristate acetate (PMA) to T cells. (   )

23. This molecule is a transcription factor involved in the expression of several T cell activation genes activated when its bound inhibitor is phosphorylated. (   )

24. Damage to neurons in patients with multiple sclerosis (MS) may be caused by autoreactive T cells that recognize peptides derived from myelin proteins presented by self MHC molecules. These autoreactive T cells secrete interferon (IFN)-γ and promote inflammation, which damages the myelin sheath surrounding neurons. The exact immunodominant epitopes recognized by autoreactive T cells in MS patents have been identified. One potential method of therapy for patients with MS is to administer therapeutic peptides that differ from the immunodominant epitopes by one or two amino acids. Which one of the following statements best describes the basis for this therapeutic approach?

    A. The therapeutic peptides, called "altered peptide ligands," could inactivate T cells specific for myelin proteins, or drive them to differentiate into T cells that do not produce IFN-γ.
    B. The therapeutic peptides, called "altered peptide ligands," could interfere with processing of the natural myelin proteins by the patient's antigen-presenting cells.
    C. The therapeutic peptides could bind to the TCRs of myelin-specific T cells but not to the self MHC molecules, thereby blocking T cell activation.
    D. The therapeutic peptides could down-regulate MHC expression.
    E. The therapeutic peptides could replace the damaged myelin and restore neuronal function.

Answers

1. (E) CD40L is not expressed on naive T cells and is only up-regulated subsequent to activation by an antigen-presenting cell (APC). In the naive helper T cell, the TCR binds to the MHC-peptide complex whereas the CD4 coreceptor engages a conserved region on the MHC II molecule. Integrins on the T cell interact with adhesion ligands on the APC. This region of binding between the T cell and the APC is known as the immunologic synapse and also includes costimulatory interactions, such as CD28 on the T cell binding to B7 on the APC.
   CMI5 171; BI2 74, 76-80

2. (B) In general, the TCR binds to peptide-MHC complexes with lower affinity than antigen-antibody interactions. This relatively low-affinity interaction occurs briefly; thus, a T cell may need multiple engagements with the antigen-presenting cell (APC) before a threshold of activation occurs. If this threshold is not reached, the T cell may enter into an inactive state known as anergy. On any given APC, less than 1% of the MHC molecules display the same peptide.
   CMI5 173-174

3. (E) Antigen-presenting cells (APCs) are responsible for presenting peptide-MHC complexes and costimulatory molecules to naive T cells; this leads to activation of the T cells. The most potent APCs are the dendritic cells, because they constitutively express high levels of costimulatory molecules. Langerhans cells are dendritic cells found in epidermis. Other APCs include macrophages and B cells. Kupffer cells are a type of macrophage found in the liver. Neither neutrophils nor follicular dendritic cells (FDCs) are involved in antigen presentation to T cells. FDCs are unrelated to dendritic cells and are found within the germinal centers of lymph nodes.
   CMI5 163-164; BI2 46

4. (D) IL-2 is involved in the proliferation of both CD4$^+$ and CD8$^+$ T cells. Activation of the naive T cell results in signals transduced via the TCR (signal 1) and CD28 (signal 2). This signaling results in the activation of transcription factors, such as Fos, Jun, and NFAT, which increase transcription of the IL-2 gene. IL-2 is then secreted and acts as both a paracrine and autocrine growth factor for T cells by binding to the IL-2 receptor (one component of which is CD25). In addition to its growth factor activity, IL-2 also "primes" T cells for apoptotic death, and this role for IL-2 is important in homeostasis of the immune system.
   CMI5 165-167; BI2 92-94

5. (C) Memory T cells are not actively proliferating and do not express high levels of IL-2 receptors. Instead, these cells are functionally quiescent and are not performing effector functions after a primary immune response. Effector T cells continue to survive in the periphery via proliferative signals from MHC-antigen binding to the TCR. Effector helper T cells can then activate macrophages and other lymphocytes via release of cytokines such as IFN-γ, as well as through CD40 ligand on the cell surface. On elimination of the infection, the effector T cells die by apoptosis.
   CMI5 168; BI2 99

6. (C) The temporal patterns of B7-1 and B7-2 expression differ. B7-2 is expressed constitutively at low levels and induced early after activation of antigen-presenting cells (APCs), whereas B7-1 is not expressed constitutively and is induced hours or days later. The expression of B7-1 and B7-2 on APCs is induced by "danger signals" of infection. These signals are mediated by binding of lipopolysaccharide (LPS), unmethylated CpG DNA, and other ligands of Toll-like receptors.

Signals mediated through cytokines, such as interferon (IFN)-γ, as well as through CD40 ligand, can also up-regulate B7-1 and B7-2 expression on APCs. Both B7-1 and B7-2 bind to CD28 on naive T cells, thus providing the second signal needed for activation of T cells.
CMI5 170; BI2 89-92

7. (D) CD40 ligand, a membrane-bound protein in the tumor necrosis factor (TNF) family of proteins, is expressed after T cell activation. When it binds to its receptor CD40, a TNF-receptor family member expressed on macrophages, and other antigen-presenting cells, signals are transmitted that enhance costimulator and cytokine expression (as well as other functions of macrophages). This serves to amplify the T cell response and enhance the killing of microbes ingested by macrophages. Antibodies are not required to activate T cells. CD40 does not transduce pro-apoptotic signals. CD40 ligand is not involved in T cell maturation and does not bind to B7-1 or B7-2.
CMI5 172-173; BI2 95-96,112-115

8. (E) All of these proteins are involved in the activation of T cells. However, Ras is not a transcription factor but a guanosine triphosphate (GTP)-binding protein present in the cytosol and in association with the plasma membrane. On exchange of guanosine diphosphate (GDP) for GTP, the Ras protein becomes functional and acts as an allosteric activator of MAP kinases, which leads the transcription of Fos.
CMI5 180-181; BI2 100-103

9. (E) PI-3 kinase is responsible for the phosphorylation of PIP2 to PIP3, leading to the activation of Itk in T cells and Btk in B cells.
CMI5 175, 180; BI2 100-103

10. (A) The patient shows signaling defects in TCR-mediated T cell activation, as well as defects in CD8$^+$ T cell maturation. Zap-70 is a tyrosine kinase required for TCR-mediated T cell activation. Mutations in Zap-70 result in impaired TCR signaling, with abnormal tyrosine phosphorylation of downstream signaling molecules, and also a defect in CD8$^+$ T cell maturation. It is not known why CD8$^+$ maturation is selectively impaired in Zap-70 deficiency. VDJ recombination, and therefore RAG-1 function, must still be intact because TCR-expressing CD4$^+$ T cells do mature. CD3, pre-Tα, and TCRα are also required for maturation of CD4$^+$ T cells, and therefore these molecules must all be expressed by this patient.
CMI5 175-180

11. (A) Btk is a Tec family protein tyrosine kinase that is particularly important in pre-B cell receptor complex signaling, and therefore in B cell maturation and activation. Mutations in Btk are responsible for X-linked agammaglobulinemia. Itk and Tec are other members of the Tec family that are important in T cells. PI-3 kinase is a phospholipid

kinase involved in signaling in many cell types, including B and T cells, and Zap-70 is a protein tyrosine kinase particularly important in TCR signaling in T cells.
CMI5 177-178; BI2 100-103

12. (B) The supramolecular activation complex (SAC), or immunologic synapse, is an organized cell-cell junction between T lymphocytes and antigen-presenting cells. It is composed of an adhesion ring, where integrins are located (the peripheral supramolecular activation cluster [pSMAC]), and a central T cell receptor cluster (the central supramolecular activation cluster [cSMAC]). The T cell proteins in the cSMAC are found within specialized domains in the T cell membrane with altered lipid contact, called lipid rafts. Immune complexes are unrelated to T cell activation and are composed of antibodies and bound antigens. Excitatory synapses are found between neurons, not immune cells.
CMI5 174-177; BI2 101

13. (C) On binding of the TCR complex with MHC-associated peptides on an antigen-presenting cell (APC), several T cell surface proteins and intracellular signaling molecules are rapidly mobilized to the site of contact, known as the immunologic synapse. Molecules that are recruited to the central supramolecular activation cluster, or center of the synapse, include the TCR complex (TCR, CD3, and ζ chains), CD4 or CD8 coreceptors, and costimulatory molecules (CD28). The clustering of signaling molecules results in the phosphorylation of ITAMs on CD3 by CD4- or CD8-associated Lck. Integrins remain at the peripheral zone of the synapse and stabilize the binding of the T cell to the APC. LAT is a transmembrane adaptor molecule recruited to the synapse whose cytoplasmic tail forms part of a scaffold of signaling molecules.
CMI5 174

14. (C) In this experiment, the mutant Zap-70 can still bind to the phosphorylated ζ chains but cannot phosphorylate LAT. This suggests that the SH2 domains are normal but that the SH1 kinase domain has been mutated. Zap-70 does not contain a PH, PR, or SH3 domain. The PH domain allows proteins to localize to the membrane by binding to PIP3. PR domains mediate protein-protein interactions via binding to SH3 domains.
CMI5 175-180

15. (A) Activated Zap-70 phosphorylates the transmembrane adapter protein LAT at tyrosine residues, which serve as docking sites for SH2 domains of other proteins. In one pathway, the SH2 domain of Grb-2 binds to phosphorylated LAT. Grb-2 is then able to recruit Sos to the membrane. Sos catalyzes GDP/GTP exchange on Ras, a G protein that is active when guanosine triphosphate (GTP) is bound and inactive when guanosine diphosphate (GDP) is bound. Active Ras functions as an allosteric activator of mitogen-activated

protein kinases (MAPK), leading to downstream activation of Erk through phosphorylation. Activated Erk stimulates the transcription of Fos (through intermediate activation of a protein called Elk). In a second pathway, PLCγ binds directly to activated LAT and is then phosphorylated by Zap-70. Activated PLCγ leads to the cleavage of PIP2 to IP_3 and DAG. Although DAG activates protein kinase C (PKC), it is IP3 that causes a release of calcium into the cytosol.
CMI5 180-182; BI2 100-103

16. (L) NFAT is a transcription factor required by T cells for the expression of interleukin (IL)-2, IL-4, tumor necrosis factor (TNF), and other cytokine genes. NFAT is present in an inactive, phosphorylated form in the cytosol of resting T cells. On dephosphorylation by calcineurin, a nuclear localization sequence is uncovered that permits NFAT to translocate to the nucleus. Once in the nucleus, NFAT induces transcription of these genes.
CMI5 184; BI2 100-103

17. (E) *Ras* was one of the first proto-oncogenes characterized. Normal *ras* is involved in TCR signaling pathways. On mutation to a constitutively active state, *ras* promotes the survival and proliferation of malignant cells.
CMI5 181; BI2 100-103

18. (N) Fos combines with phosphorylated Jun to form activation protein-1 (AP-1). AP-1 is the name for a family of DNA-binding factors composed of dimers of two different proteins. Transcription of *fos* is enhanced by the Erk pathway, whereas phosphorylation of preexisting Jun is induced through the Vav/Rac pathway. AP-1 physically associates with other transcription factors in the nucleus, and together they activate transcription of cytokine genes essential for T cell activation.
CMI5 184; BI2 100-103

19. (M) On phosphorylation, c-Jun translocates to the nucleus and binds to Fos to form AP-1.
CMI5 183; BI2 100-103

20. (K) Calcineurin is responsible for the dephosphorylation of NFAT, which is an essential transcription factor for the activation of T and B cells. The immunosuppressive drugs cyclosporine and FK506 function by inhibiting calcineurin. These drugs are commonly used to prevent transplant rejection.
CMI5 184; BI2 100-103

21. (I) IP3 is generated from the cleavage of PIP2 in the membrane to DAG and IP3 by the enzyme PLCγ, and it stimulates release of calcium into the cytosol.
CMI5 182; BI2 100-103

22. (J) Both DAG and pharmacologic agents such as phorbol myristate acetate (PMA) activate protein kinase C (PKC). PKC has many substrates and is a potent activator of many transcription factors in T cells.
CMI5 182

23. (O) NF-κB is present in the cytoplasm and is bound to an inhibitor called I-κB. On stimulation with antigen, I-κB becomes phosphorylated, dissociates from NF-κB, and is degraded by the ubiquitin-proteosomal pathway. NF-κB then translocates to the nucleus, where it participates in transcriptional activation of several genes.
CMI5 180-181; BI2 100-103

24. (A) Altered peptide ligands are synthetic peptides in which the TCR contact residues have been changed, so that the peptide induces only partial responses by the responding T cell. These peptides still bind to the same MHC molecules as the original peptides, but they can cause T cell inactivation (anergy) or change in the cytokines the T cell produces. Altered peptide ligands do not interfere with processing of the natural proteins nor can they bind to TCRs without being presented by MHC molecules. There is no basis to say that peptides can down-regulate major MHC expression or replace damaged proteins in the myelin sheath.
CMI5 187

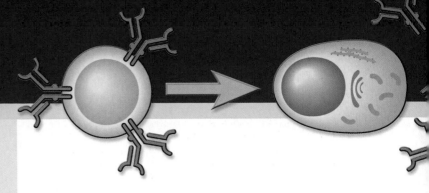

Chapter 9

B Cell Activation and Antibody Production

Cellular and Molecular Immunology, 5/E: Chapter 9—B Cell Activation and Antibody Production

Basic Immunology, 2/E: Chapter 9— Humoral Immune Responses

1. Which one of the following statements about primary and secondary antibody responses is NOT true?

   A. Antibodies in primary responses generally have lower affinity for antigen than those produced in secondary responses.
   B. Secondary responses reach peak levels more quickly than primary responses.
   C. Primary responses require higher concentrations of antigen for initiation than secondary responses.
   D. Primary responses occur to all types of antigens, but secondary responses mostly occur only to protein antigens.
   E. Primary responses are characterized by IgG antibodies, whereas secondary responses are dominated by IgM antibodies.

2. Which one of the following statements about humoral immune responses is true?

   A. Naive B cells are required for initiation of primary responses and memory B cells are required for initiation of secondary responses.
   B. Antibody responses to bacterial polysaccharide antigens require CD4$^+$ helper T cells.
   C. Heavy chain isotype switching typically occurs in response to bacterial polysaccharide antigens.
   D. Affinity maturation does not require helper T cells.
   E. Antibody-secreting cells generated during a humoral immune response live for only a few hours.

3. All of the following assays are used to detect antibody production EXCEPT:

   A. BrdU (bromodeoxyuridine) assay
   B. Enzyme-linked immunosorbent assay (ELISA)
   C. ELISPOT assay
   D. Hemolytic plaque assay
   E. Radioimmunoassay (RIA)

Questions 4-6

A 5-year-old boy has a history of recurrent pneumococcal pneumonia, *Pneumocystis carinii* pneumonia (PCP), and bacterial ear infections. His maternal uncle and an older brother experienced the same symptoms, but he has an older sister who is healthy. Laboratory studies indicate normal numbers of B cells and T cells, and the serum contains mostly IgM and very little IgG.

4. Which of the following abnormalities would NOT be likely in this patient?

   A. The IgG antibodies that are present are of lower affinity for antigen than of those of a healthy individual.
   B. Lymph nodes are without well-developed follicles containing germinal centers.
   C. Macrophage killing of intracellular microbes is impaired.
   D. There is limited diversity in the repertoire of IgM antibodies produced.
   E. There is no evidence of somatic mutation of IgM variable regions.

5. Which of the following genes most likely contains a mutation in this patient?

   A. *AID* (activation-induced deaminase)
   B. *CD40*
   C. *CD40L*
   D. *CD28*
   E. *CTLA-4*

6. If this patient did have a sister affected with the same condition, which of the following genes would most likely contain a mutation?

   A. *AID* (activation-induced deaminase)
   B. *CD40*
   C. *CD40L*
   D. *CD28*
   E. *CTLA-4*

Questions 7-10

For each of the descriptions in questions 7-10, select the B cell signaling molecule (A-I) that most closely matches it.

   A. Igα
   B. Igβ
   C. C3b
   D. C3d
   E. CR2
   F. CD19
   G. CD81
   H. Fyn
   I. Syk

7. A protein tyrosine kinase homologous to Zap-70, which phosphorylates several adaptor proteins and enzymes (   )

8. An Src family kinase that phosphorylates ITAMs in the cytoplasmic tails of B cell receptor complex proteins (   )

9. A protein that is the cell surface receptor for Epstein-Barr virus (   )

10. A protein that covalently binds to microbes and serves as a ligand for a coreceptor that enhances B cell responses to antigen (   )

11. The B cell receptor (BCR) complex and the signaling cascades to which it is linked share many similarities with the T cell receptor (TCR) complex and its linked signaling cascades. Which of the following comparisons between BCR and TCR signaling is NOT true?

    A. There are ITAMs in the cytoplasmic tails of CD3 in the TCR complex and in the cytoplasmic tails of Igα and Igβ in the BCR complex.
    B. The cytoplasmic tails of membrane Ig and TCR αβ antigen receptors are very short and lack intrinsic signaling functionality.
    C. Early signaling events induced by antigen binding to both BCR and TCR involve both Src family and Zap-70 family protein tyrosine kinases.
    D. Phospholipase C–mediated generation of IP_3 and DAG occurs downstream of both BCR and TCR signaling.
    E. CD4/CD8 coreceptors in T cells and the CR2 coreceptor in B cells both enhance responses to antigen by a PI3 kinase–dependent mechanism.

12. The initial cellular events that are induced by antigen-mediated cross-linking of the B cell receptor (BCR) complex include all of the following EXCEPT:

    A. Increased percentage of time spent in mitosis, resulting in rapid proliferation
    B. Increased expression of B7, resulting in enhanced APC function
    C. Increased expression of bcl-2, resulting in improved survival
    D. Increased expression of CCR7, promoting migration into lymph node follicles
    E. Increased expression of the interleukin-2 receptor, resulting in enhanced proliferation and response to T cell signals

13. Which one of the following statements accurately describes antigen recognition events in a lymph node during a helper T cell–dependent antibody response to a protein antigen?

    A. Naive B cells and naive T cells simultaneously recognize the intact protein antigen.
    B. Naive B cells recognize intact proteins, generate peptide fragments of these proteins, and present them in complexes with major histo-

compatibility complex (MHC) molecules to naive helper T cells.

C. Naive B cells recognize intact proteins, generate peptide fragments of these proteins, and present them in complexes with MHC molecules to differentiated helper T cells.

D. Naive T cells recognize peptides bound to MHC molecules presented by dendritic cells, and naive B cells recognize the intact protein antigen bound to the surface of follicular dendritic cells.

E. Differentiated helper T cells recognize peptides bound to MHC molecules on dendritic cells, and the T cells secrete cytokines that promote antibody production by any nearby B cells that have recognized different protein antigens.

14. Which one of the following B cell responses is NOT stimulated by CD40 ligand?

A. Association of TRAFs with the cytoplasmic tails of CD40 molecules
B. Activation of NF-κB
C. Enhanced expression of B7-1 and B7-2
D. Enhanced Ig isotype switch recombinase activity
E. Enhanced production of membrane Ig

15. Which of the following mechanisms contributes to the change from B cell production of membrane Ig to secreted Ig?

A. V(D)J recombinase-mediated deletion of the exon encoding the transmembrane domain
B. Alternative processing of primary RNA transcripts to remove the transmembrane domain and include a secretory tail piece
C. Increased vesicular exocytosis of intracellular stores of the secretory form of Ig
D. Switch recombinase-mediated recombination of the heavy chain locus to juxtapose the V(D)J segment with the exon encoding a secretory tail piece
E. Up-regulation of ectoenzymes that proteolytically cleave membrane Ig heavy chains just proximal to the membrane

16. Which of the following statements about Ig isotype switching is NOT true?

A. Interleukin-4 promotes switching to the IgE isotype by increasing germline transcription of the Cε exon.
B. Isotype switching involves recombination of a V(D)J complex with downstream C region genes and the deletion of intervening DNA including other C region genes.
C. Activation-induced deaminase (AID) is required for switch recombination.
D. The enzymes that mediate isotype switching recognize conserved heptamer and nonamer DNA sequences adjacent to the constant region exons.
E. The same recombined V(D)J gene complex is used to encode the antigen-binding region of the antibodies produced by a B cell before and after isotype switching.

Questions 17-21

For each of descriptions in questions 17-21, select the letter of the Ig isotype (A-E) that most closely matches it. Answers may be used more than once.

A. IgM
B. IgD
C. IgG
D. IgE
E. IgA

17. An allergy attack (   )

18. Phagocytosis (   )

19. Unclear functional role (   )

20. Binds to receptors in the gastrointestinal tract of infants for absorption into the serum (   )

21. T cell–independent antigens (   )

22. Which one of the following molecules is important for the production of IgE antibodies?

A. CD28
B. CD40
C. IFN-γ
D. IL-2
E. TGF-β

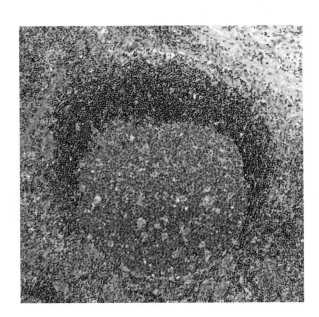

23. The figure above shows a histologic section of a follicle of a lymph node. Based on the appearance of the biopsy specimen, which of the following descriptions of the patient from whom the specimen was taken is most accurate?

A. Has a CD40 ligand deficiency
B. Is undergoing an antibody response to a bacterial polysaccharide
C. Is undergoing an antibody response to a viral capsid protein
D. Is in an immunologically quiescent state
E. Has Burkitt's lymphoma

24. Which of the following events does NOT occur within germinal centers?

    A. Somatic mutation of Ig V genes
    B. Generation of memory B cells
    C. B cell proliferation
    D. Affinity maturation
    E. Ig gene V(D)J recombination

25. Which of the following descriptions about affinity maturation is correct?

    A. Depends on somatic mutation of V genes
    B. Depends on negative selection of B cells that can bind antigen in the germinal center
    C. Depends on antigen processing and presentation by dendritic cells within the germinal center
    D. Depends on the autoimmune regulator (AIRE) gene
    E. Depends on somatic recombination of Ig V genes

26. Which of the following antigenic structures might activate B cell antibody production without the aid of T cells?

    A. Lysozyme
    B. Benzene
    C. Glucose-6-phosphate
    D. ABO blood group antigen
    E. Rh factor antigen

27. Antibody feedback is mediated by which of the following molecules?

    A. Ig FcγRIIB
    B. Ig Fcε
    C. Ig FcγRI
    D. CR1
    E. IgM

Answers

1. (E) In a primary immune response, IgM antibodies are initially produced against antigens. IgG production requires T cell–dependent isotype switching and is seen predominantly in secondary responses. Primary antibody responses can be mounted to any type of antigen, but secondary responses usually require CD4$^+$ T cell help, and therefore the antigen must be a protein. Primary responses do require higher concentrations of antigen for initiation. The affinity of membrane Ig for antigen is lower on naive B cells, which are responsible for primary responses, compared with memory B cells, which are responsible for secondary responses. Secondary responses develop more quickly and produce higher peak levels of antibody as compared with primary responses.
CMI5 190-191; BI2 125-126

2. (A) Humoral responses require antigen-dependent activation of B cells through binding of the antigen to membrane Ig on naive B cells or on memory B cells, for primary or secondary responses, respectively. In most cases, nonprotein antigens do not stimulate isotype switching or affinity maturation because these changes require T cell help, and only protein antigens can stimulate T cells. For both nonprotein and protein antigens, antibody-secreting cells that are generated may live for months, often in the bone marrow.
CMI5 189-191; BI2 123-126

3. (A) BrdU (bromodeoxyuridine) is a thymidine analogue that is used to measure cellular proliferation in vivo. BrdU is injected into the organism, and tissues are subsequently stained with anti-BrdU antibody to quantify the extent of BrdU incorporation into cellular DNA. The other assays listed all can be used to detect antibody production.
CMI5 193

4. (D) This is a common presentation of hyper-IgM syndrome. Patients with this disease have B cells that are unable to undergo isotype switching, and therefore contain only IgM in the serum but very low levels of IgG, IgA, and IgE. Clinically, these patients are susceptible to bacterial infections and often present with a history of recurrent pneumonia, otitis media, and gastrointestinal infections. Mutations in genes coding for CD40L, CD40, and activation-induced deaminase (AID) have been identified in these patients. During an immune response, T cell interactions with B cells via CD40L-CD40, as well as active AID, are both essential for numerous processes, including isotype switching, somatic mutation, and germinal center formation. Thus, patients with hyper-IgM syndrome produce antibodies that typically have a lower affinity for antigen (due to the lack of somatic mutation) and do not develop large follicles containing a light zone and dark zone (germinal center) within lymph nodes. Mechanisms of generation of diversity of the Ig repertoire should not be impaired in this patient. Although somatic mutation of variable regions will be impaired, this will not be manifest in IgM antibodies. In addition, patients with either CD40L or CD40 mutations, but not AID mutations, will have an increased susceptibility to certain intracellular infections (such as *Pneumocystic carinii* pneumonia), because the microbicidal activity of macrophages is partially dependent on CD40-mediated signals.
CMI5 201, 204-210, 459; BI2 133, 213

5. (C) Because both a maternal uncle and an older brother, but not the patient's sister, are affected, the inheritance pattern is most likely X-linked recessive. The *CD40L* gene is located on the X-chromosome.
CMI5 201, 204-210, 459; BI2 133, 213

6. (B) If the patient's sister is also affected with hyper-IgM syndrome, then the inheritance pattern is autosomal recessive. Both the *AID* and *CD40* genes are located on autosomal chromosomes, and mutations in both have been identified as causes of hyper-IgM syndrome. However, only a mutation in *CD40* will result in reduced macrophage function and susceptibility to *Pneumocystis carinii* pneumonia, as is observed in this patient.
CMI5 201, 204-210, 459; BI2 133, 213

7. (I) The tyrosine kinase Syk binds through its SH2 domains to the phosphotyrosine residues on the cytoplasmic tails of Igα and Igβ. On activation, Syk, in turn, activates numerous downstream signaling molecules, including B cell linker protein (BLNK). BLNK serves as a scaffolding protein for the activation of different pathways, including the Ras-MAP kinase pathway, the phospholipase C pathway with calcium release, and Btk activation. Ultimately, the same transcription factors that are important players in T cell activation also mediate B cell activation, including NFAT, AP-1, and NF-κB.
CMI5 192-194; BI2 127

8. (H) On antigen-mediated cross-linking of the B cell receptor (BCR), the ITAMs of Igα and Igβ are phosphorylated by Src family kinases, including Fyn, Lyn, and Blk. This initiates the signaling cascade for B cell activation.
CMI5 192; BI2 127

9. (E) Complement receptor 2 (CR2; gp140) is the cell surface receptor for Epstein-Barr virus (EBV) and mediates EBV entry into the cell. CR2 also serves as a coreceptor with the B cell receptor, mediating complement-dependent enhancement of B cell activation.
CMI5 195; BI2 128-129

10. (D) C3d is a complement protein fragment that binds covalently to microbial surfaces. C3d serves as the link between the BCR, which binds directly to the microbe, and the CR2 coreceptor. This cross-linking between the BCR and CR2 serves to amplify the B cell response 1000-fold when compared with immune responses in which CR2 is not recruited. CR2 forms a complex with two other proteins, CD19 and CD81, on the B cell surface. When CD19 is brought into proximity with BCR-associated kinases, the cytoplasmic tail of CD19 is rapidly phosphorylated. CD19 then activates several signaling pathways, including PI3-kinase.
CMI5 195; BI2 128-129

11. (E) The CR2 coreceptor, in association with CD19 and CD81, activates PI3-kinase. CD4 and CD8 do not activate PI3-kinase but, rather, bring the Src family tyrosine kinase Lck into proximity of the TCR complex.
CMI5 192-195; BI2 128-129

12. (D) In the initial events after antigen binding to the B cell receptor, B cells migrate out of, not into, the lymph node follicles and toward the T cell zones by increasing expression of CCR7, a chemokine receptor that responds to chemokines produced in the T cell zone. Helper T cells play an important role in the activation of B cells, inducing proliferation, isotype switching, and somatic mutation both by the release of cytokines as well as through direct interactions with the B cell via CD40L. T cell–mediated activation of B cells can only occur in the presence of protein antigens. Other early events that occur in B cell activation include increased proliferation and time spent in mitosis, increased expression of B7 to enhance the B cell's ability to activate T cells, increased expression of the anti-apoptotic protein bcl-2 to promote survival, and increased expression of cytokine receptors to enhance survival and proliferative signals coming from T cells.
CMI5 196-198; BI2 129

13. (C) T cells and B cells cannot recognize the same protein antigen molecule simultaneously because T cells only recognize peptide-MHC complexes. B cells bind intact proteins, internalize them via surface Ig, and then present peptide-MHC complexes to helper T cells, not to naive T cells. The helper T cells specific for the peptide-MHC complexes have been differentiated from naive T cells that recognized the same peptide-MHC complexes presented by dendritic cells. Follicular dendritic cells display intact protein antigens to previously activated (but not naive) B cells during the germinal center reaction. Collaboration of T cells and B cells requires direct contact of T cells and B cells specific for the same antigen, even though the antigen recognition events are not simultaneous, because the bidirectional activation requires membrane-bound molecules (i.e., CD40 ligand on the T cells and CD40 on the B cells).
CMI5 196-201; BI2 130-131

14. (E) CD40 ligand binding to B cell CD40 enhances production of secreted, not membrane, Ig. CD40 signaling involves recruitment of signaling intermediates, called tumor necrosis factor–receptor associated factors (TRAFs), to the cytoplasmic tails of CD40 and the downstream activation of NF-κB, as well as other transcription factors. The signaling cascades result in increased expression of various genes, including B7 costimulators, and increased Ig isotype switching, which is mediated by switch recombinases.
CMI5 201-203; BI2 133

15. (B) Primary transcripts of Ig genes include sequences encoding both transmembrane and secretory tail piece domains. Alternative splicing of these transcripts determines which form of Ig is ultimately made. V(D)J recombinases are not involved in modifications of Ig heavy chain expression, and switch recombinases are only involved in changes in DNA related to isotype switching. Membrane Ig is not cleaved to form secretory Ig.
CMI5 203-204

16. (D) Heptamer and nonamer sequences are part of the recombination signal sequences recognized by V(D)J recombinases, and not by the enzymes that mediate switch recombination. I exons and S (switch) regions are the DNA "landmarks" just upstream of each constant region gene that dictates where switch recombination will occur. Switch recombination is incompletely understood, but requires AID as well as other enzymes that gain access to the S regions when germline transcription through the I, S, and C exons is induced by cytokines. The same V(D)J unit is used to encode the antigen-binding site after switch

recombination, and this preserves antigen specificity of the antibodies produced while effector functions of the antibodies change.
CMI5 204-207; BI2 133-136

17. (D) IgE antibodies play an essential role in immediate-type hypersensitivity reactions (e.g., allergies), asthma, and helminthic infections. In allergic reactions, mast cells express Fcε receptors, which are bound to IgE antibodies specific for the allergen (these IgE antibodies were created after a prior exposure to the allergen). On re-exposure to allergen that binds to the IgE antibodies, the mast cells are induced to degranulate and release large quantities of histamine and other vasoactive substances.
CMI5 205; BI2 134

18. (C) Phagocytosis is primarily mediated by neutrophils and macrophages during an immune response to an infection. Both of these cell types express Fcγ receptors that bind to the constant regions on IgG antibodies and phagocytose the antigen-coated microbes.
CMI5 205; BI2 134

19. (B) IgD is expressed only as a membrane Ig on naive B cells, but its function is unclear.
CMI5 205; BI2 134

20. (C) Neonatal immunity is mediated in part by antibodies in breast milk, which are absorbed in the gastrointestinal tract by specific Fc receptors. These receptors are specific for the IgG isotype and are called FcγRN (N for "neonatal"). Absorption of antibodies from the mother's breast milk is a primary mode of immunity for the first 6 months of life, before the infant has produced significant amounts of antibody on its own.
CMI5 205; BI2 134

21. (A) B cells do not undergo isotype switching in response to T cell–independent antigens. The primary isotype is therefore IgM.
CMI5 211; BI2 134

22. (B) Cytokines play essential roles in regulating the switch to particular heavy chain isotypes. IFN-γ is important in switching to the IgG isotype (specifically IgG3), whereas TGF-β is a stimulator of IgA production. The cytokine that promotes IgE production is IL-4, but this is not an answer choice. However, the process of isotype switching in general is known to depend on signaling through CD40L-CD40, and is also dependent on the activity of the enzyme activation-induced deaminase (AID). CD28 is a costimulatory molecule that is important for T cell activation and CD40L up-regulation. However, other costimulatory molecules are also present on T cells that can cause up-regulation of CD40L. IL-2 is a growth factor cytokine for T cells.
CMI5 204; BI2 134-136

23. (C) The image shows a follicle with an active germinal center reaction (indicated by the eccentric pale area). Germinal center reactions are stimu-lated by protein antigens and CD4+ helper T cells specific for those antigens. They depend on CD40 ligand on the T cell, which binds to CD40 on the B cells. Although there is vigorous proliferation of one or a few clones of the B cells, the germinal center reaction is not neoplastic, and most of the B cells will die within the follicle.
CMI5 208

24. (E) V(D)J recombination to form functional Ig genes occurs only in developing B cells, mostly in the bone marrow. Germinal centers are sites of differentiation of mature B cells, in response to T cell–dependent protein antigens. The germinal center "reaction" begins with helper T cell signals delivered to B cells via CD40 ligand and cytokines. This results in B cell movement back into the follicle and brisk B cell proliferation of one or a few clones of B cells specific for an inciting antigen. The proliferating B cells undergo somatic mutation of the variable genes, at which point mutations are introduced that may alter the affinity of the encoded antibodies for their antigens. Antigens are displayed in limited concentrations on the surfaces of follicular dendritic cells in the germinal center, and only B cells whose high-affinity Ig receptors can bind these antigens are selected to survive. Some of these cells become antibody-secreting cells, and others become memory B cells.
CMI5 206-210; BI2 136-139

25. (A) Somatic mutation of V genes is the basis for production of immunoglobulins with different affinities, which are then positively selected in the germinal center; B cells that cannot bind antigen with high affinity die through a default pathway of apoptosis. Antigen processing and presentation by dendritic cells are required to generate helper T cells outside the follicle, but not to activate B cells in the follicle. Autoimmune regulator (AIRE) is involved in thymic expression of tissue antigens but is not involved in affinity maturation. Somatic recombination of V genes is involved in producing functional Ig genes during B cell development, but it is not involved in germinal center reactions.
CMI5 206-210; BI2 134

26. (D) T cell–independent antigens consist of polysaccharides, glycolipids, and nucleic acids with multiple repeated epitopes, so that maximal cross-linking of the B cell receptor is induced, thus bypassing the need for T cell help. Of the answer choices, the best choice is the ABO blood group antigen, because of its polyvalent glycolipid structure. Lysozyme and the Rh factor are protein antigens. Benzene and glucose-6-phosphate are not polyvalent.
CMI5 211-212; BI2 139-140

27. (A) Antibody feedback is the mechanism of regulation of humoral immune responses and is mediated by the Ig FcγRIIB receptor, which delivers inhibitory signals into the B cells on binding the Fc portion of IgG.
CMI5 213-214; BI2 140-141

Chapter 10

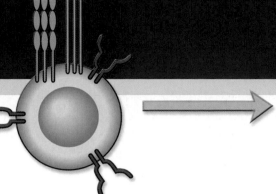

Immunologic Tolerance

Cellular and Molecular Immunology, 5/E: Chapter 10—Immunologic Tolerance

Basic Immunology, 2/E: Chapter 9—Immunologic Tolerance and Autoimmunity

1. Immunologic tolerance is defined as:

   A. The removal of an antigen, or the microbes expressing the antigen, by the immune system, so that the host can tolerate the infection
   B. Activation of only B cells, and not T cells, on exposure to an antigen
   C. Unresponsiveness of the immune system to an antigen, which is induced by previous exposure to that antigen
   D. The production of memory B cells and T cells on primary exposure to an antigen, which allows the host to tolerate a secondary exposure to the antigen
   E. Vaccination of individuals against particular pathogens to prevent subsequent infections

2. Failure of self-tolerance is the cause of which one of the following types of diseases?

   A. Allograft rejection
   B. Autoimmunity
   C. Atopy
   D. Anergy
   E. Acne

3. Which of the following statements about induction or maintenance of T cell tolerance is NOT true?

   A. Central tolerance is induced when immature developing T cells in bone marrow or thymus encounter self antigens.
   B. Peripheral T cell tolerance results when mature naive T cells recognize antigens without adequate B7-1– or B7-2–mediated costimulation.

C. Peripheral T cell tolerance results when T cells recognize antigen in the setting of an innate immune response to the antigen.

D. Peripheral T cell tolerance to some antigens is induced when mature T cells recognize antigen and bind B7-1 or B7-2 via the inhibitory CTLA-4 receptor.

E. Peripheral T cell tolerance to an antigen may be induced by persistent and repeated stimulation of lymphocytes by that antigen in tissues.

4. Which one of the following is NOT a mechanism of T cell tolerance?

A. Inhibition of T cell activation by interleukin-12 from regulatory T cells.

B. Apoptosis induced by Fas ligand binding to Fas.

C. Anergy induced by B7-1 or B7-2 binding to CTLA-4.

D. Anergy induced by peptide-major histocompatibility complex (MHC) binding to T cell receptors (TCRs) without B7-1 or B7-2 binding to CD28.

E. TCR-mediated up-regulation of Bim or similar pro-apoptotic proteins.

5. Transgenic mouse lines have been very useful for the study of mechanisms of self-tolerance. In one such line, transgenes were introduced encoding a T cell receptor (TCR) specific for the H-Y antigen, which is a protein expressed by many cell types only in male mice. When these transgenic mice were analyzed, researchers found that T cells expressing the H-Y–specific TCR developed normally in female mice but not in male mice. This finding illustrates which of the following mechanism of self tolerance?

A. Peripheral anergy

B. Central (thymic) deletion

C. Clonal ignorance

D. Regulatory T cell–mediated suppression

E. Peripheral deletion

6. Autoimmune polyendocrinopathy-candidiasis-ecto-dermal dystrophy (APECED) is a rare disease in which there is autoimmune destruction of several endocrine organs. This disease is caused by mutations in the autoimmune regulator gene called *AIRE*. *AIRE* is normally expressed primarily in the thymus and serves as a transcription factor in thymic epithelial cells. A failure to produce *AIRE* leads to a failure in tolerance to several self-proteins. Which ONE of the following statements best explains the influence of AIRE on self tolerance?

A. *AIRE* up-regulates expression of proteins that induce proliferation of thymic epithelial cells, allowing greater self antigen presentation to T cells.

B. *AIRE* up-regulates expression of cytokines that inhibit activation of T cells.

C. *AIRE* up-regulates expression of MHC proteins, allowing for greater self antigen presentation to developing T cells.

D. *AIRE* up-regulates expression of proteins usually expressed only in peripheral organs, allowing presentation of the proteins to developing T cells.

E. *AIRE* up-regulates expression of Fas ligand on thymic epithelial cells to induce apoptosis in self-reactive T cells.

7. Which one of the following statements regarding positive and negative selection of T cells is NOT true?

A. Thymic epithelial cells present self-peptide-MHC to developing T cells undergoing the selection process.

B. T cells that do not recognize self-peptide-MHC die by neglect.

C. T cells that bind too strongly to self-peptide-MHC die by Fas ligand-mediated apoptosis.

D. During positive selection, developing T cells express higher levels of anti-apoptotic proteins such as bcl-2.

E. A breakdown in negative selection may result in the development of some autoimmune diseases.

8. A genetic deficiency in the ability to produce which of the following molecules results in autoimmunity?

A. B7-1

B. CD28

C. CD40L

D. Interferon-γ

E. Interleukin-2

9. Which of the following molecules does NOT promote lymphocyte apoptosis?

A. Bid

B. Caspase-8

C. FADD

D. FLIP

E. Glucocorticoid

10. Many tumors are found to overexpress bcl-2, which favors survival of the transformed cells. Which of the following best describes the function of bcl-2?

A. Direct inhibition of caspase-8

B. Direct inhibition of caspase-9

C. Up-regulates expression of DNA repair enzymes

D. Reduces the leakiness of the mitochondrial membrane

E. Inhibits the activity of granzymes released from cytotoxic T lymphocytes

11. Which of the following terms best describes the mechanism by which effector T cells are deleted by repeated stimulation by persistent antigen?

A. Passive cell death

B. Central tolerance

C. Peripheral tolerance

D. Death by neglect

E. Activation-induced cell death

12. All of the following describe features of apoptosis EXCEPT:

    A. Caspase activation
    B. Membrane blebbing
    C. Inflammation
    D. Nuclear fragmentation
    E. DNA cleavage

13. Which of the following is NOT a property of regulatory T cells?

    A. Interleukin-2 receptor (CD25) expression
    B. Secretion of transforming growth factor-β
    C. Maturation in the thymus
    D. Secretion of interferon-γ
    E. Inhibition of function of other T cells

14. Which one of the following factors generally favors tolerance to an antigen and not stimulation of an immune response?

    A. High doses of antigen
    B. Short-lived persistence of antigen
    C. Cutaneous portal of entry
    D. Presence of adjuvant
    E. Costimulator expression on antigen-presenting cells

15. Which of the following factors generally favors stimulation of an adaptive immune response to an antigen, and not tolerance?

    A. Intravenous portal of entry of antigen
    B. Presence of antigen in generative lymphoid organs
    C. Absence of costimulatory molecules on antigen-presenting cells
    D. Innate immune response to the antigen
    E. Presence of antigen during the neonatal period

16. Which of the following statements about B cell tolerance is NOT true?

    A. Negative signaling induced by monovalent antigens is a mechanism of central B cell tolerance.
    B. Exclusion of B cells from follicles is a mechanism of peripheral B cell tolerance.
    C. Functional anergy is a mechanism of peripheral B cell tolerance.
    D. Receptor editing is a mechanism of central B cell tolerance.
    E. Down-regulation of antigen receptor expression is a mechanism of central B cell tolerance.

Questions 17-23

For each feature of self-tolerance described in questions 17-23, choose the term (letters A-K) that most closely matches it.

    A. Immature (IgM⁺IgD⁻)
    B. Thymic cortex
    C. Bone marrow
    D. Antigen recognition without T cell help
    E. Receptor editing
    F. Activation-induced cell death
    G. Regulatory T cell–mediated suppression
    H. Antigen recognition with costimulation
    I. Double positive (CD4⁺CD8⁺)
    J. Anergy
    K. Thymic medulla

17. Tolerance-sensitive stage of T cell maturation (   )

18. Mechanism of peripheral tolerance for T cells but not B cells (   )

19. Mechanism of central tolerance of B cells (   )

20. Mechanism of peripheral tolerance induction of B cells but not T cells (   )

21. Tolerance-sensitive stage of B cell maturation (   )

22. Mechanism of peripheral tolerance of B cells and T cells (   )

23. Site of central T cell tolerance induction (   )

24. The adaptive immune system has mechanisms of homeostasis that serve to terminate immune responses and return the immune system to a basal resting state. Which of the following is LEAST likely to be involved in lymphocyte homeostasis?

    A. CTLA-4
    B. Fas ligand
    C. CD28
    D. B cell Ig Fc receptors
    E. Anti-idiotypic antibodies

Answers

1. (C) Immunologic tolerance refers to the unresponsiveness of the immune system to particular antigens and develops on previous exposure to the antigen. Although the exact requirements for inducing tolerance have not been clearly defined, factors that do influence tolerance include the concentration of antigen, the mode of administration of the antigen, and the presence of costimulatory molecules on antigen-presenting cells for peptide antigens.
CMI5 216; BI2 161

2. (B) Autoimmunity is an immune reaction against self (autologous) antigens. For this reaction to occur, normal mechanisms of tolerance must fail. Allograft rejection is an immune reaction against allogeneic, not autologous, antigens. Atopy is the name for allergic diseases, which are caused by IgE and mast cell–mediated immune responses to foreign antigens. Acne is an infection of hair follicles in the skin and was included as a choice because it begins with the letter A; it is not an autoimmune disease.
CMI5 217; BI2 162

3. (C) Innate immune responses are usually required for induction of adaptive immune responses and may actually contribute to breaking tolerance to self antigens. Central tolerance occurs because of the susceptibility of immature lymphocytes to death in response to antigen receptor signals. Autoreactive

lymphocytes that are not deleted during development must be regulated by a mechanism of peripheral tolerance, which is induced in T cells by antigen receptor stimulation without costimulation, with CTLA-4–mediated negative signaling, by repeated and persistent stimulation by antigen, and by suppression by regulatory T cells.
CMI5 218-219; BI2 162-168

4. **(A)** Regulatory T lymphocytes secrete transforming growth factor-β and interleukin (IL)-10, which act as immunosuppressive cytokines. IL-12 is a proinflammatory cytokine produced mainly by activated macrophages and dendritic cells; it promotes effector T cell differentiation and interferon-γ production. T cell anergy can be induced by lack of B7-costimulation or by B7-binding to CTLA-4. Activation-induced cell death is apoptosis induced by Fas signals or by T cell receptor signals that enhance Fas-independent pro-apoptotic pathways in T cells.
CMI5 219, 222-232; BI2 166-171

5. **(B)** The failure of the male antigen-specific T cells to develop in male mice reflects negative selection by central deletion of the developing self-reactive T cells. Peripheral anergy describes inactivation of fully developed mature T cells outside the thymus. Clonal ignorance is a peripheral mechanism in which already developed T cells fail to see self antigen outside the thymus. Regulatory T cell suppression will not impair T cell development. Peripheral deletion occurs after self-reactive T cells develop and leave the thymus.
CMI5 221; BI2 163-164

6. **(D)** In autoimmune polyendocrinopathy-candidiasis-ectodermal dystrophy (APECED), there is an autoimmune attack of specific peripheral organs such as the pancreas, adrenals, and thyroid gland. Because the mutation occurs in a protein primarily expressed in the thymus, the underlying pathophysiology of the disease most likely represents a breakdown in central tolerance. Self-reactive T cells that are negatively selected in normal individuals instead survive in patients with autoimmune regulator gene (*AIRE*) mutations. Because specific organs are always involved in the disease, this is not just a general reduction in antigen presentation to developing T cells. *AIRE* functions to up-regulate intrathymic expression of certain proteins expressed in peripheral organs, so that these peptides can be presented to developing T cells. In this way, T cells specific for these peripheral self peptides can be deleted. Inhibitory cytokines play a role in tolerance mainly in the periphery. Fas ligand is not involved in the negative selection of T cells in the thymus, but it does play a role in peripheral T cell tolerance.
CMI5 221-222; BI2 163-164

7. **(C)** Developing T cells that bind with high avidity to self peptide–major histocompatability complex (MHC) in the thymus are deleted by negative selection. This process is mediated by signaling through the T cell receptor via a poorly understood pathway, but it does not involve the Fas ligand. Thymic epithelial cells, as well as professional antigen-presenting cells in the thymus, present peptide-MHC to developing T cells, generating signals that promote survival. This is called "positive selection" and results in increased expression of bcl-2. Rare autoimmune diseases, such as autoimmune poly-endocrinopathy-candidiasis-ectodermal dystrophy (APECED), may result from failure of central negative selection.
CMI5 220-222, 228-230; BI2 163-166

8. **(E)** Although interleukin (IL)-2 is a growth-promoting cytokine for T cells, knockout mice lacking IL-2 develop autoimmunity due to the failure of regulatory T cell function and failure of Fas-mediated apoptosis of self-reactive T cells in the periphery. Signaling via IL-2 is essential for the Fas ligand–mediated apoptotic pathway in activated T cells as well as for the development and function of regulatory T cells. B7-1, CD28, and interferon-γ all contribute to stimulating T cell differentiation and activation; deficiencies in these molecules are more likely to result in immunodeficiency than in autoimmunity.
CMI5 231; BI2 168

9. **(D)** FLIP is an inhibitor of the Fas-dependent activation-induced cell death pathway and works by blocking the interaction between FADD and caspase-8, thereby inhibiting the activation of the latter. Bid is a pro-apoptotic protein involved in a non–Fas-dependent pathway, and glucocorticoids promote T cell apoptosis.
CMI5 227-231; BI2 168

10. **(D)** Bcl-2 is an anti-apoptotic protein that functions by inhibiting the formation of channels in the mitochondrial membrane, thus preventing the release of cytochrome c into the cytosol. Cytochrome c, when released from the mitochondria, is a potent activator of apoptosis that binds to Apaf-1. Together, this complex activates procaspase-9, which in turn activates procaspase-3 and subsequently leads to DNA cleavage. FLIP is a direct inhibitor of procaspase-8 activation. Bcl-2 is not an inhibitor of caspase-9 or of granzymes.
CMI5 227-231

11. **(E)** After repeated stimulation by antigen during an immune response, effector T cells undergo apoptosis because the Fas-Fas ligand pathway is up-regulated and because pro-apoptotic proteins, such as Bim, are up-regulated. The net effect is that the population of mature lymphocytes is depleted of T cells specific for the antigen that induced repeated stimulation. This is known as activation-induced cell death and serves to clear effector T cells close to the end of an immune response, as well as to delete autoreactive T cells. Passive cell death refers

to a loss of survival stimuli resulting in the intrinsic, or mitochondrial, pathway of apoptosis. Peripheral tolerance refers to the deletion or anergy induced in self-reactive lymphocytes in nongenerative organs (e.g., not the bone marrow or the thymus). Death by neglect is the fate of developing T cells in the thymus, whose T cell receptors do not bind any self MHC-peptide complexes.
CMI5 225-226

12. (C) Apoptotic cells are phagocytosed by macrophages without causing inflammation. Apoptosis is usually induced by activation of a cascade of enzymes inside the cell, called caspases, which ultimately stimulates DNA cleaving enzymes. The result is nuclear fragmentation and secondary membrane changes, such as blebbing.
CMI5 227; BI2 168

13. (D) Regulatory T cells mature in the thymus, usually express CD25, and function to suppress the function of other T cells, either by direct interactions with antigen-presenting cells or T cells or by secreting immunosuppressive cytokines, such as interleukin-10 or transforming growth factor-β. They do not secrete proinflammatory cytokines such as interferon-γ.
CMI5 232; BI2 168-170

14. (A) High doses of antigens favor thymic deletion (if the antigen is a self-antigen) or peripheral deletion by activation-induced cell death. Antigens that induce immune responses are often present for short durations, enter through skin, and are associated with adjuvants that enhance antigen presentation and costimulatory molecule expression.
CMI5 233; BI2 170-171

15. (D) Innate immune responses enhance the ability of antigen to activate naive B cells and T cells in various ways, such as by inducing costimulatory molecules on the antigen-presenting cells. The presence of antigen within generative lymphoid organs (bone marrow, thymus) favors central tolerance. Neonatal exposure to antigen favors neonatal tolerance. Both intravenous administration of antigen and lack of costimulators favor peripheral tolerance.
CMI5 233; BI2 170-171

16. (A) Central B cell tolerance is most likely to be induced by multivalent antigens that can cross-link multiple membrane Ig molecules and thereby deliver strong signals to developing B cells. This may result in B cell apoptosis, antigen receptor down-regulation, or receptor editing, whereby V(D)J recombination is reinitiated and light chain gene usage is altered. In peripheral B cell tolerance, B cells may become anergic or they may be excluded from entry into follicles, owing in part to failure of expression of CCR5 chemokine receptors.
CMI5 234; BI2 171-172

17. (I) Central T cell tolerance is induced largely by clonal deletion (negative selection) in the thymus at the CD4$^+$CD8$^+$ stage of T cell maturation.
CMI5 236; BI2 80-82, 163-166

18. (G) Regulatory T cells are known to suppress T cells but not B cells. Helper T cell–dependent B cell responses may be indirectly suppressed by this mechanism.
CMI5 231-232, 236; BI2 168-170

19. (E) If an immature B cell in the bone marrow recognizes self-antigen, *RAG* gene expression may be induced and additional Ig light chain V(D)J recombination events may occur. This will change the antigen specificity of the expressed Ig.
CMI5 150, 236; BI2 171-172

20. (D) B cell recognition of antigen in the periphery without concomitant helper T cell–derived signals may render the B cells anergic or unable to enter follicles for further differentiation.
CMI5 234, 236; BI2 172

21. (A) Tolerance induction of B cells and T cells requires antigen receptor expression, but it occurs most readily before full maturation is completed. For B cells, IgM$^+$ IgD$^-$ immature B cells are the most sensitive to tolerance induction.
CMI5 234, 236; BI2 171-172

22. (J) Anergy, which is a block in signaling that prevents full activation of lymphocytes, is a mechanism of peripheral tolerance for both B and T lymphocytes.
CMI5 223-225, 234-235, 236; BI2 166-168, 172

23. (B) Double-positive T cells, which are the cells susceptible to central T cell tolerance induction, are found in the thymic cortex. The developing T cells that are not deleted at the double-positive stage mature into single-positive (CD4$^+$ or CD8$^+$) thymocytes and migrate into the medulla before exiting the thymus.
CMI5 153-154, 160, 236; BI2 80-82, 163-166

24. (C) CD28 binds to B7-1 or B7-2 and provides activating signals to T cells during the initiation of T cell responses, not self-regulating signals during the waning of an immune response. Although mechanisms of homeostasis in normal immune responses to foreign antigens are not well defined, they may include the same mechanisms that are important for self-tolerance, such as CTLA-4–mediated T cell inhibition and Fas-Fas ligand–mediated lymphocyte apoptosis. B cell homeostasis is mediated in part by antibody feedback inhibition, via FcγRIIB, and by anti-idiotypic antibodies that are induced during immune responses and are specific for the unique antigen-binding regions of other antibodies.
CMI5 213-214, 237-238

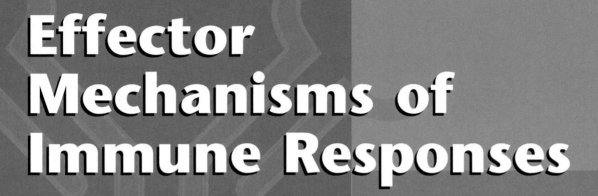

Effector Mechanisms of Immune Responses

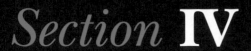

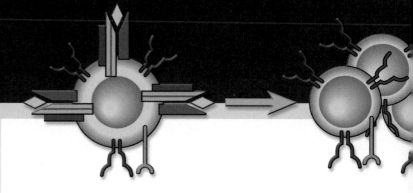

Chapter 11

Cytokines

Cellular and Molecular Immunology, 5/E: Chapter 11—Cytokines

Basic Immunology, 2/E: Chapter 2—Innate Immunity; and Chapter 5—Cell-Mediated Immune Responses

1. Which one of the following statements about cytokines is NOT true?

   A. Some cytokines are lipid mediators of inflammation.

   B. Cytokines are often produced by cells in the innate immune response to microbial infection.

   C. Multiple cytokines may have the same biologic effects (i.e., there is redundancy in the cytokine system).

   D. An individual cytokine may have pleiotropic effects (i.e., act in different ways on several different cell types).

   E. Cytokine production by a cell is usually a brief, self-limited event.

2. Interleukin (IL)-2 is a cytokine produced by T lymphocytes that acts as a growth factor for T lymphocytes. A T cell may bind and respond to the same IL-2 molecules it secretes. Which of the following terms best describes this mode of action of a cytokine?

   A. Endocrine
   B. Paracrine
   C. Autocrine
   D. Autoimmune
   E. Holocrine

3. Janus kinases (JAKs) are tyrosine kinases linked to certain cytokine receptors, and they phosphorylate signal transducers and activators of transcription (STATs). Which one of the following cytokines does NOT bind to receptors that use JAK-STAT signaling pathways?

   A. Tumor necrosis factor-α
   B. Interleukin (IL)-12

C. IL-4

D. IL-6

E. Interferon-γ

4. All of the following are properties of type I (hemopoietin family) cytokine receptors EXCEPT:

A. They contain tryptophan-serine-X-tryptophan-serine (WSXWS) motifs.

B. They bind cytokines that fold into four α-helical strands.

C. They often employ separate cytokine binding chains and signaling chains.

D. They bind cytokines of both adaptive and innate immunity.

E. They employ seven-membrane spanning, G protein–linked signal transduction pathways.

5. Which one of the following pairs of cytokines has the most redundant functions in innate immune responses?

A. Interleukin (IL)-12 and tumor necrosis factor (TNF)

B. TNF and IL-1

C. Interferon (IFN)-γ and IL-10

D. IFN-α and IFN-γ

E. IL-1 and IL-4

6. Anti–tumor necrosis factor (TNF) antibodies are now used in the treatment of patients with rheumatoid arthritis. A complication of this therapy, seen in a subset of patients, is infections with various microorganisms, including bacteria and fungi. Which of the following is a function of TNF that is important in the defense against infections and is likely to be impaired in the setting of TNF blockade?

A. Induction of fever

B. Reduction in cardiac output

C. Enhanced procoagulant activity of endothelial cells

D. Enhanced glucose utilization by muscle cells

E. Induction of E-selectin expression on endothelial cells

Questions 7-11

The tumor necrosis factor (TNF) family of proteins includes several soluble and membrane proteins that share structural homologies. All members of this family bind to members of the TNF-receptor family of molecules expressed on cell surfaces. TNF-R family members are structurally homologous to one another and utilize similar signal transduction pathways.

For each description of a TNF or a TNF-R family member in questions 7-11, select the term listed in options A-E that best matches it.

A. TNF-RI

B. CD40

C. Fas ligand

D. RANK

E. Lymphotoxin

7. Produced by T cells and binds to the same receptors as does TNF-α produced by macrophages ( )

8. Expressed on macrophages and B lymphocytes, this receptor plays an important role in the helper T cell–mediated effector functions. ( )

9. Expressed on osteoclasts, this receptor is important in remodeling bone. ( )

10. Expressed on many cells types, its cytoplasmic tail includes a death domain, binds TNF-receptor associated death domain (TRADD), and initiates a pro-apoptotic signaling cascade. ( )

11. Expressed as a membrane molecule on the surface of activated T cells, it binds to a receptor found on many cell types, including T cells, and induces apoptosis. ( )

12. IL-1 is a cytokine that shares many of the same biologic effects as tumor necrosis factor (TNF)-α. Which of the following properties of TNF-α is NOT shared by interleukin-1?

A. Produced by macrophage in response to lipopolysaccharide (LPS)

B. Stimulates acute phase reactant synthesis in the liver

C. Binding to its receptor activates the NF-κB transcription factor

D. Induces apoptotic death of cells

E. Enhances endothelial expression of leukocyte adhesion molecules

13. Interleukin (IL)-1 receptor antagonist (IL-1ra) is a protein structurally homologous to IL-1. Which one of the following is a property of IL-1ra?

A. Binds to a distinct receptor from IL-1, which delivers signals that block IL-1 receptor signals

B. Is an effective treatment for septic shock

C. Is produced by T cells but not macrophages

D. Binds to type I IL-1 receptors and acts as a competitive inhibitor of IL-1

E. Induces apoptosis of cells, unlike IL-1

14. Which of the following is NOT a property of a typical chemokine?

A. Small polypeptide ranging in size from 8 to 12 kD

B. Contains two conserved cysteine residues

C. Binds to seven-membrane spanning, G protein–linked receptors

D. Stimulates leukocyte migration from blood into tissues

E. Produced exclusively by vascular endothelial cells

Questions 15-19

For each of the following descriptions (questions 15-19) of a chemokine or chemokine receptor, select the chemokine or chemokine receptor (A-G) that most closely matches it.

A. CXCL8 (IL-8)

B. CXCL10 (IP-10)

C. CCL19 (ELC)

D. CCL11 (Eotaxin)

E. CCR5

F. CXCR1

G. CX3CL1 (Fractalkine)

15. Mediates neutrophil recruitment into tissues ( )

16. Binds to interleukin-8 ( )

17. Binds chemokines important in T cell recruitment into peripheral inflammatory sites ( )

18. Important in dendritic cell and T cell localization in lymph nodes ( )

19. Important mediator of inflammatory component of immediate hypersensitivity reactions ( )

20. Chemokine receptors are involved in all of the following processes EXCEPT:

    A. Embryonic development of heart and brain
    B. Stimulation of apoptosis in neutrophils
    C. Activation of cell-surface integrins
    D. Stimulation of polymerization and depolymerization of cytoplasmic actin filaments
    E. Entry of human immunodeficiency virus (HIV) into cells

21. One of the principal functions of interleukin (IL)-12 is to enhance the production of which of the following cytokines by natural killer (NK) cells and T lymphocytes?

    A. IL-4
    B. Tumor necrosis factor
    C. IL-10
    D. IL-2
    E. Interferon-γ

22. A 19-year-old woman sees the physician because of severe systemic *Mycobacterium avium-intracellulare* infections. She had a history of three similar mycobacterial infections between the ages of 4 and 17 years and severe systemic *Salmonella* type B infections when she was 4, 7, and 14 years of age. No abnormalities in numbers or cell surface markers of T cells, B cells, natural killer cells, or macrophage cells were detectable. Mononuclear cells from the patient's blood produced very little interferon-γ in response to various stimuli when compared with cells from a healthy donor. The patient responded well to treatment with antibiotic therapy. Which of the following is the most likely explanation for this patient's medical history?

    A. Defect in interleukin (IL)-12 receptor signaling
    B. Defect in IL-4 receptor signaling
    C. Defect in cytolytic T lymphocyte function
    D. Defect in B cell antibody production
    E. Defect in IL-7 receptor expression

23. Which of the following is a mechanism by which the type I interferons IFN-α and IFN-β function to eradicate viral infections?

    A. Enhance class II MHC expression
    B. Enhance IFN-γ production by macrophages
    C. Induce apoptosis of virally infected cells
    D. Enhance class I MHC expression
    E. Enhance expression of terminal deoxynucleotidyl transferase (TdT)

24. Inflammatory bowel disease (IBD) is characterized by a dysregulated inflammatory response in the intestinal mucosa, including abnormally high expression of various inflammatory cytokines by macrophages. Which one of the following cytokines is the most logical choice as a potential therapeutic agent for IBD?

    A. Interleukin (IL)-1
    B. IL-10
    C. IL-12
    D. IL-6
    E. IL-2

25. Which of the following cytokines is NOT a product of antigen-activated T cells?

    A. Interleukin (IL)-2
    B. IL-4
    C. IL-5
    D. Interferon (IFN)-γ
    E. IFN-α

26. A 3-month-old boy is taken to the pediatrician because of diarrhea, failure to thrive, mucocutaneous candidiasis, and respiratory syncytial virus infection. Laboratory analyses indicate an absence of T cells, normal numbers of B cells, but very low immunoglobulin levels. This clinical presentation is consistent with a mutation in the gene encoding a signaling chain shared by which of the following groups of cytokine receptors?

    A. Receptors for interleukin (IL)-2, IL-4, and IL-7
    B. Receptors for granulocyte-macrophage colony-stimulating factor (GM-CSF), IL-3, and IL-5
    C. Receptors for IL-6 and IL-11
    D. Receptors for interferon (IFN)-γ and IFN-α
    E. Receptors for IL-12 and IL-23

27. Which of the following is NOT a biologic function of interleukin (IL)-2?

    A. Proliferation of antigen-stimulated CD4+ cells
    B. Proliferation of neutrophils
    C. Proliferation of antigen-stimulated CD8+ T cells
    D. Potentiation of apoptotic death of antigen-stimulated T cells
    E. Differentiation of cytolytic function of natural killer cells

Questions 28-31

For each of the descriptions of a biologic function in questions 28-31, select the T cell–derived cytokine (A-E) that matches it.

    A. Interferon-γ
    B. Interleukin (IL)-4
    C. IL-5
    D. Transforming growth factor-β
    E. Lymphotoxin

28. Stimulates growth and activation of eosinophils ( )

29. Induces B cell isotype switching to IgE production ( )

30. Stimulates expression of class II MHC on various cell types (   )

31. Inhibits proliferation and differentiation of T cells and the activation of macrophages (   )

32. A 29-year-old woman with Hodgkin's lymphoma was treated with anti-neoplastic chemotherapy. As a complication of the therapy, she became severely neutropenic. Which of the following cytokines is the appropriate reagent to administer to this patient?

    A. Monocyte colony-stimulating factor
    B. Interleukin-7
    C. Erythropoietin
    D. Interferon-γ
    E. Granulocyte-macrophage colony-stimulating factor

Answers

1. (A) All cytokines are proteins. Although many cells do produce lipid mediators of inflammation, such as arachidonic acid metabolites, these are not called cytokines. Cells of the innate immune system often produce cytokines in direct response to microbial products, such as bacterial endotoxin. Pleiotropism and redundancy are characteristics of most cytokines, which complicates therapeutic strategies based on the use of cytokines or cytokine blockers.
   CMI5 244; BI2 93

2. (C) When a cell itself responds to the cytokines it produces, the cytokine is acting in an *autocrine* manner. *Paracrine* describes actions of a cytokine on cells near to the cell that produces them. *Endocrine* refers to the actions of cytokines (or hormones) on cells distant to the cells that produce them, and requires transport of the cytokine through the bloodstream. *Autoimmune* does not refer to cytokine actions, but rather, to the recognition of self molecules by the adaptive immune system. *Holocrine* is not an immunologic term but refers to secretions from a gland composed of parts of cells.
   CMI5 244-245; BI2 93

3. (A) Tumor necrosis factor (TNF)-α binds to receptors that are members of the TNF receptor (TNF-R) family. TNF-R family receptors signal via adapter proteins, such as TNF receptor-associated death domain (TRADD) and TNF receptor-associated factors (TRAFs), and lead to activation of the NF-κB and AP-1 transcription factors. Interleukin (IL)-12, IL-4, IL-6, and interferon (IFN)-γ, as well as several other cytokines, all bind to receptors that activate JAK-STAT pathways. The particular JAK and STAT proteins may vary depending on the cytokine and cytokine receptor involved.
   CMI5 246-248

4. (E) Chemokines are the only cytokines that bind to seven-membrane–spanning, calcium-mobilizing receptors. The members of the type I cytokine receptor family, which includes receptors for interleukin (IL)-2, IL-4, IL-6, IL-12, and granulocyte-macrophage colony-stimulating factor (GM-CSF), employ JAK-STAT signal transduction pathways. Often, the JAK kinases are associated with a specialized signaling chain of the receptor, distinct from the cytokine-binding chain. Membership in the family is based on the presence of certain common structural motifs in the extracellular portions of the cytokine-binding chain, including conserved cysteine residues and the tryptophan-serine-X-tryptophan-serine (WSXWS) motif. These conserved features contribute to the affinity of the type I receptors for cytokines that fold into four α-helices.
   CMI5 246-247

5. (B) Tumor necrosis factor (TNF) and interleukin (IL)-1, two of the most important proinflammatory cytokines of the innate immune system, share many of the same biologic properties, including endothelial activation, fever induction, and stimulation of acute phase reactant synthesis. Both TNF and IL-1 are also produced by many of the same cell types in response to similar stimuli such as microbial products that bind to Toll-like receptors. IL-12, which may also be produced in response to the same signals that induce TNF and IL-1, has a more limited set of actions, mainly on T cells and natural killer (NK) cells. Interferon (IFN)-γ is a proinflammatory cytokine that activates macrophages, whereas IL-10 is anti-inflammatory and inhibits macrophage activation. IFN-α (and IFN-β) shares some functions with IFN-γ, such as induction of class I major histocompatibility complex (MHC) expression on target cells, but the major activity of IFN-α is induction of antiviral states in cells. The major activity of IFN-γ is macrophage activation. IL-4 is not a cytokine of innate immunity, but rather, a product of T_H2 T cells, which promotes IgE synthesis by B cells.
   CMI5 249-254; BI2 34-36

6. (E) Rheumatoid arthritis is an autoimmune inflammatory disease that affects joints. Tumor necrosis factor (TNF) is present in the inflamed joints of patients with this disease. TNF stimulates synthesis of endothelial adhesion molecules, including E-selectin, which are important in the recruitment of neutrophils and other leukocytes into tissues. Neutrophil recruitment is essential in defense against many microorganisms. TNF can also directly activate the microbicidal activities of neutrophils. It is not clear if fever has beneficial effects in combatting infection. Reduced cardiac output, enhanced procoagulant activity of endothelial cells, and enhanced muscle glucose metabolism are all maladaptive responses to very high circulating levels of TNF associated with septic shock.
   CMI5 252-253; BI2 34-36

7. (E) Lymphotoxin (LT), also known as tumor necrosis factor (TNF)-β, shares 30% sequence homology

with TNF-α made by macrophages; it binds to the same receptors as TNF-α, and thus has the same biologic effects. The quantity of LT secreted by antigen-stimulated T cells is much less than TNF-α secreted by activated macrophages, and therefore LT does not have systemic effects. LT is considered to be an important link between T cell activation and acute inflammation, and it is also critical for the architectural development of lymphoid organs. CMI5 270

8. (B) CD40 is a member of the tumor necrosis factor receptor family expressed by B cells, macrophages, and other cell types. CD40 binds CD40 ligand on activated helper T cells, and ligand binding initiates signaling pathways that activate macrophages and B lymphocytes. CD40-mediated macrophage activation leads to enhanced phagocytic and microbicidal functions, and CD40-mediated B cell activation is essential for helper T cell–dependent Ig isotype switching and affinity maturation. CMI5 201-203, 253, 311-312; BI2 90, 95, 112-113

9. (D) RANK, also known as osteoprotegerin receptor, is a tumor necrosis factor receptor family member expressed on osteoclasts and some macrophages. RANK is involved in bone resorption, both in health and in disease states such as rheumatoid arthritis. CMI5 253

10. (A) Tumor necrosis factor (TNF)-RI is one of two receptors for TNF-α expressed on a wide variety of cell types. TNF-RI, like Fas, is directly linked to apoptotic pathways because it contains a death domain in the cytoplasmic tail. CMI5 250-251

11. (C) Fas ligand (FasL) is a member of the tumor necrosis factor family and binds Fas on T cells and other cell types. Fas-Fas ligand-dependent apoptosis of T cells is important for T cell homeostasis; deficiencies in Fas or FasL cause autoimmune disease. CMI5 226-231, 250; BI2 168

12. (D) Unlike tumor necrosis factor (TNF)-α, interleukin (IL)-1 does not activate apoptotic pathways in cells, reflecting a difference in signal transduction pathways linked to the TNF and IL-1 receptors. IL-1 is also not capable, on its own, of causing the tissue injury and systemic pathology seen in septic shock, whereas TNF-α is. Both TNF and IL-1 are produced in response to activation of macrophages by LPS or other microbial products. Although TNF-R and IL-1 receptor signaling differ, they both lead to NF-κB activation, which partially explains why the two cytokines do induce many of the same biologic responses, such as hepatic acute phase reactant synthesis and endothelial adhesion molecule expression. CMI5 253-255; BI2 34-36

13. (D) Interleukin (IL)-1ra is produced by activated macrophages and binds to the same IL-1 receptor

that mediates the actions of IL-1. Unlike IL-1, IL-1ra does not stimulate signal transduction through the receptor and therefore acts as a competitive IL-1 inhibitor. Clinical trials of IL-1ra as a treatment for septic shock have not been successful, likely reflecting the multiplicity of factors that mediate septic shock. IL-1ra has been shown to be an effective treatment for rheumatoid arthritis. IL-1ra does not induce apoptosis. CMI5 254

14. (E) Chemokines are made by many cell types, including endothelial cells, lymphocytes, mononuclear phagocytes, and many types of epithelial cells. Production may be induced by inflammatory cytokines, such as interleukin-1 and tumor necrosis factor, or may be constitutive in many tissues. All chemokines are 8-12 kD polypeptides with two conserved cysteine residues, which are either adjacent or separated by one or three amino acids. The spacing of these cysteine residues determines to which subfamily a chemokine belongs. Chemokines bind to seven-membrane, G protein–coupled chemokine receptors, which are divided into subfamilies depending on the subfamily of chemokines that bind to them. A major biologic activity of chemokines is stimulation of leukocyte migration into tissues, but chemokines also regulate tissue morphogenesis and distribution of cells within lymphoid tissues. CMI5 254-255; BI2 35

15. (A) Interleukin-8, a CXC family chemokine, is one of the major chemokines that attracts neutrophils into tissues. Neutrophils respond to several other CXC chemokines but not CC chemokines. CMI5 256

16. (F) CXCR1, the only CXCR family receptor listed, binds interleukin-8, a CXC family chemokine. CMI5 256

17. (E) CCR5 is expressed on T_H1 T cells and binds at least three CC chemokines, including RANTES (CCL5), MIP-1α (CCL3), and MIP-1β (CCL4), which are produced at sites of infection. CMI5 256

18. (C) ELC (CCL19) and SLC are produced by stromal cells in the parafollicular zones of lymph nodes. Dendritic cells and T cells express the CCR7 receptor that binds these chemokines. CMI5 36-37, 256

19. (D) Eotaxin (CCL11) is produced at sites of allergic inflammation and binds to CCR3 on eosinophils, thereby stimulating eosinophil migration into these sites. CMI5 256, 444

20. (B) Chemokine receptors are not linked to apoptosis pathways and are not involved in neutrophil death. Chemokine receptors do promote neutrophil and other leukocyte movement into tissues by increasing the strength of leukocyte integrin binding

to their endothelial ligands, and by stimulating actin filament polymerization and depolymerization required for leukocyte movement. Gene knockout studies in mice indicate that chemokine receptors are involved in the development of the heart and brain. Certain chemokine receptors, including CCR5 and CXCR4, are cofactors for human immunodeficiency virus (HIV) entry into cells.
CMI5 254-255; BI2 25-27, 108

21. (E) Interleukin (IL)-12 stimulates the production of interferon (INF)-γ by natural killer (NK) cells and T lymphocytes. In a typical sequence of events, microbes stimulate macrophages and dendritic cells to secrete IL-12; IL-12 stimulates T cells and NK cells to secrete INF-γ; IFN-γ activates macrophages to kill the microbes. IL-12 does not directly enhance TNF production, but IFN-γ does synergize with microbial products to enhance TNF production by macrophages. IL-4 and IL-10, which are produced by some T cells, but not NK cells, are not induced by IL-12. IL-2 is a T cell growth factor synthesized by T cells in response to antigen and costimulatory signals but not in response to IL-12.
CMI5 254-255; BI2 35-36, 95-99

22. (A) This patient is susceptible to infection by bacteria that live and replicate within phagolysosomes in macrophages, such as *Mycobacterium* and *Salmonella* species. Defense against such organisms requires macrophage activation by interferon (INF)-γ, which is dependent on interleukin (IL)-12 produced during the innate immune response to such organisms. Therefore, a defect in IL-12 receptor expression would fit this clinical picture. Several individuals with genetic defects in the expression of the signaling chain of the IL-12 receptor (IL-12Rβ1) have been identified after presenting with intracellular bacterial infections. IL-23, which has overlapping function with IL-12, also binds a receptor that utilizes the same IL-12Rβ1 signaling chain, and therefore the consequences of IL-12Rβ1 deficiency may in part be related to a lack of response to IL-23. A defect in IL-4 receptor signaling would result in diminished T_H2 responses, including reduced IgE production, which would not impair defense against intracellular bacteria. Defects in antibody production also would not impact the eradication of intracellular microbes. A cytolytic T lymphocyte functional defect would be expected to result in susceptibility to viral infections as well as to intracellular bacterial infections. IL-7 is required for lymphocyte development, and therefore a lack of IL-7 receptor expression would lead to reduced numbers of both T and B lymphocytes.
CMI5 259-260; BI2 97-98

23. (D) A major mechanism by which the adaptive immune system eradicates viral infections is by cytolytic T lymphocyte (CTL)-mediated killing of infected cells. CTL recognition of viral antigens is class I MHC-restricted. Type I interferons enhance CTL killing of virally infected cells by up-regulating expression of class I MHC, thereby enhancing presentation of viral peptides to the CTL. Type I interferons do not up-regulate expression of class II MHC or interferon (IFN)-γ, although IFN-γ does up-regulate class II MHC. Terminal deoxynucleotidyl transferase (TdT), an enzyme involved in generation of junctional diversity of antigen receptors, is not up-regulated by type I interferons. IFN-α and IFN-β do up-regulate expression of other enzymes, such as 2′,5′ oligoadenylate synthetase, which interfere with viral genome replication.
CMI5 260-261; BI2 34-35

24. (B) Interleukin (IL)-10 inhibits many of the functions of macrophages, including production of IL-12 and tumor necrosis factor (TNF); IL-10 gene knockout mice develop inflammatory bowel disease (IBD). IL-10 therapy for IBD is in the experimental stage. IL-1, IL-12, and IL-6 are all proinflammatory and would not be expected to be beneficial in IBD. IL-2 promotes T cell growth and susceptibility to apoptosis. Although IL-2 deficiency in mice is associated with an IBD-like disease, this may be related to impaired T cell tolerance. There is no basis to predict that administering IL-2 would improve IBD in humans.
CMI5 261-262; BI2 34-35

25. (E) Interferon (IFN)-α, an innate immune system cytokine with antiviral functions, is a product of microbe-stimulated macrophages. Interleukin (IL)-2 is synthesized by T cells in response to antigen stimulation and acts as an autocrine growth factor. IL-4 and IL-5 are produced mainly by antigen-activated T_H2 T cells, and promote IgE- and eosinophil-mediated defense mechanisms. Interferon (IFN)-γ is produced by antigen-activated T_H1 T cells and promotes macrophage-mediated (and some antibody-mediated) defense mechanisms. IFN-γ may also be produced by natural killer (NK) cells during innate immune responses.
CMI5 264; BI2 93-94

26. (A) This boy suffers from severe combined immunodeficiency disease (SCID). The majority of males with SCID have mutations in the common signaling γ chain ($γ_c$) utilized by receptors for interleukin (IL)-2, IL-4, IL-7, IL-9, and IL-15. The profound defect in T cell development and lack of B cell function is mostly attributable to lack of IL-7 receptor signaling. Genetic deficiencies in the common β chain required for signaling of the granulocyte-macrophage colony-stimulating factor (GM-CSF) and IL-3 and IL-5 receptors result in a form of respiratory failure called pulmonary alveolar proteinosis, but these patients do not have SCID. Receptors for IL-6 and IL-11 share a common gp130 signaling chain, but there are no known genetic deficiencies in this protein. Receptors for interferon (IFN)-γ and IFN-α do not share signaling chains. Receptors for IL-12 and IL-23 share the β1 signaling chain, and genetic deficiencies in this

protein result in an immunodeficiency state characterized by intracellular bacterial infections.
CMI5 248, 266, 455-466; BI2 211

27. (B) Neutrophils are a terminally differentiated cell type that is incapable of cell division. Interleukin (IL)-2 does promote cell cycle progression and proliferation of antigen-activated $CD4^+$ and $CD8^+$ T cells. IL-2 also contributes to the acquisition of cytolytic function of $CD8^+$ T cells and natural killer (NK) cells, although NK cells require higher concentrations of IL-2 than do T cells. In addition to its growth promoting and differentiation activities, IL-2 enhances T cell susceptibility to apoptosis, and this function is important for homeostasis of immune responses.
CMI5 265-266; BI2 93-95

28. (C) Interleukin-5 (IL-5) is secreted by helper T cells of the T_H2 subset and promotes inflammatory responses rich in eosinophils. The protective function of eosinophils is against helminth infections, but, more commonly, eosinophils are associated with allergic disease.
CMI5 268; BI2 96-97

29. (B) Interleukin (IL)-4 is secreted by helper T cells of the T_H2 subset and promotes IgE production by B cells. IgE contributes to antigen-induced mast cell degranulation and immediate hypersensitivity reactions. Therefore, IL-4 production contributes to allergic disease.
CMI5 266-268; BI2 96-98

30. (A) Interferon (IFN)-γ is a proinflammatory cytokine secreted by helper T cells of the T_H1 subset and natural killer (NK) cells. This cytokine induces class II MHC expression on various cell types, thereby enhancing antigen presentation to $CD4^+$ T cells. Other important biologic activities of IFN-γ are induction of class I MHC expression, macrophage activation, and B cell Ig isotype switching.
CMI5 268-269; BI2 95-98

31. (D) Transforming growth factor (TGF)-β is produced by antigen-activated effector T cells and regulatory T cells. The principal function of TGF-β is inhibition of T cell differentiation and proliferation, as well as inhibition of macrophage activation. TGF-β is also an IgA isotype switch factor.
CMI5 269-279; BI2 169

32. (E) GM-CSF (granulocyte-macrophage colony-stimulating factor) is a hematopoietic cytokine, which, in recombinant form, enhances the production and half life of neutrophils and monocytes/macrophages and enhances the microbicidal activity of these cells. GM-CSF therapy is used in the setting of bone marrow suppression due to chemotherapy and in AIDS. M-CSF (monocyte colony-stimulating factor) enhances monocyte development in bone marrow but not in neutrophils. Interleukin-7 supports lymphocyte development, but it would not help to increase neutrophil production. Erythropoietin specifically enhances red blood cell development.
CMI5 271-272

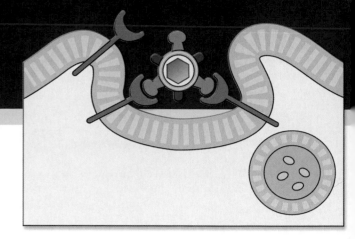

Chapter 12

Innate Immunity

Cellular and Molecular Immunology, 5/E: Chapter 12—Innate Immunity

Basic Immunology, 2/E: Chapter 2—Innate Immunity

1. Which of the following statements about the innate immune system is NOT true?

   A. Innate immunity is present in all multicellular organisms, including plants and insects.
   B. Deficiencies in innate immunity markedly increase host susceptibility to infection, even in the setting of an intact adaptive immune response.
   C. Innate immunity is better suited for eliminating virulent, resistant microbes than is adaptive immunity.
   D. The innate immune response can be divided into recognition, activation, and effector phases.
   E. The innate immune response against microbes influences the type of adaptive immune response that develops.

2. A 4-year-old girl stepped on a rusty nail in her backyard. Two days later, she is taken to the pediatrician because her heel is painful, red, and swollen and is warm to the touch. All of the following are mechanisms of innate immunity that may be protecting the patient against pathogenic microbes in the heel wound EXCEPT:

   A. Epithelial barrier function of the skin of her foot
   B. Intraepithelial lymphocytes present in the skin
   C. Circulating neutrophils migrating to the site of the wound
   D. Soluble cytokines that induce a local inflammatory response
   E. Circulating anti-tetanus toxin antibodies

3. Which of the following comparisons of the innate and adaptive immune systems is FALSE?

    A. The innate immune system is more likely to recognize normal self, and therefore cause autoimmunity, than is the adaptive immune system.
    B. Receptors used for recognition in innate immunity are encoded in the germline, whereas those of the adaptive immune system are encoded by genes generated via somatic recombination of germline receptor gene loci.
    C. The innate and adaptive immune systems share some of the same effector mechanisms.
    D. Both the innate and adaptive immune systems can recognize nonmicrobial substances.
    E. The innate immune system does not have memory but the adaptive immune system does.

4. Toll-like receptors (TLRs) are a family of homologous receptors expressed on many cell types and are involved in innate immune responses. Ten different mammalian TLRs have been identified, and several ligands for many of these receptors are known. Which of the following is a TLR ligand?

    A. Single-stranded RNA
    B. Transfer RNA
    C. Double-stranded DNA
    D. Unmethylated CpG DNA
    E. Heterochromatin

5. A 67-year-old homeless man is brought to the emergency department after being found behind a neighborhood bar in freezing weather. On arrival, he has a shaking chill, fever, and cough productive of blood-tinged sputum. A chest radiograph shows lobar consolidations consistent with bacterial pneumonia. Blood cultures are positive for *Streptococcus pneumoniae*. Which of the following molecular patterns recognized by Toll-like receptors expressed on the surface of this patient's phagocytes is important for activating his innate immune system against this gram-positive bacterial infection?

    A. Peptidoglycan
    B. Double-stranded RNA
    C. Lipopolysaccharide (LPS)
    D. Lipoarabinomannan
    E. Phosphatidylinositol dimannoside

6. The signaling pathways triggered by Toll-like receptors typically result in activation of which of the following pairs of transcription factors?

    A. NFAT and T-bet
    B. AP-1 and GATA-3
    C. Fos and STAT-6
    D. NFκB and AP-1
    E. Lck and Jun

7. Toll-like receptors and other receptors are potent activators of various components of the innate immune system. All of the following proteins are expressed in response to signaling by these receptors EXCEPT:

    A. Interleukin-12
    B. E-selectin
    C. Tumor necrosis factor
    D. Inducible nitric oxide synthase (iNOS)
    E. CD28

8. Which of the following is a receptor on macrophages that is specific for a structure produced by bacteria but not by mammalian cells?

    A. CD36 (scavenger receptor)
    B. Fc receptor
    C. Complement receptor
    D. Mannose receptor
    E. ICAM-1

9. Which one of the following comparisons between neutrophils and macrophages is true?

    A. Neutrophils that enter inflammatory sites can survive for days, but macrophages are very short lived and only survive for hours.
    B. Both neutrophils and macrophages are phagocytic and can kill internalized microbes.
    C. Neutrophils proliferate at inflammatory sites, but macrophages are terminally differentiated and cannot proliferate.
    D. Neutrophils, but not macrophages, express the high-affinity FcγRI receptor, which recognizes specific opsonins bound to microbes and facilitates phagocytosis.
    E. Both neutrophils and macrophages contain abundant cytoplasmic granules containing lysozyme, collagenase, and elastase.

10. A 43-year-old man with a history of kidney transplantation is on immunosuppressive drugs. He presents to the emergency department 84 days after transplantation with a slight fever, accompanied by violent shaking chills, rapid heart rate, and dangerously low blood pressure. Blood cultures are positive for gram-negative bacteria, including *Klebsiella* and *Pseudomonas*. Although the patient was initially alert and responsive to fluids and antibiotic therapy, his condition rapidly deteriorates into disseminated intravascular coagulation (DIC), hypoglycemia, and cardiovascular failure. Which of the following is an essential mediator of this patient's condition?

    A. Transforming growth factor-β
    B. Tumor necrosis factor-α
    C. Interleukin (IL)-2
    D. IL-10
    E. IL-3

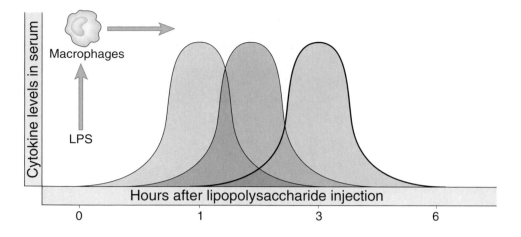

11. The figure above summarizes the temporal cytokine cascade in sepsis. Peaks 1, 2, and 3 correspond to which of the following cytokines?

   A. Interleukin (IL)-10, tumor necrosis factor (TNF), IL-12
   B. IL-15, IL-1, transforming growth factor-β (TGF-β)
   C. TNF, IL-1, IL-12
   D. IL-10, IL-15, TNF
   E. TGF-β, IL-12, IL-15

12. Macrophages and neutrophils express several enzymes that are involved in biochemical mechanisms that kill ingested microbes. Which of the following is NOT an enzyme expressed by these cells?

   A. Inducible nitric oxide synthase (iNOS)
   B. Granzyme B
   C. Phagocyte oxidase
   D. Myeloperoxidase
   E. Lysozyme

13. All of the following molecules are opsonins that facilitate efficient phagocytosis of microbes by neutrophils and macrophages EXCEPT:

   A. C3b
   B. C5a
   C. C-reactive protein
   D. IgG
   E. Mannose-binding lectin

14. A 3-year-old boy, who is small for his age, has a history of pyogenic (pus-producing) infections and cutaneous skin abscesses. Physical examination is remarkable for high fever, enlarged liver and spleen, and swollen cervical lymph nodes. A culture from an abscess on his arm reveals *Staphylococcus aureus*, a gram-positive bacteria that is also catalase-positive. Immunoglobulin and complement levels are normal. Results of the nitroblue tetrazolium test are consistent with a diagnosis of chronic granulomatous disease (CGD). The boy's immunodeficiency involves impaired generation of which of the following?

   A. C5a
   B. C-reactive protein
   C. Mannose-binding lectin
   D. Reactive oxygen intermediates
   E. Membrane attack complex

15. A 4-year-old-girl sees her physician because of a severe necrotizing, oropharyngeal herpes simplex viral (HSV) infection. She has a past medical history of cytomegalovirus (CMV) pneumonitis and cutaneous HSV infection. Phenotypic analysis of her blood cells shows an absence of CD56+ and CD16+ cells. There are normal numbers of CD4+ and CD8+ cells in the blood, and serum antibody titers are normal. The patient's CD8+ T cells were able to kill virally infected target cells in vitro. Which of the following is NOT characteristic of this girl's immunodeficiency disease?

   A. Lack of cells whose activation is normally inhibited by self class I major histocompatibility complex (MHC)
   B. Impaired granzyme B–dependent killing of virally infected target cells
   C. Lack of cells that are activated by IL-15
   D. Impaired interferon (IFN)-γ production during early phases of viral infection
   E. Failure to form viral peptide-class I MHC complexes

16. Which one of the following statements about inhibitory receptors on natural killer (NK) cells is true?

   A. Inhibitory receptors on NK cells express ITAM motifs in their cytoplasmic tails.
   B. Some inhibitory receptors on NK cells recognize HLA-A or HLA-C.
   C. Some inhibitory receptors on NK cells are members of the integrin family.
   D. Some inhibitory receptors on NK cells are members of the Toll-like receptor family.
   E. Inhibitory receptors on NK cells are not expressed on the same NK cells that express activating receptors.

17. Complement activation in the innate immune system can be initiated in the absence of antibody. Which of the following molecular components of the complement system is involved in initiation of antibody-independent complement activation?

    A. C1
    B. C9
    C. Mannose binding lectin
    D. CR2
    E. Mannose receptor

18. Which of the following is an example of how the innate immune response stimulates or modifies adaptive immunity?

    A. Tumor necrosis factor (TNF) secreted by helper T cells enhances adhesion molecules on endothelial cells and promotes recruitment of inflammatory cells.
    B. Interferon (IFN)-γ produced by T helper cells is a potent activator of macrophages, allowing killing of phagocytosed microbes.
    C. B7-1 expression on antigen-presenting cells is up-regulated in response to signaling through Toll-like receptors, thus enabling costimulation of T cells.
    D. Infected cells coated by IgG3 are recognized by Fc receptors on natural killer cells, allowing efficient killing of the infected cells.
    E. Double-stranded RNA of replicating viruses potently stimulates IFN-β expression by fibroblasts, inducing an "antiviral state" in neighboring, uninfected cells.

Questions 19-23

For each of the descriptions of a component of the innate immune system in questions 19-23, select the term that best matches it from the list below (A-J).

    A. Defensin
    B. Opsonin
    C. Natural antibody
    D. Adjuvant
    E. Complement
    F. Inflammation
    G. C-reactive protein
    H. Mannose-binding lectin
    I. Reactive oxygen intermediate
    J. Inducible nitric oxide synthase

19. Superoxide anion, hydroxyl radical, or hydrogen peroxide, produced by activated phagocytes (   )

20. Plasma protein that serves as a soluble pattern recognition receptor binding to microbial cells but not to mammalian cells (   )

21. Produced by B-1 cells, protects against microbes that succeed in penetrating epithelial barriers (   )

22. Acute-phase reactant produced by the liver and released into blood (   )

23. Broad-spectrum antibiotic present in the skin and in neutrophil granules; its synthesis is increased in response to inflammatory cytokines (   )

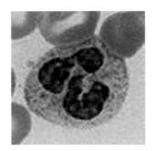

24. Which of the following is NOT a typical property of the cell type shown above?

    A. Phagocytic
    B. Expresses myeloperoxidase
    C. Binds to E-selectin on activated endothelial cells
    D. Expresses Fc receptors for IgG
    E. Presents antigen to CD4⁺ T cells

Answers

1. (C) Innate immunity is the first line of defense against infections, yet many pathogenic microbes have evolved strategies to resist innate immunity. Adaptive immunity, being more potent and specialized, plays a critical role in defending against these virulent microbes. Innate immunity is the phylogenetically oldest mechanism of microbial defense, and it is present in all multicellular organisms, including plants and insects. Studies have shown that hampering effector mechanisms of innate immunity renders hosts much more susceptible to infection, even with a functional adaptive immune system. It is also true that, like the adaptive response, the innate immune response consists of recognition, activation, and effector phases. Although it provides the initial, rapid response against microbes, innate immunity can influence adaptive immune responses to tailor them against particular microbes.
CMI5 275-276; BI2 21-22

2. (E) Secreted antibodies against protein antigens are effectors of humoral immunity, a component of the adaptive immune system. All other mechanisms listed are part of the innate immune system. Intact epithelial surfaces prevent microbial entry, and epithelial cells express anti-microbial factors, such as defensins. Neutrophils are effector cells that function in early phagocytosis and killing of microbes. Cytokines that mediate inflammation (e.g., tumor necrosis factor, interleukin-1, chemokines) are components of innate immunity. Intraepithelial T lymphocytes present in the epidermis and mucosal epithelia express a limited diversity of antigen receptors; as such, they are considered effector cells of innate immunity and function in host defense by secreting cytokines, activating phagocytes, and killing infected cells.
CMI5 279; BI2 24-32

3. (A) Innate immune system receptors are encoded by germline genes that have evolved to recognize microbial structures or molecules produced by stressed self, and therefore there is little chance of innate immune responses to normal self. Because the specificities of adaptive immune system receptors (Ig or T cell receptor molecules) are randomly generated by somatic recombination and junctional-diversity mechanisms, there is a greater chance that the adaptive immune system receptors may recognize normal self molecules, leading to autoimmunity. Mechanisms of tolerance minimize this possibility, but these mechanisms can fail. The adaptive immune system receptors can recognize nonmicrobial structures. Although most innate immune system receptors recognize microbial structures, some Toll-like receptors and activating receptors of natural killer cells do recognize nonmicrobial self proteins expressed by stressed, damaged, or infected cells. Memory is a unique property of the adaptive and not the innate immune system.
CMI5 276-277; BI2 22-24

4. (D) More than 10 mammalian Toll-like receptors (TLRs) have been identified, and each appears to recognize a different set of structures that are found in pathogenic microbes but not in mammalian cells. Such structures are called pathogen-associated molecular patterns (PAMPs). Unmethylated cytosine guanosine (CpG) motifs are typical of bacterial and protozoan DNA, but not mammalian DNA, and are therefore PAMPs. TLR9 binds CpG DNA. Transfer RNA, single-stranded RNA, double-stranded DNA, and heterochromatin are all normal components of mammalian cells and are not recognized by TLRs. Double-stranded RNA is produced by some viruses but not by mammalian cells and is recognized by TLR3.
CMI5 283-284; BI2 27

5. (A) Gram-positive bacteria contain cell walls rich in peptidoglycan. When shed by bacteria such as *Streptococcus pneumoniae*, peptidoglycan serves as a ligand that binds Toll-like receptor 2 (TLR2), stimulating an innate immune response. The other choices listed are also ligands that stimulate TLRs, but they are not present in gram-positive bacteria. Double-stranded RNA is found in replicating viruses, lipopolysaccharide (LPS) is a component of the outer cell wall of gram-negative bacteria, and both lipoarabinomannan and phosphatidylinositol dimannoside are present in mycobacteria.
CMI5 283-284; BI2 27

6. (D) The predominant signaling pathway used by Toll-like receptors (TLRs) results in the activation of the NF-κB transcription factor. Ligand binding to the TLR at the cell surface leads to recruitment of several cytoplasmic signaling molecules through specific domain-domain interactions, resulting in degradation of IκB and subsequent activation of NFκB. In some cell types, certain TLRs also engage other signaling pathways, such as the MAP kinase cascade, leading to activation of the AP-1 transcription factor. T-bet and GATA-3 are transcriptional regulators involved in helper T cell differentiation. Fos is a component of AP-1, and STAT-6 is a transcription factor activated by IL-4 binding to cells. Lck is not a transcription factor, but rather a tyrosine protein kinase involved in antigen-receptor signaling in T cells.
CMI5 283; BI2 27

7. (E) CD28, the activating receptor for B7-1 and B7-2 costimulatory molecules, is constitutively expressed on the surface of many T cells and is not induced by Toll-like receptor (TLR) signaling. TLR signaling does induce expression of B7-1 and B7-2 on antigen-presenting cells. Other genes expressed in response to TLR signaling encode proteins important in many different components of innate immune responses. These include inflammatory cytokines such as tumor necrosis factor-α (TNF-α), interleukin-1 (IL-1), and IL-12; endothelial adhesion molecules such as E-selectin; and proteins involved in microbial killing mechanisms, including inducible nitric oxide synthase (iNOS). The specific genes expressed depend on the cell type of the responding cell.
CMI5 283, 296; BI2 27-30

8. (D) The macrophage mannose receptor binds to terminal mannose and fucose residues on bacterial glycoproteins and glycolipids. Mammalian cells do not typically contain these residues. CD36 binds many different ligands, including microbial and self molecules. Fc receptors, complement receptors, and ICAM-1 are receptors for mammalian complement fragments, Ig, and LFA-1, respectively.
CMI5 282; BI2 28-29

9. (B) Neutrophils and macrophages can both actively phagocytose and kill microbes, and both express opsonin receptors, such as FcγRI or complement receptors that enhance phagocytosis. Neutrophils are short lived, whereas macrophages can survive for days or weeks. Macrophages are not terminally differentiated and can undergo cell division at inflammatory sites, but neutrophils cannot. Only neutrophils have cytoplasmic granules filled with enzymes, including lysozyme, collagenase, and elastases; these are called specific granules.
CMI5 279-280, 282; BI2 25-27

10. (B) This patient is suffering from septic shock, characterized by the clinical triad of disseminated intravascular coagulation (DIC), hypoglycemia, and cardiovascular failure. This condition is most often initiated by endotoxin, also known as lipopolysaccharide (LPS), a component of the outer cell walls of gram-negative bacteria. LPS is a potent stimulus for tumor necrosis factor (TNF)-α secretion by mononuclear phagocytes and other cell types. Most of the biologic effects of LPS are mediated through TNF-α. Transforming growth factor-β (TGF-β) and interleukin (IL)-10 are anti-

inflammatory cytokines, IL-2 is a T cell growth factor, and IL-3 is a hematopoietic cytokine. These cytokines are not mediators of septic shock.
CMI5 285-286; BI2 36

11. (C) Endotoxin activates macrophages to secrete multiple cytokines, particularly tumor necrosis factor (TNF), interleukin-1 (IL-1), and IL-12. TNF is a major mediator of endotoxin-induced injury to the host, and TNF concentrations in serum rise first. TNF, in turn, induces IL-1 synthesis. TNF and IL-1 act on vascular endothelium to produce other cytokines and activate adhesion molecules. Macrophages also respond by secreting IL-12, which induces local production of interferon-γ (IFN-γ). IFN-γ causes further TNF secretion by endotoxin-activated macrophages. In this way, successive waves of these cytokines are produced, with associated damage to host tissues.
CMI5 263, 285; BI2 36

12. (B) Granzyme B, a proteolytic enzyme component of cytolytic T lymphocyte (CTL) and natural killer (NK) cell granules, is involved in initiating caspase-dependent CTL killing of target cells. Granzyme B is not involved in phagocyte killing of ingested microbes. Inducible nitric oxide synthase (iNOS) generates NO in macrophages, and NO is toxic to microbes. Phagocyte oxidase and myeloperoxidase are involved in generating free radical species that kill ingested microbes in phagocytes. Lysozyme is a proteolytic enzyme in neutrophil granules that contributes to microbial killing.
CMI5 286-288; BI2 28-30

13. (B) C5a is a peptide released after cleavage of C5 protein during the complement cascade. It stimulates the influx of neutrophils to the site of infection, thus acting as a chemoattractant, not as an opsonin. C3b (covalently bound to microbes on which complement activation has taken place) and IgG bound to antigen, are particularly potent opsonins, because phagocytes have receptors for both C3b and the Fc region of IgG. C-reactive protein and mannose-binding lectin also can coat microbes and be recognized by phagocyte receptors; thus they serve as opsonins.
CMI5 282, 293; BI2 28, 146, 152

14. (D) Chronic granulomatous disease (CGD) is a rare, inherited immunodeficiency disease associated with a defective intracellular respiratory burst in phagocytes. It consists of a group of heterogeneous disorders of oxidative metabolism in which the pathways required for generation of toxic reactive oxygen species (ROIs) are impaired. In patients with CGD, phagocytosis occurs normally, but the engulfed microbes are not killed and they multiply within the cell. In this way, patients are susceptible to recurrent infections with organisms such as *Staphylococcus,* which are of low virulence in normal hosts.
CMI5 287; BI2 29, 215

15. (E) The presence of normal numbers of CD8+ T cells and the ability of these cells to kill virally infected target cells indicates that the class I major histocompatibility complex (MHC) pathway of viral peptide antigen presentation is intact. The patient's immunodeficiency is due to a lack of natural killer (NK) cells. NK cells express CD56 and/or CD16. NK cells are activated by interleukin-15 (IL-15) and IL-12, are normally inhibited by recognizing class I MHC on other cells, kill target cells with altered class I MHC expression through a granzyme B–dependent mechanisms (similar to cytolytic T lymphocyte killing), and produce interferon-γ as part of the early innate response to viral infection.
CMI5 289-293; BI2 30-32

16. (B) Natural killing (NK) inhibitory receptors recognize class I MHC molecules that are normally and constitutively expressed, including various alleles of HLA-A and HLA-C. The cytoplasmic tails of NK inhibitory receptors contain immunoreceptor tyrosine-based inhibitory motifs (ITIMs), but not immunoreceptor tyrosine-based activation motifs (ITAMs). Some inhibitory receptors on NK cells are members of the Ig superfamily, but not the integrin or TLR families. NK cells usually express both activating and inhibitory receptors, and activation is regulated by a balance between signals generated from both types of receptors. The inhibitory receptors on NK cells bind to self class I MHC molecules, which are expressed on most normal cells. When activating and inhibitory receptors are simultaneously engaged, the inhibitory receptor signals dominate and the NK cell is not activated.
CMI5 291-292; BI2 30-32

17. (C) Mannose-binding lectin (MBL) is a soluble serum component that is structurally similar to C1 of the classical complement pathway. MBL binds to mannan residues on microbial surfaces and triggers proteolytic cleavage and activation of downstream components of the complement system. C9 is not involved in initiation of complement activation but is part of the common final membrane attack complex (MAC) pathway. CR2 is a cell surface receptor for complement fragments. A mannose receptor is a cell surface receptor on phagocytes that binds mannan residues and promotes phagocytosis of microbes.
CMI5 293-294; BI2 32-34

18. (C) Innate immune responses are important stimulators of adaptive immunity. Increased expression of B7-1 and B7-2 on antigen-presenting cells after microbial activation of Toll-like receptors (innate immunity) is critical in providing costimulatory signals for T cell activation (adaptive immunity) via binding to CD28 receptors on T cells. T helper cell–mediated endothelial or macrophage activation is an example of adaptive immunity using the effector mechanisms of innate immunity. Neither IgG3 opsonization facilitating natural killer cytolytic

activity nor double-stranded RNA stimulating interferon-β secretion involve innate immunity enhancing adaptive immunity.
CMI5 260, 293, 296; BI2 36-38

19. (I) Reactive oxygen intermediates (ROIs) are generated by enzymes in phagocytes, such as phagocyte oxidase and myeloperoxidase. They have unpaired electrons in their outer orbitals and induce oxidative damage to cellular membranes and DNA. ROIs can kill microbes, but they also damage host cells.
CMI5 287; BI2 28-30

20. (H) Mannose-binding lectin is a C-type lectin found in the serum that binds microbial surface carbohydrates with terminal mannose residues and mediates phagocytosis and activation of the lectin complement pathway.
CMI5 294; BI2 36

21. (C) Natural antibodies are IgM antibodies produced by B1 B cells. They have very limited diversity and bind to commonly encountered microbial structures, such as phosphoryl choline.
CMI5 279; BI2 25

22. (G) C-reactive protein, a member of the pentraxin family of plasma proteins, is an acute phase reactant that is rapidly up-regulated by hepatocytes in response to inflammatory cytokines, such as interleukin (IL)-1, IL-6, and tumor necrosis factor-α.
CMI5 294; BI2 36

23. (A) Defensins are a family of vertebrate antimicrobial peptides found in epithelial barrier cells and neutrophil granules. They are toxic to a wide variety of microorganisms and may work by perturbing the permeability of limiting membranes of microbes.
CMI5 278; BI2 24

24. (E) The cell type shown is a neutrophil (polymorphonuclear leukocyte). This innate immune system effector cell is a major component of acute inflammatory infiltrates, but it does not express class II MHC molecules and is therefore not an antigen-presenting cell for CD4$^+$ T cells.
CMI5 280; BI2 25

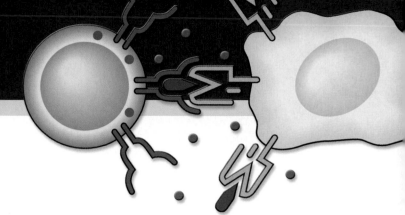

Chapter 13

Effector Mechanisms of Cell-Mediated Immunity

Cellular and Molecular Immunology, 5/E: Chapter 13—Effector Mechanisms of Cell-Mediated Immunity

Basic Immunology, 2/E: Chapter 5—Cell-Mediated Immune Responses; and Chapter 6—Effector Mechanisms of Cell-Mediated Immunity

1. Which of the following statements about cell-mediated immunity (CMI) is NOT true?

   A. Deficiencies in CMI result in susceptibility to infections by viruses and intracellular bacteria.
   B. CMI can be adoptively transferred by injecting serum from one individual to another.
   C. Delayed-type hypersensitivity (DTH) is not a protective response against intracellular bacteria such as *Mycobacterium tuberculosis.*
   D. The principal form of CMI that protects against viral infections is mediated by CD8+ cytolytic T lymphocytes.
   E. Phagocytes are essential in the effector phase of CMI responses to bacteria such as *Listeria monocytogenes.*

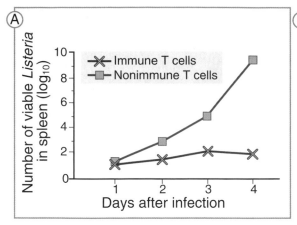

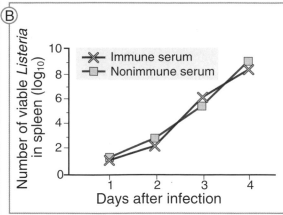

2. The graphs above show the effectiveness of passive transfer of T cells (A) or serum (B) in controlling a bacterial infection in mice. T cells or sera were taken from mice that had previously recovered from infection with *Listeria monocytogenes* ("immune") or from previously uninfected mice ("nonimmune"), and these T cells or sera were transferred to previously uninfected mice. The recipient mice were then infected with *Listeria monocytogenes*. The number of viable organisms in the spleens of the recipient mice was determined between 1 and 4 days after infection. Based on the results shown, which of the following statements is NOT correct?

A. *Listeria monocytogenes* is an intracellular bacterium that can live within phagocytes.
B. Antibodies are not effective in clearing an established infection by *Listeria monocytogenes*.
C. Innate immune responses appear to be sufficient in controlling *Listeria monocytogenes*.
D. Effector or memory T cells specific for *Listeria monocytogenes* are important in clearing infection by this organism.
E. Protective immunity to *Listeria monocytogenes* can be passively transferred.

3. The induction phase of a cell-mediated immune response includes which of the following events?

A. CD4$^+$ T cell secretion of interferon-γ leading to macrophage activation
B. CD8$^+$ T cell lysis of a virally infected cell
C. Clonal expansion of CD8$^+$ T cells within a lymph node
D. Migration of CD4$^+$ effector T cells from blood vessels into a tissue site of infection
E. Migration of a naive CD4$^+$ T cell from the thymic medulla into the circulation

4. Which of the following comparisons between T$_H$1 and T$_H$2 cells is true?

A. T$_H$1 cells produce interleukin (IL)-1 but not IL-2, and T$_H$2 cells produce IL-2 but not IL-1.
B. T$_H$1 cells are class I major histocompatibility complex (MHC) restricted, and T$_H$2 cells are class II MHC restricted.

C. The chemokine receptors CXCR3 and CCR5 are more highly expressed on T$_H$2 cells than on T$_H$1 cells.
D. T$_H$2 cells are more likely to bind to E-selectin and P-selectin on endothelial cells than are T$_H$1 cells.
E. T$_H$1 cells produce interferon (IFN)-γ but not IL-4, and T$_H$2 cells produce IL-4 but not IFN-γ.

5. Differentiation of T$_H$2 cells from naive precursor cells is dependent on which of the following?

A. Toll-like receptor (TLR) ligands
B. T-bet
C. Interleukin-12
D. GATA-3
E. Interferon-α

Questions 6-9
Match descriptions of cell-mediated immune responses in questions 6-9, with the appropriate molecule (A-H) from the following list.

A. Interferon-γ
B. Interleukin (IL)-10
C. IL-12
D. CD40L
E. CD40
F. STAT6
G. STAT4
H. IL-5

6. This intracellular signaling molecule and transcription factor is activated by IL-12. ( )

7. This membrane molecule is expressed on the surface of activated T$_H$1 cells and promotes macrophage activation. ( )

8. This product of T$_H$2 cells promotes immunity to helminthic infections. ( )

9. This intracellular signaling molecule and transcription factor is required for differentiation of T$_H$2 cells and for responses of other cells to T$_H$2 cells. ( )

10. The mechanisms by which T$_H$1 cells protect against microbes include all of the following EXCEPT:

A. Secretion of interferon (IFN)-γ, which activates microbicidal functions of macrophages

B. Expression of CD40 ligand, which binds to CD40 on macrophages and activates them

C. Secretion of IFN-γ, which promotes B cell production of opsonizing antibodies

D. Secretion of lymphotoxin and tumor necrosis factor, which enhance neutrophil killing of ingested microbes

E. Release of granzyme B, which stimulates apoptosis of bacteria

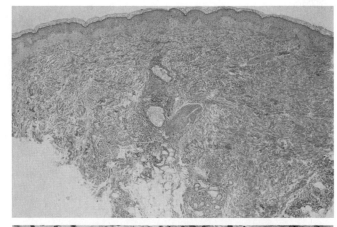

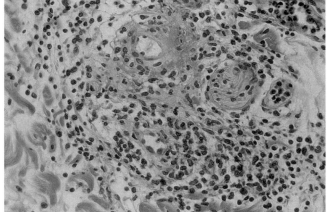

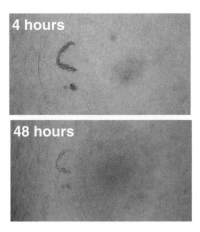

11. A 3-year-old boy with a history of multiple bacterial and fungal infections is seen by an immunologist for evaluation of immunodeficiency disease. In one test, the boy was given three separate intradermal injections of tetanus toxoid, mumps antigen, and *Candida* antigen at three different sites. After 4 hours, and again at 48 hours, each of the injection sites appeared as shown in the figure above. Each site felt firm to the touch. Which of the following conclusions can be properly made based on this test result?

A. The boy is allergic to multiple protein antigens.

B. The boy is capable of producing antibodies specific for tetanus toxoid, mumps antigen, and *Candida* antigen.

C. The boy has functioning CD4+ T cells.

D. The boy has a defect in macrophage-dependent clearance of antigens.

E. The boy was not immunized against tetanus toxoid or mumps.

12. A histologic section of a positive PPD skin test for tuberculosis is shown above. Which of the following accurately describes the histopathology and/or the immunologic process?

A. There is a persistent delayed-type hypersensitivity response to *Mycobacterium tuberculosis* organisms at the skin test site.

B. There are numerous T cells that have responded to *Mycobacterium tuberculosis* antigens and macrophages that have been activated by the responding T cells.

C. There is vasculitis caused by immune complex deposition in blood vessel walls.

D. The site is inflamed due to injury from the needle puncture, but no morphologic evidence of the T cell response can be seen by light microscopy.

E. The test site is infiltrated with eosinophils, and resident mast cells have been activated.

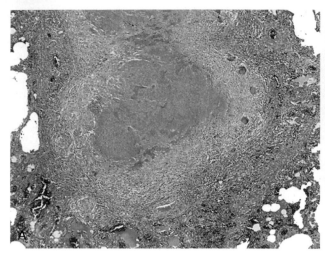
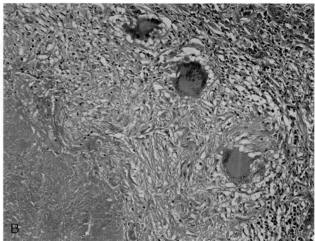

Questions 13 and 14

A 36-year-old immigrant from India goes to the emergency department because of cough and hemoptysis. The patient reports a recent bout of night sweats as well as weight loss. A chest radiograph shows three distinct nodular masses localized to the lung apices. A lung biopsy is performed, and the histologic sections, shown above, reveal nodular collections of activated macrophages, some forming multinucleated giant cells, abundant lymphocytes, and central necrosis.

13. Which of the following is the most likely diagnosis of this type of immune inflammatory response?

   A. Granulomatous inflammation
   B. Acute inflammation
   C. Ischemic necrosis
   D. Immune complex disease
   E. Immediate hypersensitivity

14. Which of the following statements about the form of inflammation shown in the figure is NOT correct?

   A. It is a form of chronic delayed-type hypersensitivity.
   B. It occurs when microorganisms persist within phagocytic vesicles in macrophages.
   C. Interleukin (IL)-12 and IL-18 contribute to the inflammatory process.
   D. $CD4^+$ T cells of the T_H1 phenotype are involved in this form of inflammation.
   E. This type of inflammatory response serves to clear infections by certain microorganism without leaving scar tissue.

Questions 15-20

For each of the descriptions in questions 15-20, select the molecule involved in T cell traffic (A-L).

   A. P-selectin
   B. L-selectin
   C. CCR8
   D. Tumor necrosis factor (TNF)
   E. VCAM-1
   F. LFA-1
   G. CCR5
   H. CCR4
   I. $\alpha4\beta7$
   J. Cutaneous lymphocyte antigen (CLA)
   K. Mip1-α
   L. VLA-4

15. Mediates naive $CD4^+$ T cell migration into lymph nodes (   )

16. Induces expression of endothelial selectins and Ig superfamily adhesion molecules, promoting effector T cell migration into inflammatory sites (   )

17. A ligand on a subset of T cells that binds to E-selectin

18. Mediates homing of a subset of T cells into the intestinal mucosa (   )

19. A membrane molecule expressed on T cells that promotes migration of T_H2 cells into certain inflammatory sites (   )

20. A T cell adhesion molecule that binds to fibronectin in extracellular matrices (   )

21. Activated macrophages perform all of the following functions EXCEPT:

   A. Inhibition of fibroblast proliferation and angiogenesis within damaged tissues
   B. Production of lysosomal enzymes and reactive oxygen species that kill phagocytosed microbes
   C. Presentation of antigen to helper T cells
   D. Secretion of inflammatory cytokines such as tumor necrosis factor and interleukin-1
   E. Production of nitric oxide, which helps kill microorganisms

22. Which of the following molecules is NOT important in the interaction between a cytolytic T lymphocyte and a target cell?

   A. B7-1
   B. ICAM-1
   C. LFA-1
   D. T cell receptor
   E. Class I MHC

23. Which pair of molecules is a component of cytolytic T lymphocyte (CTL) granules and is important in the mechanism of CTL killing of target cells?

    A. Perforin and Fas ligand
    B. P-selectin and tumor necrosis factor
    C. Major basic protein and granzyme B
    D. C9 and interferon-γ
    E. Perforin and granzyme B

24. Which of the following mechanisms does NOT contribute to the generation of a cytolytic T lymphocyte (CTL) response to a viral infection?

    A. Dendritic cells phagocytose infected cells or viral particles and present them to naive CD8$^+$ T cells via the class I MHC pathway.
    B. Dendritic cells are infected with the virus and present viral peptides to naive CD8$^+$ T cells via the class I MHC pathway.
    C. CTLs are directly activated by CD40L expressed on activated helper T cells through CD40.
    D. Helper T cells secrete cytokines, such as interleukin-2, that promote the proliferation and differentiation of CD8$^+$ T cells.
    E. Helper T cells activate infected antigen-presenting cells (APCs) via the CD40 ligand-CD40 pathway, and the activated APCs present viral peptides to naive CD8$^+$ T cells via the class I MHC pathway.

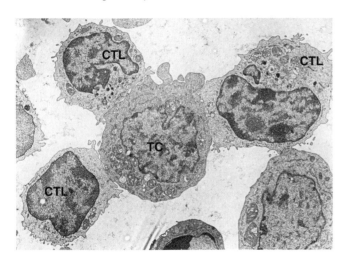

25. The figure above is an electron microscopic view of three cytolytic T lymphocytes (CTLs) in contact with a target cell. Assume that the CTLs are specific for a viral peptide derived from Epstein-Barr virus (EBV) bound to an HLA-A2 MHC molecule, and the target cell is an EBV–infected HLA-A2–expressing cell. Which of the following statements about the interaction between the CTLs and the target cell is true?

    A. The target cell will become necrotic as a result of recognition by the CTLs.
    B. Both the CTLs and the target cell will die as a result of their mutual interactions.
    C. The CTLs will detach from the target cell and survive, before the target cell dies by apoptosis.

    D. The naive CD8$^+$ T cell precursors to the CTLs shown were restricted by a class I MHC allele different from HLA-A2.
    E. The adhesion of the CTLs to the target cell depends on E-selectin.

26. A 23-year-old man who was recently infected by the HIV virus volunteered for investigative studies of his immune response to the virus. Investigators identified cytolytic T lymphocytes (CTLs) in the patient's blood that recognized a particular peptide derived from a protein encoded by the HIV *gag* gene. Six months later, viral isolates from the patient showed point mutations in the *gag* gene sequence encoding that peptide. Which of the following statements about the HIV *gag* mutations is most likely to be correct?

    A. The patient's CTL response to the virus provided selective pressure for the emergence of virus carrying the mutation.
    B. The CTL that recognized the original *gag*-encoded peptide will still be able to recognize the mutated Gag peptide.
    C. The CTLs specific for the original Gag peptide were incapable of killing HIV-infected cells.
    D. The *gag* mutation will enhance the ability of natural killer cells to recognize and kill HIV infected cells.
    E. The *gag* mutations have more relevance to the viral evasion of the antibody response rather than the CTL response.

Answers

1. (B) The original definition of cell-mediated immunity (CMI), which is still valid, is protection against infection that can be transferred by T cells but not by serum. Serum is a cell-free fraction of blood that includes antibodies, and therefore serum transfer can provide passive humoral immunity. CMI is required for protection against microbes that can reside within cells and therefore are inaccessible to antibodies. These organisms include microbes that are phagocytosed and viruses that replicate in the cytoplasm. Immunodeficiency states in which CMI is impaired (e.g., AIDS) result in infections by viruses and intracellular bacteria or fungi. Delayed-type hypersensitivity (DTH), like all hypersensitivity reactions, causes tissue damage and disease, but not protection. It is true that DTH reactions involve the same cells and molecules as does CMI.
   CMI5 298-299; BI2 105-106

2. (C) Control of infection appears to rely on previous exposure and immunization, since nonimmune T cells or sera afforded no protection. Therefore, innate immunity is not sufficient for control of infection and adaptive immunity is required. Since immune sera, which contain antibodies, did not protect, but immune T cells did, it is likely that the

organisms replicate within cells and are inaccessible to antibodies.
CMI5 299-300; BI2 112

3. (C) The induction phase of cell-mediated immune responses occurs in lymphoid tissues and includes antigen presentation to naive T cells, leading to clonal expansion and differentiation of those T cells into effector cells. Migration into infection sites and interferon-γ secretion by CD4$^+$ helper T cells, as well as target cell killing by CD8$^+$CTL, are part of the effector phases of cell-mediated immune responses. Naive T cell migration out of the thymus is the last step in T cell maturation and occurs regardless of the presence of antigen.
CMI5 301-303; BI2 105-111

4. (E) The signature cytokines of T$_H$1 and T$_H$2 cells are interferon-γ and interleukin (IL)-4, respectively. IL-5 and IL-13 are also very specific for T$_H$2 cells. IL-1 is not typically produced by helper T cells of either subset. IL-2 is produced by naive T cells and T$_H$1 cells. Both T$_H$1 and T$_H$2 cells are CD4$^+$ helper T cells, and therefore are both restricted to recognizing peptide antigens bound to class II MHC molecules. The trafficking patterns of T$_H$1 and T$_H$2 cells differ, and this is related to differences in the expression of adhesion molecules and chemokine receptors. T$_H$1 cells express abundant functional ligands for E-selectin and P-selectin and the chemokine receptors CXCR3 and CCR5, which bind to various chemokines found at sites of active innate immune responses. T$_H$2 cells bind poorly to endothelial selectins and express less CXCR3 and CCR5.
CMI5 303-304; BI2 111-112

5. (D) GATA-3 is a transcription factor that is expressed during differentiation and is required for T$_H$2 differentiation. T-bet is a protein that regulates genetic changes required for T$_H$1 differentiation. In general, innate immune responses, many of which are stimulated microbial products binding Toll-like receptors (TLRs) on antigen-presenting cells (APCs), promote T$_H$1 differentiation. In part, the positive influence of innate immune responses on T$_H$1 differentiation is mediated by cytokines secreted by activated APCs, including interleukin-12 and type I interferons (IFN-α and IFN-β).
CMI5 304-306; BI2 95-99

6. (G) Interleukin (IL)-12 binding to its receptors on T cells and natural killer (NK) cells activates the Janus kinase Tyk2, which phosphorylates and activates STAT4. The functional responses of cells to IL-12 are dependent on STAT4-dependent gene transcription. Therefore, T$_H$1 differentiation, which requires IL-12 stimulation of naive T cells, is dependent on STAT4.
CMI5 257-259, 304-306; BI2 100-103

7. (D) CD40L (CD154), a member of the tumor necrosis factor (TNF) family of proteins, is expressed on T$_H$1 cell after antigen-induced activation and binds to CD40, a member of the TNF receptor family, on macrophages. The signals generated by CD40 promote macrophage activation as well as B cell differentiation. Interferon-γ, also produced by helper T cells, synergizes with CD40 ligand in activating macrophages.
CMI5 306; BI2 112-114

8. (H) Interleukin (IL)-5 is a cytokine produced by T$_H$2 cells that stimulates production of eosinophils in the bone marrow and promotes eosinophil activation. Eosinophil granules contain molecules, such as major basic protein, that are particularly toxic to helminths.
CMI5 306; 313-314; BI2 115-116

9. (F) STAT6 is an intracellular signaling molecule that is activated by interleukin (IL)-4, via JAK3 and JAK4. IL-4 activation of STAT6 is required for the differentiation of naive T cells into the T$_H$2 phenotype, as well as for the effects of IL-4 on other cell types, such as isotype switching to IgE in B cells.
CMI5 304-306

10. (E) Granzyme B, a product of CD8$^+$ cytolytic T lymphocytes, promotes death of infected host cells, but not of extracellular microbes. The principal function of T$_H$1 cells is to enhance phagocyte defense against intracellular infections. Interferon (IFN)-γ and CD40 ligand, produced by T$_H$1 cells, enhance killing of microbes ingested by macrophages, in part by stimulating the production of inducible nitric oxide synthase and phagocyte oxidase. IFN-γ, produced by T$_H$1 cells, is an isotype switch factor, promoting the production of IgG subtypes that bind to Fc receptors on phagocytes and fix complement. Therefore, these opsonizing IgG subtypes facilitate the phagocytosis of the microbes to which they bind. T$_H$1 cells also secrete tumor necrosis factor and lymphotoxin, two cytokines that can activate neutrophil killing of internalized microbes.
CMI5 306-307, 312; BI2 96-97, 112-113

11. (C) The test performed on the 3-year-old boy was a cutaneous delayed-type hypersensitivity (DTH) assay of cellular immunity. This test determines if an individual can mount a memory T cell response to antigens to which he or she has previously been exposed. Tetanus toxoid and mumps antigens are given in routine childhood vaccines, and *Candida* antigens are ubiquitous in the environment. The redness and swelling produced by the injections indicate that the protein antigens have been processed and presented to memory CD4$^+$ helper T cells specific for these antigens. These T cells became activated and produced cytokines, which promoted the subsequent recruitment and activation of monocytes and macrophages. The delayed-type hypersensitivity (DTH) responses should not be confused with an IgE- and mast cell-mediated immediate hypersensitivity (allergic) response, which can also be tested for by intradermal injections. The DTH response does not require antibodies; however, it is possible that the boy has

antibodies specific for the test antigens. The positive test result suggests that macrophage function, as well as T cell function, is normal.
CMI5 310-311; BI2 112-113

12. (B) The figure shows a typical delayed-type hypersensitivity (DTH) response in which there are perivascular mononuclear cell infiltrates in the dermis consisting of activated lymphocytes and macrophages. The infiltrates surround blood vessels in which the endothelial cells are activated. In DTH sites, T cells specific for the inciting antigen are activated, proliferate, and cause the activation of macrophages as well as the recruitment of other lymphocytes and monocytes. No *Mycobacterium tuberculosis* organisms are administered in the PPD test, just purified proteins derived from the organisms. Although the inflammation surrounds blood vessels, there is no vasculitis, and immune complexes do not contribute to this type of reaction. The needle used to administer the PPD test is very small, and inflammation due to the needle puncture is minimal. Eosinophils and mast cell deregulation are typical of immediate hypersensitivity reactions but not DTH.
CMI5 310-311; BI2 112-113

13. (A) The figure shows a granuloma consisting of a nodule with central necrosis surrounded by activated macrophages, many multinucleated giant cells, and lymphocytes. This is typical of granulomatous inflammation in the setting of *Mycobacterium tuberculosis* infection, and the clinical history is also typical of active pulmonary tuberculosis. Granulomas also may form in response to infections with other microorganisms, including other bacteria and fungi that live within macrophages. Central necrosis is not always present in granulomas. Note that the granulomatous response is very different from a DTH response seen in a positive PPD skin test for exposure to tuberculosis, as shown in question 12. In the skin test, there are no live microbes administered and no long-term persistence of the antigen. Acute inflammation largely consists of polymorphonuclear leukocyte infiltrates and few or no lymphocytes, macrophages, or giant cells. Ischemic necrosis, which is death of tissue due to lack of sufficient blood supply, and immune complex disease usually result in acute inflammation, followed by chronic inflammation with macrophages and lymphocytes. In immediate hypersensitivity reactions, there is early edema, followed by a late phase with acute inflammation.
CMI5 313; BI2 115

14. (E) Granulomas usually lead to the formation of fibrotic scars, and in this way, granulomatous diseases impair organ function. Granulomas represent a form of chronic delayed-type hypersensitivity (DTH), owing to the persistence of microbial antigens within macrophages, and persistent activation of T lymphocytes and macrophages. As with all DTH responses, interferon-γ secreted by T_H1 cells, and

interleukin (IL)-12 and IL-18 secreted by macrophages, contribute to the inflammatory process.
CMI5 313; BI2 115

15. (B) L-selectin is expressed abundantly on naive T cells, but not effector T cells, and binds to peripheral lymph node addressin (PNAd) on high endothelial venules in lymph nodes. This adhesive interaction is required for naive T cell migration from blood into lymph nodes, a first step in the initiation of cell-mediated immune responses.
CMI5 34-36; BI2 108-109

16. (D) Tumor necrosis factor (TNF) is a cytokine secreted by mononuclear phagocytes as part of the innate immune response. One important function of TNF is to induce adhesion molecule expression on nearby vascular endothelial cells, including E-selectin, ICAM-1, and VCAM-1. These adhesion molecules contribute to the recruitment of various inflammatory cells.
CMI5 308-311; BI2 108-110

17. (J) CLA is an E-selectin ligand expressed on a subset of effector and memory CD4$^+$ and CD8$^+$ T lymphocytes; it promotes the migration of these T cells into the skin.
CMI5 310

18. (I) The integrin α4β7 is expressed on a subset of effector and memory T cells, which home to intestinal mucosa. α4β7 binds to mucosal addressin cell adhesion molecule (MAdCAM) on endothelial cells in the intestine.
CMI5 310

19. (H) CCR4 is one of the chemokine receptors that is more abundantly expressed on T_H2 cells than other T cell subsets. CCR4 binds the chemokines CCL17 and CCL22.
CMI5 304

20. (L) VLA-4 (α4β1) is an integrin expressed on T cells. In addition to binding to VCAM-1 on endothelial cells, VLA-4 also binds fibronectin in the extracellular matrix. In this way, VLA-4 contributes to movement and retention of T cells in the extravascular space.
CMI5 310-311; BI2 108

21. (A) Activated macrophages, through the secretion of growth factors, promote fibroblast proliferation and angiogenesis in an effort to repair damaged tissues.
CMI5 312-313; BI2 115

22. (A) Although naive CD8$^+$ T cells require second signals, such as B7 costimulation, in order to differentiate into effector cytolytic T lymphocyte (CTL), once differentiated, the CTL can kill a target cell that does not express costimulatory molecules. The CTL only requires one signal for killing of the target cell, which depends on the T cell receptor binding to a peptide-class I MHC complex on the surface of the target cell. Tight adhesion

between the CTL and target cell is also required, and this is often mediated by T cell integrin LFA-1 binding to target cell ICAM-1.
CMI5 314; BI2 117-118

23. (E) Perforin and granzyme B are the cytolytic T lymphocyte (CTL) granule constituents of most importance in killing of target cells. CTL granules are emptied by exocytosis into the intercellular space between the CTL and target cell. Here perforin polymerizes to form pore-like structures that insert into the target cell plasma membrane and/or in the membranes of endocytic vesicles in the target cell. Granzyme B is a proteolytic enzyme that cleaves substrates in the cytoplasm of the target cell, leading to a cascade of enzyme activation that ends in apoptosis. Granzyme B enters the target cell either through perforin pores or by receptor-mediated endocytosis. FasL is expressed on the surface of the CTL, not in granules. FasL binding to Fas on target cells may induce apoptosis of the target cells by a caspase-dependent pathway, but this is a minor mechanism of CTL killing relative to perforin- and granzyme B–dependent mechanisms. P-selectin is an endothelial adhesion molecule stored in cytoplasmic granules, and MBP is a cationic protein found in eosinophil granules. Although perforin is homologous to the complement protein C9, C9 is not present in CTL granules. CTLs do produce interferon-γ, but they do not store this cytokine in granules.
CMI5 314-316; BI2 117-118

24. (C) T cells do not express CD40, and they do not respond directly to CD40 ligand. There is clear evidence that CD8$^+$ cytolytic T lymphocyte (CTL) responses to viral infections require professional antigen-presenting cells (APCs) as well as CD4$^+$ helper T cells. How this works is complicated; all viruses do not infect professional APCs, and helper T cells are class II MHC restricted whereas CD8$^+$ CTL precursors are class I MHC restricted. Several mechanisms have been shown to contribute to naive CD8$^+$ T cell activation in experimental systems. One mechanism is cross presentation of viral peptides by professional APCs that were not infected but acquired the viral antigens from other cells. Infected APCs may present viral peptides to CD4$^+$ T cells, stimulating a helper T cell response, which then, via secreted cytokines, helps activate CD8$^+$ T cells. Helper T cells may also enhance APC function of infected cells via CD40-CD40 ligand interactions.
CMI5 302

25. (C) Cytolytic T lymphocytes (CTLs) do not die after delivery of a lethal hit to a target cell, but instead they detach and are capable of killing additional infected cells. Several mechanisms prevent the CTL from destroying itself, including expression of enzymes that inhibit perforin polymerization in the CTL membrane. The target cells do not die by necrosis, but rather by apoptosis. The T cell receptor (TCR) on a naive CD8$^+$ T cell is identical to the TCR expressed on the CTL effectors that are derived from the naive cell, and therefore the peptide-MHC complex that is recognized by naive and effector CTL is the same. Adhesion between CTLs and target cells is dependent on the integrin LFA-1, but not on E-selectin, which is exclusively an endothelial adhesion molecule.
CMI5 314-316; BI2 117-118

26. (A) Cytolytic T lymphocytes (CTLs) are highly specific for short peptide epitopes of viral proteins bound to self-MHC molecules. Random mutations in the viral genome that alter these peptide sequences will lead to escape from CTL detection. Therefore, CTLs do provide a selective pressure for such mutations. Given these selective pressures, it is most likely that the mutations that are found in the virus that has survived in the patient are no longer recognized by the CTL. Because only one or two amino acid residues of a viral peptide will contact a particular TCR, point mutations that ablate T cell recognition are likely to occur. The emergence of escape variants with mutated peptides implies that the CTLs that recognized the original peptide were capable of killing the infected cells, but mutations arose before all infected cells were killed. Natural killer cells recognize alterations in self class I MHC expression but do not recognize specific viral peptide sequences. Although antibodies may be produced specific for distinct epitopes of the same proteins that elicit CTL responses, the information given about changes in a T cell epitope implicate the relevance of the CTL response.
CMI5 357-358; BI2 118-119

Chapter 14

Effector Mechanisms of Humoral Immunity

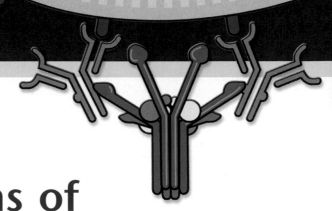

Cellular and Molecular Immunology, 5/E: Chapter 14—Effector Mechanisms of Humoral Immunity

Basic Immunology, 2/E: Chapter 7— Humoral Immune Responses

1. In 1890, Emil von Behring and Shibasaburo Kitasato demonstrated the efficacy of serum transfer at conferring infection resistance—a process now known as "passive immunity." The researchers isolated serum from animals that had recovered from infection with the diphtheria bacilli and subsequently injected the serum into other healthy animals. This procedure conferred specific resistance against the pathologic effects of diphtheria infection in the recipient animals. Which of the following immune phenomena were primarily responsible for these effects?

   A. Pathogen-specific B and T cells from the original infected animals triggered a robust immune response after re-exposure to diphtheria antigens in the recipient animal.
   B. Inflammatory cytokines in the transferred serum increased the strength and efficacy of innate immune system activity.
   C. Diphtheria-specific antibodies in the transferred serum neutralized bacillus toxins and promoted bacterial elimination by innate effector cells.
   D. Serum complement proteins in the transfer directly promoted bacterial cell lysis and phagocytosis.
   E. The recipient animal's immune response to the foreign serum further activated host immune system function, allowing greater response to the bacillus infection.

2. Which of the following anatomic regions is normally protected from pathogens only by humoral immune responses and not by cell-mediated immune responses?

A. Skin
B. Intestinal lumen
C. Intestinal epithelium
D. Central nervous system
E. Spleen

3. Up to half of the IgG found in the serum of a normal individual is produced by which of the following cells?

A. Naive B cells in lymph nodes
B. Activated B cells in the spleen
C. B cells in germinal centers of lymph nodes
D. B lymphocytes in the gastrointestinal tract
E. Long-lived plasma cells in the bone marrow

4. Treatment of antibodies with the enzyme papain under conditions of limited proteolysis results in hinge-region cleavage, yielding monovalent antigen-binding Fab fragments that lack a constant region. Which effector function of antibodies would Fab fragments be able to perform?

A. Complement pathway activation
B. Antibody-dependent cell-mediated cytotoxicity
C. Opsonization
D. Antigen cross-linking and precipitation
E. Microbe neutralization

5. Most effective vaccines that are currently in widespread use are specific for pathogenic viruses, and the immunity induced by the vaccines is mediated largely by antibodies. Which of the following statements accurately describes the major mechanism by which these vaccine-dependent antibody responses function?

A. The antibodies bind extracellular viral particles and prevent them from infecting cells.
B. The antibodies bind to viral antigens on the surface of infected cells and promote phagocytosis of the cells.
C. The antibodies bind to viral antigens on the surface of infected cells and promote complement-mediated lysis of the cells.
D. The antibodies bind to extracellular viral particles and target Fc receptor-expressing cytolytic T lymphocytes to kill the viruses.
E. The antibodies bind to viral envelope proteins and induce signals that inhibit viral replication.

6. Which of the following binds to and is readily phagocytosed by mononuclear phagocytes and neutrophils?

A. Antigen-IgM complexes
B. Bound complement protein C3b
C. Free serum IgG
D. IgE bound to a helminthic parasite
E. Mannose-binding lectin (MBL)

7. An 8-month-old boy infant with a 3-month history of recurrent upper and lower respiratory tract infections is admitted to the hospital. The physicians consider the possibility of a hereditary immune disorder and run several tests, eventually determining that the patient has undetectable levels of serum IgA. The infant is treated with strong antibiotics and recovers. Which of the following is NOT a medical problem likely to occur in this patient as he gets older?

A. Anaphylactic reactions to blood transfusions
B. Chronic gastrointestinal infections
C. Lactose and wheat gluten intolerance
D. Inflammatory skin disease
E. Recurrent nasal sinus congestion

8. Which of the following statements about Ig Fc receptors is NOT true?

A. Some Fc receptors or Fc receptor–associated signaling chains contain ITAMs in their cytoplasmic tails.
B. Some Fc receptors are linked to signal transduction pathways that cause granule exocytosis.
C. There are Fc receptors specific for all common Ig isotypes.
D. Some Fc receptors with ITIMs in their cytoplasmic tails transduce inhibitory signals.
E. Fc receptor signaling may enhance generation of reactive oxygen intermediates in phagocytes.

Questions 9-12
For each of the following descriptions in questions 9-12, select the Fc receptor (A-G) that best matches it.

A. FcγRI (CD64)
B. FcγRIIB (CD32)
C. FcγRIIIA (CD16)
D. FcεRI
E. FcεRII (CD23)
F. FcαR (CD89)
G. FcRn

9. High-affinity Ig receptor on mast cells important in immediate hypersensitivity reactions ( )

10. High-affinity Ig receptor on macrophages and neutrophils important for phagocytosis and activation ( )

11. Low-affinity Ig receptor on natural killer cells that mediates antibody-dependent cell-mediated cytotoxicity ( )

12. Ig receptor on B cells that mediates feedback inhibition ( )

13. Which of the following events initiates activation of the alternative complement pathway?

A. C1q binding to a microbial surface
B. Mannose-binding lectin (MBL) binding to a microbial surface
C. Complement receptor 1 (CR1) binding of C3b
D. Factor I cleavage of C3
E. Spontaneous cleavage of C3 to C3b

14. Which of the following is NOT a property of the classical pathway C3 convertase?

A. Composed of proteolytic fragments of C4 and C2
B. Has protease activity specific for C3 to form C3b

C. Inhibited by decay acceleration factor (DAF)

D. Stabilized by C4 binding protein (C4bp)

E. Same substrate specificity as the alternative pathway C3 convertase

15. Which of the following statements about C3 is NOT correct?

A. C3 contains an internal thioester bond that participates in covalent linkage to cell surfaces.

B. C3 is the most abundant complement protein in the serum.

C. A proteolytic fragment of C3 is part of both the C3 and C5 convertases.

D. Activated C3 is a serine protease that cleaves C4.

E. C3 in the plasma is spontaneously cleaved into C3b.

Questions 16-20

For each of the functions described in questions 16-20, select the complement system protein (A-F) that best matches it.

A. C3b

B. iC3b

C. C3d

D. C5b

E. C5a

16. Generated by factor I–mediated proteolysis, this complement fragment binds to complement receptor 2 (CR2) on B cells and enhances B cell activation. ( )

17. Generated by factor I–mediated proteolysis, this opsonizing complement fragment binds to CR3 on phagocytes. ( )

18. Produced by C3 convertases, this opsonin promotes phagocytosis of microbes. ( )

19. This complement fragment is a chemoattractant for neutrophils. ( )

20. This complement fragment is a component of the membrane attack complex. ( )

21. A 17-year-old boy is taken to the emergency department because of severe abdominal and lumbar pain. Physical examination reveals splenomegaly, and laboratory studies reveal hemoglobinemia and thrombocytopenia. A urine sample is remarkable for gross hemoglobinuria. The patient reports a history of bloody urine on multiple occasions in the past. Flow cytometric analysis of the patient's red blood cells (RBC) will most likely indicate reduced or absent expression of which pair of molecules that is normally present on RBC membranes?

A. Complement receptor 1 (CR1) and CR2

B. C1 inhibitor (C1 INH) and membrane cofactor protein (MCP, CD46)

C. Decay accelerating factor (DAF, CD55) and CD59

D. C4 binding protein (C4bp) and factor H

E. Complement receptor 3(CR3) and complement receptor 4(CR4)

22. A 15-year-old girl is brought to a pediatric clinic with severe abdominal pain, nausea, and vomiting. She does not have a fever, peritoneal signs, or an elevated white blood cell count. The symptoms resolve in 48 hours. She has a history of multiple transient episodes of facial edema without pruritus. Laboratory examination is most likely to reveal which of the following abnormalities in this patient?

A. C4 deficiency

B. Reduced levels of C1 inhibitor (C1 INH)

C. Absence of C3

D. Presence of C3 nephritic factor

E. Deficiency of factor I

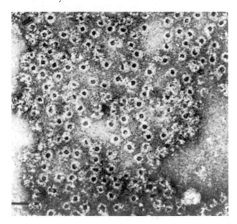

23. The figure above shows lesions in an erythrocyte membrane caused by complement activation. All of the following statements about these lesions are true EXCEPT:

A. The lesions are formed by polymerization of C9 in the membrane.

B. The lesions permit influx of water and ions into the cell.

C. The lesions are structurally similar to those caused by perforin derived from cytolytic T lymphocytes.

D. Failure to form these lesions in microbial membranes leads to serious infections by a wide variety of microbes.

E. Formation of these lesions is inhibited by CD59.

24. All of the following are accurate statements about neonatal immunity EXCEPT:

A. Transfer of maternal IgG across the placenta is mediated by an Fc receptor structurally similar to class I MHC.

B. IgA is absorbed in the gut from breast milk and re-secreted by the infant into the bronchial mucosa.

C. IgA secretion into breast milk involves transport through breast epithelial cells, and is dependent on the poly-Ig receptor.

D. Transport of IgG across the neonatal intestinal epithelium is mediated by an Fc receptor structurally similar to class I MHC.

E. Loss of maternal antibodies is partly responsible for increased frequency of infections in infants at about 6 months of age.

Answers

1. (C) The serum from infected animals contains diphtheria-specific antibodies. Some of these antibodies can bind to and neutralize diphtheria toxin, reducing symptoms of infection, whereas others interact with the bacilli themselves, inducing bacterial death by phagocytosis and complement fixation. Antibodies have a half-life of several weeks in the circulation, and therefore promote short-term disease resistance and immunity. No B cell or T cell would have been transferred with the serum, which is a cell-free fraction of blood. It is unlikely that there are inflammatory cytokines in the serum donor, because it had already recovered from infection, and cytokines alone would not impart resistance to infection. Serum transfer should not provide any complement components not already present in the recipient. Although it is possible that the foreign serum elicited an immune response to allelic differences in the transferred serum proteins, this should not impart specific resistance to diphtheria.
CMI5 8, 318; BI2 143-144

2. (B) The lumen of mucosal lined tissues, such as the intestinal and bronchial lumen, are protected by IgA, which is actively secreted at these sites. T cells do not normally migrate into these lumen and are usually involved in immune responses to organisms that breach the surface linings of these structures. The epithelial linings of mucosal tissues and the skin do contain lymphocytes that protect against invading pathogens. Both antibodies and T cells are involved in responses to infections within most other tissues.
CMI5 318-319

3. (E) During a humoral immune response, naive B cells differentiate into antibody-producing cells, and some of these migrate to the bone marrow, where they can reside and produce antibodies for years. Many of these cells are called plasma cells, based on their histologic appearance. Naive B cells do not secrete antibodies. Although activated B cells in spleen or lymph node germinal centers produce large amounts of antibody during an active humoral immune response, they do not account for most of the serum IgG normally. Intestinal B cells secrete large amount of IgA, which is transported into the lumen.
CMI5 319; BI2 137-138

4. (E) Fab fragments lack the Fc constant region and are therefore not recognized by immune effector cells or complement. In addition, they are monovalent and therefore are incapable of cross-linking antigen. However, Fab fragments are able to bind and neutralize toxins and inhibit the activity of pathogens by compromising the function of cell-surface proteins. These effects, called "neutralization" of pathogens, are the only mechanisms of antibody action that depend solely on antigen binding.
CMI5 321; BI2 146

5. (A) Antiviral vaccines work by generating long-lived antibody-producing cells and memory B cells that can secrete high affinity neutralizing antibodies, which prevent viral particles from entering host cells. The antibodies may prevent primary infection as well as prevent reinfection of cells after virions are released from an infected cell. Some vaccine-induced antiviral antibodies may opsonize viral particles and promote their phagocytosis. Antibody-dependent complement activation may also promote phagocytes or lysis of extracellular enveloped viruses. However, opsonization and lysis of virally infected host cells may not always be protective since these mechanisms could promote spread of viruses from cell to cell. Cytolytic T lymphocytes do not have Fc receptors, and they cannot directly kill virions but only kill host cells expressing viral proteins. Membrane proteins of enveloped virions are not linked to signal transduction pathways.
CMI5 321-322, 356; BI2 146-147

6. (B) Mononuclear phagocytes and neutrophils bind to complement protein C3b primarily through the CR1 receptor, which then stimulates phagocytosis of the complement-bound pathogen. Although phagocytes have Fc receptors of IgG isotypes, free IgG molecules without bound antigen do not bind tightly to these receptors to stimulate phagocytosis. There are no IgM Fc receptors and therefore antigen-IgM complexes are not phagocytosed readily, unless they have activated complement. Mannose-binding lectin (MBL) promotes complement activation on mannose-containing microbial surfaces and mannose can bind to phagocyte mannose receptors, but MBL alone does not bind to phagocyte receptors.
CMI5 335; BI2 151-152

7. (D) Lack of IgA causes decreased immune function in the respiratory and gastrointestinal mucosa, resulting in increased risk of sinus, lower respiratory tract, and gastrointestinal tract infections. In addition, IgA binds to and prevents immune responses to food constituents such as lactose and wheat gluten. Finally, the complete lack of IgA in some of these patients means that IgA itself is immunogenic. Because antibodies that are capable of interacting with IgA-like molecules are often being produced by B1 B cells, it is not uncommon to see a hypersensitivity reaction, including anaphylaxis, if these patients receive a blood transfusion. Normally, IgA is not on the skin, and there is no connection between IgA deficiency and inflammatory skin diseases.
CMI5 343; BI2 156-157

8. (C) There are no IgM-binding Fc receptors. Most Fc receptors transduce activating signals on binding Ig. The signals may be linked to many different functional responses. In phagocytes, these include generation of reactive oxygen intermediates that are toxic to ingested microbes. In mast cells,

eosinophils, and natural killer cells, Fc receptor signaling stimulates granule exocytosis. Signaling depends on recruitment of molecules to ITAM motifs that are in the cytoplasmic tails of the Ig binding polypeptide, or non–Ig-binding signaling chains that are associated with the Fc receptor. The FcγRIIB receptor on B cells transduces inhibitory signals via a tyrosine phosphatase-binding ITIM domain in its cytoplasmic tail.
CMI5 321-325; BI2 146-149

9. (D) FcεRI is a high affinity IgE receptor expressed on mast cells and basophils. Although serum IgE levels are relatively very low, FcεR1 receptors are fully occupied by IgE due to the high affinity of the receptor. Cross-linking of this receptor by allergen binding to the IgE leads to mast cell activation, which includes granule exocytosis with release of mediators such as histamine, as well as production of lipid mediators and cytokines.
CMI5 321-326; BI2 146-149

10. (A) FcγRI (CD64) is a high-affinity IgG1 and IgG3 receptor that mediates phagocytosis of opsonized organisms and delivers signals that enhance microbicidal activity of the phagocytes.
CMI5 321-326; BI2 146-149

11. (C) FcγRIIIA (CD16) is a low-affinity IgG receptor that targets natural killer (NK) cells to bind and destroy IgG-opsonized target cells and signals the NK cell to release cytotoxic granules.
CMI5 323-326; BI2 146-148

12. (B) FcγRIIB (CD32) is a low-affinity IgG receptor expressed on B lymphocytes. When antigen-IgG complexes simultaneously bind to membrane Ig and to FcγRIIB, phosphatases activated by FcγRIIB block activating signals from the B cell antigen receptor complex.
CMI5 213, 321-326; BI2 146-149

13. (E) The alternative pathway is initiated when C3b, generated by spontaneous cleavage of C3 in the fluid phase, covalently binds to a cell surface. C1q is required for initiation of the classical pathway. It does not bind directly to cell surfaces but rather to the constant regions of two Ig molecules, which may be bound to cell surface antigens. Mannose-binding lectin (MBL) binds to mannose on microbial surfaces to initiate the lectin pathway. Factor D is a constitutively active serum protease that cleaves factor B after it binds C3b in the alternative pathway. Factor I is a protease that cleaves C3b and C4b and regulates both alternative and classical pathways. CR1 on phagocytes binds C3b-opsonized microbes.
CMI5 326-333; BI2 149-152

14. (D) The classical pathway C3 convertase C4b2a cleaves C3 to generate C3b and C3a. The alternative pathway C3 convertase C3bBb has the same activity. C3 convertases are highly regulated, preventing complement activation on autologous cell surfaces. The classical pathway C3 convertase is not stabilized but is inhibited by C4bp, which competi-

tively binds C4b, displacing C2 from the complex. C4bp also acts as a cofactor for the proteolytic cleavage of C4b by factor I. DAF and complement receptor 1 (CR1) and membrane cofactor proteins (MCP) also inhibit classical pathway C3 convertase formation. Similar mechanisms exist to block alternative pathway C3 convertase formation.
CMI5 326-338; BI2 149-155

15. (D) C3, the most abundant complement protein in plasma, is not a protease. The proteolytic fragment of C3, called C3b, is a component of both classical and alternative pathways C3 convertase, which are proteolytic enzymes. An internal thioester bond in C3 becomes metastable when C3 is proteolytically cleaved and contributes to covalent linkage of C3b to cell surfaces. Spontaneous cleavage of C3 in the plasma, called C3 tickover, generates C3b, which initiates the alternative pathway.
CMI5 326-333; BI2 149-152

16. (C) C3d is covalently bound to cell surface and is produced by sequential factor I–mediated proteolytic processing of C3. It binds to CR2 on B cells simultaneously with antigen binding to membrane Ig. CR2 is part of a coreceptor complex, which also includes CD19 and CD21. CD19 transduces signals that synergize with the B cell receptor complex signals to activate the B cell.
CMI5 194-195, 340-342; BI2 128-129, 152

17. (B) iC3b is covalently bound to cell surfaces and is produced by sequential factor I-mediated proteolytic processing of C3. iC3b binds to CR3 and CR4, which are integrins expressed by phagocytes.
CMI5 335, 338-339

18. (A) C3b is the larger fragment of C3 convertase-mediated cleavage of C3, which becomes covalently bound to cell surfaces and is recognized by complement receptor 1 (CR1) on phagocytes.
CMI5 327-331, 335, 338-339; BI2 149-153, 154

19. (E) C5a is a small soluble fragment generated by C5 convertase-mediated cleavage of C5. C5a binds to a G protein–coupled serpentine receptor on neutrophils and stimulates chemokinesis. The C5a receptor is also expressed on other cell types, and C5a has several proinflammatory functions, including mast cell and endothelial cell activation. C3a and C4a have similar biologic activities as C5a, but they are not as potent. Together, C5a, C4a, and C3a are called anaphylatoxins.
CMI5 339-340; BI2 152

20. (D) C5b is the larger fragment of C5 generated by C5 convertase. It is the initial component in the formation of the membrane attack complex, which includes C5, C6, C7, C8, and several C9s.
CMI5 333, 340; BI2 151-153

21. (C) The patient's history is consistent with a diagnosis of paroxysmal nocturnal hemoglobinuria (PNH; Marchiafava-Micheli syndrome), which is

due to a genetic defect in the synthesis of glycosyl-phosphatidyl-inositol (GPI) anchors for membrane proteins. Two important regulatory proteins of the complement system, DAF (CD55) and CD59, are expressed as GPI-linked membrane proteins, and therefore their expression is reduced in PNH. DAF normally promotes dissociation of C3 convertase that spontaneously forms on blood cells at a low level. CD59 prevents assembly of poly-C9 and MAC-mediated lysis of blood cells. Without sufficient expression of CD55 and CD59, red blood cells and platelets are susceptible to complement-mediated membrane damage, causing thrombosis and hemolysis. CR1 and CR2 deficiencies have not been reported. C1 INH deficiency causes hereditary angioneurotic edema. C4bp and factor H are not membrane proteins, but rather are soluble plasma proteins that block classical and alternative C3 convertase formation, respectively. CR3 and CR4 are integrins that function as adhesion molecules on leukocytes as well as on complement receptors. Leukocyte adhesion deficiency I, caused by mutations in the gene encoding the CD18 β chain of these integrins, manifests as an immunodeficiency disease.
CMI5 338

22. **(B)** This patient's presentation and history are consistent with a diagnosis of hereditary angioneurotic edema, which is due to genetic or acquired deficiencies in C1 inhibitor (C1 INH). C1 INH normally blocks excessive C1 activation and proteolysis of C2 and C4. Reduced levels of C1 INH cause excessive proteolysis and reduced levels of C4 and C2, as well as generation of vasoactive peptides derived from C4 and C2. These peptides cause edema. Gastrointestinal symptoms are due to bowel wall edema. Laryngeal edema can be life threatening. C4 deficiency due to gene mutations, which constitutes the most common complement system deficiency, predisposes to systemic lupus erythematosus (SLE) or SLE-like illness. Deficiency of C3 is associated with severe, recurrent bacterial infections at an early age and immune complex glomerulonephritis. C3 nephritic factor is an autoantibody against the alternative pathway C3 convertase. Patients with this antibody present with an illness similar to C3 deficiency. Factor I deficiency is associated with a failure to regulate C3 convertase, so that C3 becomes depleted and patients suffer recurrent infections and glomerulonephritis.
CMI5 336-337, 341-342; BI2 155

23. **(D)** The figure shows an electron micrograph of a red blood cell membrane with multiple pores formed by the membrane attack complex (MAC) of complement. These pores are 100 Å in diameter and, once formed, cause osmotic lysis of cells. The pores are formed by C5, C6, C7, C8, and poly-C9. C9 is structurally homologous to perforin found in natural killer cells and cytolytic T lymphocyte granules, which also forms pores in target cell membranes. MAC formation is negatively regulated by the cell membrane protein CD59. Deficiencies in the components of the MAC are associated with susceptibility only to infection by *Neisseria* species (meningococcal and gonococcal).
CMI5 334, 341

24. **(B)** IgA is secreted into breast milk via poly-Ig receptor-mediated transcellular transport, but it is not reabsorbed in the infant's gut. Rather, IgA remains in the lumen of the alimentary canal as a defense against intestinal microbes. IgG from breast milk *is* reabsorbed into the circulation from the gut lumen by the class I MHC-like neonatal Fc receptor (FcRN). This same receptor also mediates transplacental transport of IgG. Passive immunity mediated by maternal antibodies wanes with time; at about 6 months, infants have a nadir of circulating antibodies because maternal antibodies are depleted and antibodies produced by the infant have not reached maximal levels. This nadir corresponds to a period of increased susceptibility to infections, which is even more exaggerated in children with immunodeficiency diseases.
CMI5 342-343

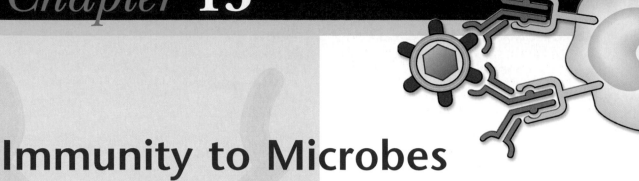

Chapter 15

Immunity to Microbes

Cellular and Molecular Immunology, 5/E: Chapter 15—Immunity to Microbes

1. A common strategy by which microbes survive their host's immune responses involves changing the structures of the molecules they produce so that they are no longer recognized by the host's immune system. This strategy, called antigenic variation, is most likely to allow evasion of which type of immune recognition?

   A. Toll-like receptor–dependent recognition of microbes by cells of the innate immune system
   B. Mannose receptor–dependent recognition of microbes by cells of the innate immune system
   C. Antibody recognition of microbial cell surface molecules
   D. Natural killer cell inhibitory receptor recognition of class I major histocompatibility complex (MHC) molecules on infected cells
   E. T cell receptor recognition of microbial cell wall lipid antigens

2. Different types of immune responses may be required to protect against different types of pathogenic microbes. For example, antibody responses and complement activation are effective in combatting extracellular bacterial infections but not intracellular bacterial infections. Which of the following species is an intracellular bacterium and is therefore not susceptible to antibody-mediated immune mechanisms?

   A. *Staphylococcus aureus*
   B. *Streptococcus pneumoniae*
   C. *Escherichia coli*
   D. *Clostridium tetani*
   E. *Legionella pneumophila*

3. Antibodies can protect against the pathogenic effects of bacterial infections by neutralizing the toxins that the bacteria produce. Vaccines composed of inactivated forms of bacterial toxins, called

toxoids, can induce the formation of protective antibodies against bacterial toxins. Which of the following pairs of bacterial species produce toxins for which there is effective vaccine prophylaxis?

A. *Staphylococcus aureus* and *Streptococcus pneumoniae*
B. *Clostridium tetani* and *Corynebacterium diphtheriae*
C. *Escherichia coli* and *Mycobacterium tuberculosis*
D. *Vibrio cholerae* and *Listeria monocytogenes*
E. *Klebsiella pneumoniae* and *Pseudomonas aeruginosa*

4. A 22-year-old woman is brought to the emergency department 2 weeks postpartum with fever, hypotension, and a widespread rash. After a thorough physical examination and laboratory tests, a diagnosis of toxic shock syndrome (TSS) is made. This disease is caused by staphylococcal infection and production of a bacterial superantigen called toxic shock syndrome toxin-1 (TSST-1). Which of the following descriptions accurately reflects the pathophysiology of TSS?

A. TSST-1 is processed into peptides and presented by the class II MHC pathway to helper T cells, resulting in a cell-mediated response to infected cells, inflammation, and tissue damage.
B. TSST-1 is "presented" by class II MHC expressing cells to T cells expressing a particular TCR Vβ gene segment, resulting in deletion of many T cells, immunodeficiency, and secondary infection, leading to septic shock.
C. TSST-1 acts as a potent growth factor for staphylococcal organisms, and the infection overwhelms the patient's immune system.
D. Antibodies to TSST-1 form immune complexes with the toxin, and these deposit in blood vessel walls, causing widespread vasculitis and tissue damage.
E. TSST-1 is "presented" by class II MHC expressing cells to T cells expressing a particular TCR Vβ gene segment, resulting in polyclonal activation of a many T cells and the release of large amounts of inflammatory cytokines.

5. Which of the following is NOT part of the innate immune response to extracellular bacteria?

A. Complement activation by lipopolysaccharide
B. Complement activation by mannose
C. Activation of phagocytes by Toll-like receptors
D. Natural killer cell activation
E. Inflammation

6. All of the following are known mechanisms by which extracellular bacteria evade the immune system EXCEPT:

A. Capsules that prevent phagocytosis
B. Inhibition of class I MHC expression
C. Genetic variation of surface antigens
D. Inhibition of complement activation
E. Scavenging of reactive oxygen intermediates

7. A particular species of microbe evades the immune system by several mechanisms, including inhibiting phagosome fusion with lysosomes, degrading reac-

tive nitrogen intermediates generated by nitric oxide synthetase, and inhibition of class II MHC expression. Which of the following is most likely to be this species of microorganism?

A. *Streptococcus pyogenes*
B. *Candida albicans*
C. *Clostridium tetani*
D. Poliovirus
E. *Mycobacterium tuberculosis*

8. All of the following are associated with immune responses to intracellular bacteria EXCEPT:

A. Interferon-γ production by bacterial-antigen-specific CD4+ T cells
B. Opsonization of infected cells by complement
C. Interleukin-12 production by macrophages
D. Granuloma formation
E. Cytotoxic T lymphocyte killing of infected macrophages

9. An emergency splenectomy was performed on a 5-year-girl because of splenic rupture due to an automobile accident. She recovered from surgery without complications, but over the course of the next year she has had three serious infections requiring hospitalization and intravenous antibiotic treatment. Which of the following microbial organisms is the most likely species to cause infections in this girl?

A. *Listeria monocytogenes*
B. *Mycobacterium tuberculosis*
C. *Vibrio cholerae*
D. *Legionella monocytogenes*
E. *Streptococcus pneumoniae*

10. A 23-year-old man who recently emigrated to the United States from Brazil visited a clinic because he noticed several macular, erythematous skin lesions on his face and trunk. The lesions were associated with a loss of sensation and first appeared 1 year ago and since that time have been continually enlarging. A lepromin skin test in which a suspension of killed *Mycobacterium leprae* was injected into uninvolved skin of the patient was performed, and the results were negative. A skin biopsy was per-

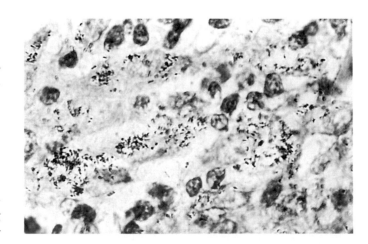

formed, and an acid-fast stain of the tissue specimen is shown at the bottom of the previous page. No granulomas were seen on the histologic sections. Which of the following statements about this patient's disease is most likely correct?

A. The patient has developed a strong cell-mediated immune response to *Mycobacterium leprae.*

B. T cells that have responded to *Mycobacterium leprae* antigens in this patient have a T_H1 phenotype.

C. Family members of this patient develop resistance and are less susceptible to infection by *Mycobacterium leprae* than unrelated persons with similar exposure.

D. Killing of *Mycobacterium leprae* organisms within macrophages in this patient is impaired.

E. The spread of the infection in this patient reflects a failure to mount an effective antibody response to *Mycobacterium leprae.*

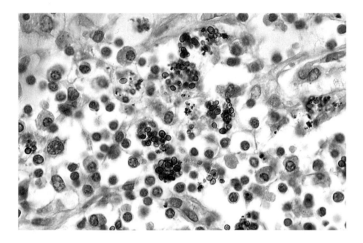

11. A 38-year-old man visited his primary care physician with fever and dyspnea. Physical examination revealed multiple palpably enlarged lymph nodes. A chest radiograph showed diffuse interstitial infiltrates and mediastinal adenopathy. A lymph node biopsy was performed. The figure above shows a histologic section of the node. Which of the following statements does NOT accurately describe this patient's infectious disease?

A. The infection has spread from the lungs to lymph nodes and may be disseminated throughout the body.

B. This disease is more likely to occur in patients with impaired $CD4^+$ T cell–mediated immunity.

C. The disease is a highly prevalent endemic mycosis found in the United States.

D. To eradicate the infection, the patient must be administered antifungal drug treatment.

E. The humoral immune response against the infectious organism provides protection against infection and dissemination.

Questions 12-15

For each of the descriptions of immune mechanisms in questions 12-15, select the immune mechanism (A-D) that correctly matches it.

A. Type I interferons (IFN-α, IFN-β)
B. $CD8^+$ cytolytic T lymphocyte
C. Antibody
D. Natural killer cell

12. Innate immunity mechanism for preventing viral infection ( )

13. Adaptive immunity mechanism for eradicating established viral infection ( )

14. Innate immunity mechanism for eradicating established viral infection ( )

15. Adaptive immunity mechanism for preventing a viral infection ( )

16. An 87-year-old man sees his doctor in March with high fever, aches and pains, and a nonproductive cough. He says that he did not get the flu vaccine this year, because he has gotten it for the past 10 years and thinks that he should be immune by now. What "immune-evasion" strategy does influenza use that requires the production and use of a new influenza vaccine each year?

A. Inhibition of antigen processing
B. Antigenic variation
C. Production of immunosuppressive cytokine
D. Infection and destruction of immune cells
E. Production of cytokine receptor homologues

17. T_H2 cells induce the production of which Ig isotype and the activation of which cell type, thereby providing defense against helminths?

A. IgA and regulatory T cells
B. IgE and natural killer cells
C. IgG and $CD8^+$ T cells
D. IgE and eosinophils
E. IgM and T_H1 T cells

18. It is postulated that an effective antimalarial vaccine must consist of combined immunogenic epitopes specific for more than one of the stages of the complex life cycle of the *Plasmodium* organism. Which stage must be targeted to prevent infection of liver cells?

A. Sporozoites
B. Merozoites
C. Trophozoites
D. Schizonts
E. Circumsporozoite

Questions 19-22

Match the description of a vaccine in questions 19-22 with the correct type of vaccine (A-G).

A. Live attenuated or killed bacteria
B. Live attenuated oral virus
C. Synthetic viral subunit vaccines
D. Conjugate vaccines
E. Recombinant viral vectors
F. DNA vaccines
G. Purified subunit vaccines

19. Good induction of mucosal immunity but risk of developing a viral disease, especially in immuno-compromised hosts (   )

20. Induction of a T cell–dependent antibody response to polysaccharides, such as *Haemophilus influenzae B* and pneumococcal capsular polysaccharides (   )

21. Composed of viral proteins synthesized from recombinant viral genes (   )

22. Composed of antigens purified from microbes or inactivated toxins, such as the tetanus toxoid vaccine (   )

23. Composed of a recombinant nonpathogenic virus carrying genes of a pathogenic virus, such as HIV (   )

Answers

1. (C) Antigenic variation allows microbes to evade adaptive immune recognition, usually by antibodies, but also by T cells. Antigenic variation usually involves mutations or recombination events in microbial genes encoding cell surface proteins or encoding enzymes involved in synthesis of cell surface sugars. The result changes microbial surface antigens. This is an effective strategy, because many of the microbial antigenic structures that the adaptive immune system recognizes, are not essential for survival or virulence of the microbe. In contrast, most structures recognized by receptors of the innate immune system (e.g., Toll-like receptor and scavenger receptor ligands) are essential for microbial survival and, as such, cannot undergo antigenic variation. Although some viruses may block class I major histocompatibility complex (MHC) expression by infected cells, this renders the cells more susceptible to natural killer cell–mediated killing and is not antigenic variation by the virus. Only a small subset of T cells recognizes lipid antigens, usually in association with CD1 molecules. There is no evidence for antigenic variation of the lipid antigens recognized by these T cells.
CMI5 346; BI2 157-158

2. (E) *Legionella pneumophila,* the causative agent of legionnaire's disease, is a gram-negative intracellular bacterium. Cell-mediated immunity is required for eradication of infection by this organism. The other bacteria listed are extracellular organisms.
CMI5 346-347

3. (B) *Clostridium tetani* produces tetanus toxin, which blocks impulse transmission across neuromuscular junctions, causing paralysis. *Corynebacterium diphtheriae* produces diphtheria toxin, which inhibits protein synthesis, causing death of respiratory mucosal epithelial cells. Combined vaccines containing both tetanus and diphtheria toxoids are routinely administered to children and provide very effective protection, mediated by antibodies.
CMI5 346-347

4. (E) Toxic shock syndrome toxin-1 (TSST-1), like other superantigens, does not need to be processed into peptides to activate T cells but instead binds to nonpolymorphic parts of class II MHC on antigen-presenting cells and simultaneously binds to conserved regions of the Vβ domain of T cell receptors encoded by particular families of Vβ genes. This results in polyclonal T cell activation, because many clones of T cells use the same Vβ gene family. The cytokines produced by the activated T cells, including tumor necrosis factor, and interferon-γ, cause widespread tissue damage. Many of the T cells that are activated by superantigens may be deleted, leading to subsequent gaps in the T cell repertoire, but this is not the cause of acute TSS.
CMI5 350; BI2 89

5. (D) Although natural killer cells are part of the innate immune system, they target infected cells, not extracellular organisms. Innate immune responses to extracellular bacteria include both the alternative complement pathway (activated by peptidoglycan and lipopolysaccharide) and the lectin pathway (activated by mannose-binding lectin). In addition, activation of phagocytes by Toll-like receptors and inflammation are key components of the innate immune response to extracellular bacteria.
CMI5 346-349

6. (B) Class I MHC restricted T cells generally are not involved in immune responses to extracellular bacteria, because these microbes rarely survive within phagocytes and do not provide antigens to the class I MHC pathway of antigen presentation. Therefore, inhibition of class I MHC expression would not be an effective evasion mechanism, although it is effective for viruses. Encapsulated bacteria, such as pneumococci, cannot be readily phagocytosed without opsonization. Antigenic variation is used by *Neisseria* species, *Escherichia coli*, and *Salmonella typhimurium* to avoid recognition by antibodies. Many bacteria produce inhibitors of complement activation. Catalase-producing staphylococci scavenge reactive oxygen species produced by activated phagocytes.
CMI5 349

7. (E) The mechanisms listed in the question would provide protection for an intracellular organism that lives within phagosomes of macrophages, such as *Mycobacterium tuberculosis.* Fusion of phagosomes with lysosomes exposes internalized microbes to a toxic environment of low pH, photolytic enzymes, and reactive oxygen intermediates. *Streptococcus pyogenes* and *Clostridium tetani* are extracellular bacteria that do survive inside phagocytes. *Candida albicans* is a fungus that also lives and grows outside of cells. Poliovirus replicates in the nucleus and cytoplasm of cells and does not reside within phagosomes.
CMI5 346-351

8. (B) Complement opsonizes extracellular microbes, not infected cells. Fragments of the complement

C3 protein that remain covalently attached to microbial surfaces, including C3b and iC3b, mediate phagocytosis of the microbes by complement receptor expressing phagocytes. Intracellular bacteria often stimulate a T_H1 response in which $CD4^+$ T cells secrete interferon (IFN)-γ. Interleukin-12 secretion by dendritic cells and infected macrophages promotes T_H1 differentiation and IFN-γ production. If the microbes successfully resist killing within phagosomes, chronic antigen stimulation leads to granuloma formation. Often, intracellular bacterial antigens will leave the phagosome and enter the cytoplasm, where they will enter the class I MHC antigen presentation pathway and stimulate a $CD8^+$ cytolytic T lymphocyte response.
CMI5 351-354

9. (E) Asplenic patients are at increased risk for serious, often disseminated infections due to polysaccharide encapsulated bacteria including *Streptococcus pneumoniae*, *Haemophilus influenzae*, and *Neisseria meningitides*. These infections are most common in children, who develop protective levels of antibodies to bacterial polysaccharides between the ages of 2 and 5 years. The spleen contributes to protection against these organisms by producing IgM and T cell–independent IgG antibodies to the bacterial polysaccharides and by phagocytosis of these organisms. *Listeria monocytogenes*, *Mycobacterium tuberculosis*, and *Legionella monocytogenes* are intracellular bacteria, and cell-mediated immunity is required for their eradication. *Vibrio cholerae* is a gram-negative extracellular intestinal bacterial pathogen. Immunity against *Vibrio cholerae* is largely mediated by mucosal IgA secretion, which is not impaired by splenectomy.
CMI5 346-348, 464

10. (D) This patient has lepromatous leprosy, caused by the intracellular bacterium *Mycobacterium leprae*. Leprosy presents as a spectrum of diseases, reflecting different immune responses to the organism. Lepromatous disease, one end of this spectrum, develops when patients fail to mount effective cell-mediated immune responses to the organism, and the disease becomes widely disseminated. There is some evidence to suggest that these patients develop T_H2 responses, in which T cells specific for the bacterial antigens produce interleukin (IL)-4 and IL-10. Macrophages phagocytose the bacteria, but in the absence of a T_H1 response they are unable to kill the organisms. The image shows multiple viable "acid-fast" bacteria within macrophages. At the other end of the spectrum is tuberculoid leprosy, in which patients mount strong T_H1 responses. Although infection is better contained in this form of the disease, persistence of antigen leads to granulomas formation and skin and nerve damage. Susceptibility to *Mycobacterium leprae* infection appears to be genetically determined, and therefore relatives of an infected individual generally are more at risk of infection than unrelated individuals with comparable exposure. Antibodies

play little role in protection against intracellular bacteria.
CMI5 352-355

11. (E) This patient has disseminated histoplasmosis. The figure shows yeast forms within phagocytes in the lymph node tissue. The fungal organism *Histoplasma capsulatum* is a facultative intracellular parasite of macrophages and is one of the most common causes of mycotic disease. Eradication of this fungus requires a T_H1 CD4 T cell response. Antibodies are not effective in protecting against *Histoplasma capsulatum*, because they do not have access to intracellular organisms. Most infections are self limited, but in the absence of adequate T cell–mediated immunity, such as in AIDS, the infection spreads and is lethal without drug therapy.
CMI5 355

12. (A) One of the key innate immunity responses that can prevent viral infection is the production of type I interferons (IFNs), which are secreted by various cell types in response to double-stranded RNA interacting with Toll-like receptors. Type I IFNs induce an antiviral state in cells, which makes them resistant to host viral replication.
CMI5 355-356

13. (B) Once viruses have infected cells, they produce cytoplasmic proteins that are processed and presented by the class I MHC pathway. $CD8^+$ cytotoxic T lymphocytes recognize viral peptide-class I MHC complexes on the surface of infected cells and kill these cells. The killing mechanism leads to apoptosis, which ensures degradation of viral DNA as well as host cell DNA.
CMI5 356-357

14. (D) Natural killer (NK) cells are innate immunity effector cells that can kill infected cells by mechanisms similar to cytotoxic T lymphocytes (CTLs). However, they are activated by different receptors than are CTLs, and they are inhibited by receptors that bind class I MHC on other cells. Viruses have the ability to evade detection by CTLs by inhibiting class I MHC expression on their host cell surfaces. When this occurs, NK cells may provide a backup defense mechanism, since they are activated by host cells that lack normal class I MHC expression.
CMI5 355-357

15. (C) Antibodies can neutralize viruses before they infect cells. Immunity imparted by many antiviral vaccines is due to antibodies.
CMI5 321, 356-357

16. (B) The influenza virus, an RNA virus in the orthomyxovirus family, uses antigenic variation to change its surface antigens and thus evade the memory cells generated during immune responses that were able to eradicate the influenza strain from the previous years. Each year a new vaccine is created that is designed to cover the most prevalent

strains for that year, based on early sentinel cases that same year.
CMI5 357

17. (D) The signature cytokines of a T_H2 cell are interleukin (IL)-4 and IL-5. IL-4 stimulates B cell class switching to IgE. IL-5 stimulates the production and activation of eosinophils. Eosinophils kill helminths by antibody-dependent cellular cytotoxicity, in which IgE specific for helminthic antigens binds to FcεR receptors on eosinophils and to the antigens on the worms. Cross-linking of the FcεR receptors causes granule exocytosis. The contents of eosinophils granule, such as major basic protein, are toxic to the worms.
CMI5 359-360

18. (A) *Plasmodium* species enter the bloodstream as sporozoites by mosquito bite and are transported to the liver, where they infect liver cells. Infected liver cells release merozoites into the blood, which infect erythrocytes. In the red blood cell (RBC), the merozoites develop into trophozoites and schizonts, and eventually the RBC releases more merozoites that can infect other RBCs. Therefore, for a vaccine to target the initial infection of liver cells, it must contain immunogenic epitopes specific for antigens expressed in the sporozoites stage.
CMI5 361

19. (B) Live attenuated viral vaccines infect recipient cells, and viral proteins are processed and presented to T cells. This method of vaccination induces good T cell–dependent antibody responses. Attenuation makes risk of serious disease from the vaccine very low. Live attenuated oral poliovirus vaccines, which induced good IgA responses in the gastrointestinal tract, are no longer used routinely in the United States because of low but definable risk of vaccine-associated cases of paralytic polio.
CMI5 363

20. (D) Conjugate vaccines are composed of bacterial capsular polysaccharides covalently coupled to proteins. This hapten-carrier arrangement promotes T cell–dependent responses to the polysaccharides, which is required for protective IgG memory responses. Polysaccharides alone do not activate T cells and therefore do not induce isotype switching or memory cell generation.
CMI5 363

21. (C) Synthetic subunit viral vaccines are composed of viral proteins synthesized from recombinant genes. The hepatitis B virus vaccine, now in widespread use, was the first synthetic viral subunit vaccine to be developed and contains the recombinant hepatitis B surface antigen (HBsAg).
CMI5 363

22. (G) The most commonly used purified subunit vaccines are the diphtheria and tetanus toxoid vaccines, which induce protective antibody responses against toxins produced by the bacteria.
CMI5 363

23. (E) Genes encoding immunodominant epitopes of a pathogenic virus can be cloned into the genome of nonpathogenic viruses, and the resulting recombinant virus can be used as a vaccine against the pathogenic virus. This is one of the approaches under development for HIV (human immunodeficiency virus) vectors, and trials of canarypox virus containing SIV (simian immunodeficiency virus) genes have been used in primates with some success.
CMI5 363

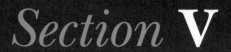

Section V

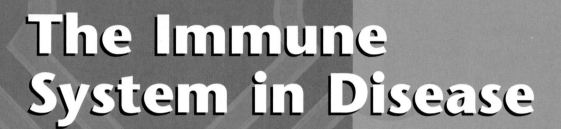

The Immune System in Disease

Chapter 16

Transplantation Immunology

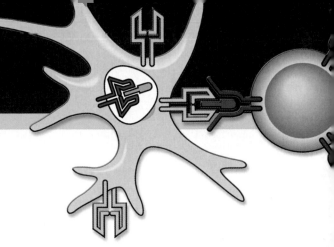

Cellular and Molecular Immunology, 5/E: Chapter 16—Transplantation Immunology

Basic Immunology, 2/E: Chapter 10—Immune Responses Against Tumors and Transplants

1. Second-set rejection may be an example of each of the following phenomena EXCEPT:

   A. Self versus non-self discrimination of the adaptive immune system
   B. B cell memory
   C. T cell memory
   D. Specificity of the adaptive immune system
   E. Self versus non-self discrimination of the innate immune system

2. A 57-year-old woman with a long-standing history of diabetes mellitus is in persistent renal failure. She has required dialysis for the past 3 years, and her clinical situation continues to deteriorate. A kidney transplant is performed from a donor who is her twin brother. Which of the following would describe the graft?

   A. Allogeneic transplant
   B. Autologous transplant
   C. Syngeneic transplant
   D. Xenogeneic transplant
   E. Congenic transplant

3. Experiments with inbred strains of mice have provided much of our knowledge of transplantation biology. All mice of one inbred strain are genetically identical to one another and homozygous for all genes. Assume that strains A and B are inbred strains that differ from each other at all MHC gene loci but at no other loci. A mating of a strain A mouse with a strain B mouse (AxB) yields AxB F1 progeny. Which of the following skin grafts would NOT be rejected?

A. AxB F_1 donor → A recipient
B. AxB F_1 donor → B recipient
C. A donor → AxB F_1 recipient
D. B donor → A recipient
E. A donor → B recipient

4. All of the following statements regarding the direct presentation of alloantigens during transplant rejection are true EXCEPT:

   A. Processing of allogenic MHC molecules is not required for T cell recognition.
   B. A high percentage (~2%) of a graft recipient's T cells are capable of directly recognizing the MHC molecules encoded by a single non-self MHC allele.
   C. All the different MHC molecules expressed on a graft cell can potentially be directly recognized by recipient T cells, even if they carry different peptides in the peptide binding grooves.
   D. Peptide bound to the directly presented foreign MHC molecule is not involved in TCR recognition.
   E. Memory T cells can be involved in direct recognition of allo-MHC molecules, even if the recipient has never been exposed to the donor MHC molecules before.

5. Which of the following observations is evidence for the indirect presentation of allogeneic MHC molecules?

   A. Allograft rejection often takes months to develop after transplantation.
   B. Antigen-presenting cells (APCs) from individual A can stimulate T cells from genetically different individual B, even if antigen processing by the APCs is inhibited.
   C. Previous grafting of tissue from a particular donor will make the recipient more susceptible to rejection of a new graft of a different tissue type taken from the same donor.
   D. Allogeneic skin grafts into class II MHC-deficient recipients can induce recipient CD4$^+$ T cell responses to the donor class II alloantigens.
   E. Human CD4$^+$ T cells from allograft recipients can be activated by peptides derived from graft MHC molecules plus APCs from the recipient.

6. The mixed leukocyte reaction (MLR) is an in vitro culture assay to test for alloreactivity between leukocytes of two individuals. In some variations of this test, cells may be "inactivated" (i.e., irradiated or treated with drugs to block their proliferation). Which of the following best describes the set up of a one-way primary MLR?

   A. Inactivated mononuclear leukocytes from one individual are cultured with inactivated mononuclear leukocytes from a second individual.
   B. Active mononuclear leukocytes from one individual are cultured with active mononuclear leukocytes from a second individual.
   C. Active mononuclear leukocytes from one individual are cultured with inactivated mononuclear leukocytes from a second individual.
   D. Inactivated mononuclear leukocytes from one individual are cultured with inactivated T cells from a second individual.
   E. Active B cells from one individual are cultured with inactivated T cells from a second individual.

7. Blood mononuclear cells are taken from donor A, irradiated so they cannot proliferate, and cultured with blood mononuclear cells from an unrelated donor B. Which of the following is most likely to occur?

   A. Donor B CD4$^+$ T cells will proliferate, but donor B CD8$^+$ T cells will not.
   B. Donor B CD8$^+$ T cells will proliferate and release cytokines, but donor B CD4$^+$ T cells will not.
   C. Donor B CD8$^+$ T cells taken from the culture at 7 days will be able to specifically kill cells from a third unrelated donor.
   D. Donor A CD8$^+$ T cells taken from the culture at 7 days will be able to specifically kill cells from donor B.
   E. Donor B CD4$^+$ T cells taken from the culture at 7 days will secrete effector cytokines, such as interferon-γ, when cultured again with donor A mononuclear cells.

8. Which of the following is NOT considered a likely mechanism of protection for the fetus against the maternal immune system?

   A. Trophoblast cells do not express paternal class II MHC molecules.
   B. Uterine decidua is an immunologically privileged site.
   C. Decidual tryptophan levels are maintained above the levels that allow T cell activation.
   D. HLA-G may protect trophoblast cells from maternal natural killer cell–mediated lysis.
   E. High levels of complement inhibitor Crry prevent complement-mediated damage to the trophoblast.

9. A 35-year-old woman with end-stage renal disease received a kidney transplant from a living related donor, and, within minutes of resumption of blood flow, the kidney turned blue and failed to produce urine. Histopathologic examination of a biopsy specimen of the failed graft revealed platelet and thrombin thrombi in the glomerular capillaries, thrombosis in arteries, and ischemic necrosis (tissue death due to lack of blood supply) of tubules. Which of the following statements about this type of graft failure is accurate?

A. There was acute rejection, mediated by cytolytic T lymphocytes, with damage to graft endothelial cells.

B. The patient had pre-formed antibodies specific for alloantigens on graft endothelial cells.

C. The connections between the recipient and graft blood vessels were defective.

D. There was acute rejection, owing to a humoral immune response to alloantigens expressed on the graft endothelial cells.

E. There is no reliable test that can be performed to indicate the risk of this type of rejection.

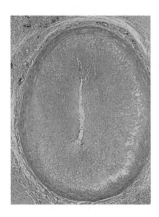

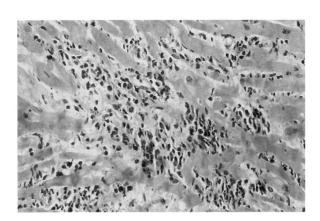

10. A 42-year-old man with a history of viral myocarditis and dilated cardiomyopathy received a heart transplant. He recovered from surgery and was doing well. Biopsy specimens of the myocardium at 1, 3, 6, and 10 weeks showed no pathologic changes. A biopsy specimen taken 14 weeks after transplantation is shown in the figure above. The pathologic diagnosis was rejection. Which of the following statements about this type of rejection is most likely true?

A. Immunosuppressive dugs, such as cyclosporine, are effective in preventing or treating this type of rejection.

B. The inflammatory infiltrate in the myocardium is a reaction to dying cardiac muscle cells, which have lost their blood supply due to blood vessel damage.

C. The patient's T cells have likely responded to minor histocompatibility antigens and not allogenic MHC antigens, because the donor was chosen to match the recipient's MHC.

D. The inflammatory infiltrate in the heart is composed largely of CD4$^+$ T cells, and not CD8$^+$ T cells, because heart transplants must be matched for class II MHC compatibility.

E. Given the long delay between transplantation and rejection, this type of rejection is called chronic rejection.

11. Six years after cardiac allograft transplantation, the patient described in Question 10 began experiencing shortness of breath. Imaging studies revealed left ventricular dilation. An endomyocardial biopsy specimen showed areas of ischemic necrosis. He then developed congestive heart failure, which was refractory to treatment, and died. A section of a coronary artery from the allograft, sampled at autopsy, is shown in the figure above. Which of the following statements most accurately describes the mechanism underlying graft failure in this patient at this time?

A. The immunosuppressive drugs that the patient took raised serum cholesterol levels, resulting in coronary artery atherosclerosis and inadequate blood supply to the myocardium.

B. The immunosuppressive drugs that the patient took caused damage to kidney tubules, resulting in renal failure and secondary strain on the heart due to excess fluid retention.

C. The rejection process, originally observed in the biopsy specimen taken 14 weeks after transplantation, was not adequately treated and enough myocardial fibers were destroyed to compromise cardiac function.

D. Chronic rejection resulted in smooth muscle cell proliferation in the intima of the coronary arteries, resulting in inadequate blood supply to the myocardium.

E. Tolerance to alloantigen in the heart was broken 6 years after the transplantation, and acute rejection ensued, damaging the myocardium.

Questions 12-16

For each of the descriptions in questions 12-16, choose the blood group antigen (A-E) that best matches it.

A. A
B. B
C. O
D. RhD
E. Lewis

12. Formed by a glycosyltransferase enzyme that adds a terminal *N*-acetylgalactosamine residue to the H antigen (   )

13. Common glycan that is fucosylated to form the H antigen ( )

14. Formation requires fucosyltransferase activity ( )

15. Nonglycosylated red cell membrane protein missing or mutated in 15% of humans ( )

16. Formed by a glycosyltransferase enzyme that adds a terminal galactose residue to the H antigen ( )

17. A 28-year-old trauma patient with blood type O received a blood transfusion in the emergency department and within 30 minutes developed shaking chills and flank pain, and his urine collected from a Foley catheter was brown. The physician discovered that type B blood was used for the transfusion owing to a clerical error. Which of the following statements about the transfusion reaction is correct?

   A. The transfusion reaction is likely not due to an ABO incompatibility, because type O individuals will not produce either anti-A or anti-B antibodies.
   B. The transfusion reaction is mediated by pre-formed IgG antibodies in the patient that recognize B antigen on the transfused erythrocytes.
   C. The transfusion reaction is mediated by IgM antibodies in the transfused blood that recognize O antigen on the patient's erythrocytes.
   D. The transfusion reaction is mediated by pre-formed IgG antibodies in the transfused blood that recognize O antigen on the patient's erythrocytes.
   E. The transfusion reaction is mediated by IgM antibodies in the patient that recognize B antigen on the transfused erythrocytes.

Questions 18-22

For each of the descriptions in questions 18-22, choose the immunosuppressive or tolerance induction therapy for allograft rejection (A-I) that best matches it.

   A. Azathioprine
   B. Cyclosporine
   C. Mycophenolate mofetil
   D. Rapamycin
   E. Anti-CD40L antibody
   F. Anti-IL-2R antibody
   G. CTLA4-Ig
   H. OKT3
   I. Corticosteroids

18. Inhibits a lymphocyte-specific isoform of inosine monophosphate dehydrogenase, an enzyme that is required for the synthesis of guanine nucleotides ( )

19. Blocks calcineurin-dependent activation of NFAT ( )

20. Inhibits macrophage cytokine secretion ( )

21. Binds FKBP and inhibits cell cycle progression in T cells ( )

22. Can induce anergy in T cells through inhibition of costimulatory signaling ( )

23. A 58-year-old man is 10 years post kidney transplantation and has been continuously treated with immunosuppressive drugs. He sees his physician because of a 4-cm hard, painless neck mass, as well as a recent history of weight loss. He is afebrile and has a normal white blood cell count. Biopsy of the mass reveals a lymph node replaced by sheets of B cells but very few T cells. The patient denies any fevers. Which of the following is the most likely mechanism for the development of this lesion?

   A. Direct carcinogenic effects of cyclosporine
   B. Cytomegalovirus infection with a strong humoral immune response
   C. Bacterial infection secondary to immune compromise from medication
   D. Chronic rejection response with prominent anti-allograft antibody response
   E. Unchecked Epstein-Barr virus infection leading to development of B cell lymphoma

24. Which of the following tests is NOT part of donor-recipient compatibility testing before transplantation?

   A. HLA matching of tissues
   B. Crossmatching
   C. ABO blood group matching
   D. Karyotyping
   E. Screening for pre-formed anti-HLA antibodies

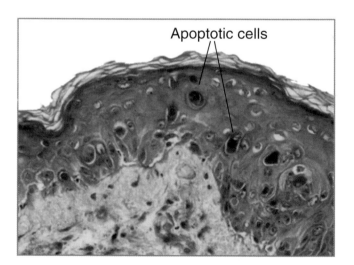

25. A 57-year-old man with a diagnosis of acute leukemia was treated by radiation and chemotherapy to ablate his bone marrow and was then transfused with bone marrow harvested from his brother. Four weeks after the bone marrow transplantation, the patient developed a severe maculopapular rash on the neck, hands, and feet. A histologic section from the biopsy is shown in the figure above. Which of the following is an accurate description of the disease process causing the patient's rash?

   A. In addition to skin, epithelial cells in the liver and gastrointestinal tract are often involved.

B. It is caused by the patient's innate immune system rejecting bone marrow–derived dendritic cells in the skin.

C. It never occurs with MHC-identical bone marrow transplantations.

D. It is due to herpesvirus infection.

E. It occurs only in the setting of hematopoietic cell transplantations.

Answers

1. (E) First-set rejection is the process by which a transplanted graft between genetically unrelated individuals is rejected by a recipient who has never been grafted or otherwise exposed to alloantigens from the graft donor before. This type of rejection takes 7 to 10 days to occur and is due to a primary adaptive immune response against the graft. Rejection of a subsequent graft transplantation between the same two individuals is known as second-set rejection, which represents a secondary immune response. This response to nonself antigens occurs much more rapidly owing to the development of immunologic memory from the previous primary response. Both antibody producing B cells and effector T cells may mediate second set rejection. The features of second set rejection are not characteristic of innate immune responses.
CMI5 369-370, 378-380; BI2

2. (A) Allografts are grafts between genetically distinct members of the same species. The twins are not identical (one brother, one sister); they are genetically different individuals and, therefore, the transplant is allogeneic. Autologous grafts, also called autografts, are organs or tissues removed from an individual and transplanted back to that same individual. Autologous skin grafts are performed on burn patients, and autologous bone marrow transplantation is performed in some cancer treatment protocols. Syngeneic grafts are between genetically identical members of the same species, such as identical twins or inbred mice. Xenogeneic transplantation occurs between individuals of different species. *Congenic* is a term used to describe two inbred strains of animals that differ genetically at only one particular locus, as a result of selective breeding. Mice congenic at MHC loci have been useful tools to study graft rejection.
CMI5 371; BI2 185

3. (C) The MHC molecules are responsible for almost all strong rejection reactions. The offspring of a mating between two different inbred strains will typically not reject grafts from either parent because all the MHC alleles of both parents are inherited by the offspring, and therefore their products are seen as self. Thus, an AxB recipient will not reject grafts from an A or B donor. However, a graft derived from an AxB F_1 animal will be rejected by either an A or a B parent, because half the MHC gene products in the graft are foreign to either A or B strains. A or B recipients will reject grafts from B or A donors, respectively, because of MCH disparities.
CMI5 372

4. (D) The direct presentation of allogenic MHC molecules involves a cross-reaction of a T cell receptor selected to recognize self-MHC with a bound nonself peptide. This can occur because an allogeneic MHC molecule with a bound peptide can mimic the structures formed by self-MHC with bound foreign peptides. Peptides bound to allo-MHC contribute to the direct pathway of presentation in two ways. First, peptides are required for assembly and surface expression of MHC molecules. Second, peptides from graft cells may contribute to the structure seen by the recipient's alloreactive T cells, even if they are from nonpolymorphic proteins found in the recipient. In such cases, it is the combination of the peptide and polymorphic residues of the MHC molecule that is recognized. As many as 2% of an individual's T cells are capable of directly recognizing a single foreign MHC molecule, and such a high frequency of reactive T cells helps to engender a strong immune response. This is known as the determinate frequency hypothesis. In addition, all of the MHC molecules on an allogeneic antigen-presenting cell are foreign to a recipient and therefore can be recognized by T cells, contributing to a strong rejection response. This is known as the determinate density hypothesis. Many of these alloreactive T cells are memory T cells that were generated during previous exposure to other foreign antigens, hence making the initial response to alloantigens stronger and faster than primary immune responses to foreign microbes.
CMI5 372-374; BI2 187-188

5. (E) In the indirect pathway, donor MHC molecules are processed and presented by recipient antigen-presenting cells (APCs) in the same conventional manner that foreign protein antigens are presented. In a graft recipient the detectable presence of CD4+ T cells that recognize donor MHC-derived peptides presented by recipient class II MHC molecules is evidence that the indirect pathway has occurred and caused clonal expansion of the foreign peptide plus self MHC specific CD4+ T cells. Allostimulation of T cells by APCs that cannot process antigen is evidence of the direct pathway of alloantigen presentation, in which intact surface MHC molecules are recognized as foreign. Sensitizing an individual for rejection of tissue from a particular donor is not necessarily tissue-specific because the same MHC alleles are expressed in different tissues, and this sensitization theoretically may occur by either direct or indirect pathways. Class II MHC-deficient recipients will not develop CD4+ T cells owing to a lack of positive selection in the thymus. On the other hand, an alloantigen-specific CD4+ T cell response to a class II MHC-deficient graft indicates that indirect alloantigen

presentation has taken place, since the graft cells will have no class II MHC molecules to present directly to the host's CD4⁺ T cells.
CMI5 374-375

6. (C) The one-way primary mixed leukocyte reaction is performed to assess the potential for T cell–mediated graft rejection and requires coculturing blood mononuclear leukocytes from the recipient with inactivated mononuclear leukocytes from the donor. The proliferative response of the recipient cells is then measured.
CMI5 375-376

7. (E) In the one way mixed leukocyte reaction are described, the responder cells from donor B will likely differ at both class I and class II MHC alleles from the stimulator cells of unrelated donor A. Therefore, both CD4⁺ and CD8⁺ T cells from donor B will proliferate. The CD4⁺ T cells will also differentiate into effector cells that will secrete cytokines on re-stimulation by the same MHC products that stimulated them in the primary culture. Although effector CD8⁺ cytolytic T lymphocytes will also be generated from donor B cells in this culture, they will only be able to recognize and kill target cells, which share class I MHC alleles with the donor A stimulator cells. The inactivated donor A cells will not differentiate into cytotoxic T lymphocytes.
CMI5 375-376; BI2 188

8. (C) Despite expressing paternally derived antigens that are allogeneic to the mother, the fetus is not rejected in utero. Multiple phenomena have been shown to contribute to this protection of the fetus from the mother's immune system. First, trophoblastic cells have no detectable levels of paternal class II MHC molecules and only express a nonpolymorphic class I MHC molecules called HLA-G, thus preventing the activation of both T cells and natural killer cells. In addition, the uterine decidua is thought to be an immunologically privileged site owing to the presence of high concentrations of inhibitory cytokines such as transforming growth factor-β. The trophoblast and decidua also appear to be resistant to complement-mediated destruction because of high levels of the complement inhibitor Crry. However, tryptophan at high levels is thought to activate immune responses and decidual tryptophan levels are normally maintained below the level required for T cell activation by the enzyme indolamine 2,3-dioxygenase.
CMI5 377

9. (B) The type of graft failure described is hyperacute rejection, which is caused by preformed antibodies specific for graft alloantigens. These antibodies are already present in the recipient's blood before transplantation and may recognize blood group antigens (if there is a blood type mismatch), allogeneic MHC proteins, or other alloantigens expressed on graft endothelial cells. The antibodies bind to the graft endothelium and

activate complement, and this leads to endothelial damage, thrombus formation, and vascular occlusion. Problems with blood vessel connections between recipient and graft could cause ischemic necrosis of the graft but not endothelial damage and thrombotic occlusion of small vessels. The crossmatch test, which is routinely performed before transplantation, detects the presence of recipient antibodies that bind to blood cells expressing donor alloantigens. Blood typing and cross-matching can prevent most potential cases of hyperacute rejection. Acute rejection, which can be mediated by both antibodies and T cells, takes at least 1 week to develop because it requires that host B and T cells become activated by the graft and produce effector cells and antibodies.
CMI5 378-381; BI2 188-189

10. (A) The biopsy specimen shows acute rejection, in which there are lymphocytes within the myocardium and dead muscle fibers. Acute rejection can occur any time 1 week after transplantation and may occur for the first time months or even years after transplantation. Acute rejection is mediated by both CD8⁺ and CD4⁺ T cells specific for alloantigens in the heart. Because cardiac allografts are taken from cadavers, and there is a shortage of supply, no MHC matching is performed. Currently used immunosuppressive drugs are able to reduce the incidence and severity of acute rejection episodes.
CMI5 380, 383; BI2 188-191, 292-294

11. (D) The figure shows concentric intimal hyperplasia (abnormal growth of cells below the endothelial layer) and critical narrowing of the lumen of a coronary artery. This is the typical pattern of graft-associated arteriosclerosis, which is caused by smooth muscle cell proliferation in the intima and is a form of chronic allograft rejection. Although hypercholesterolemia may be a complication of immunosuppressive drugs, graft arterial disease is distinct from atherosclerosis related to hypercholesterolemia, in which cholesterol deposits, cholesterol-laden "foam cells," and chronic inflammation are all present in eccentric intimal lesions. Graft arteriosclerosis is the major cause of cardiac and renal allograft failure. Immunosuppressive drugs, although effective in treating acute rejection, are not effective in preventing chronic rejection. These drugs may have renal toxicity, but secondary heart failure related to renal disease would not be associated with the coronary artery changes seen in this patient's heart. The patient is not likely to have been tolerant to the graft alloantigens; the graft did survive for 6 years because of pharmacologic immunosuppression.
CMI5 381; BI2 188-191, 292-294

12. (A) The ABO blood group system includes glycosphingolipid antigens whose synthesis requires the action of glycosyltransferase enzymes. A glycosyltransferase encoded by a gene on chromosome

9 modifies the common H antigen. The A allele of this gene adds a terminal *N*-acetylgalactosamine residue to the H antigen to form the A antigen.
CMI5 380

13. (C) The O antigen is a common glycan attached to membrane sphingolipids, which is modified by a fucosyltransferase to form the H antigen in most people. Individuals who are type O do not further modify the H antigen.
CMI5 380

14. (E) Lewis antigens are formed by fucose additions to side chains of glycosphingolipids.
CMI5 380

15. (D) About 15% of individuals do not express the RhD protein, and therefore mount immune responses to RhD⁺ cells introduced by transfusion or during pregnancy. RhD is the major antigen associated with hemolytic disease of the newborn.
CMI5 380

16. (B) The B allele glycosyltransferase adds a terminal galactose residue to the H antigen to form the B antigen.
CMI5 380

17. (E) ABO blood group antigens are T cell–independent glycosphingolipid antigens. Individuals who express A antigen (blood type A), B antigen (blood type B), or both A and B (blood type AB) do not produce antibodies specific for A, B, or both antigens, respectively, because of tolerance. Individuals who do not express A antigen (blood type B), B antigen (blood type A), or either A and B (blood type O) do produce antibodies specific for B, A, or both A and B, respectively. The antibodies are IgM natural antibodies produced by B1 B cells or marginal zone B cells in the spleen. Bacterial antigens found in intestinal flora cross react with the ABO antigens and are thought to be the antigens that stimulate these anti-ABO specific B cells. Transfusion of red blood cells with A or B antigens on their surface into an individual with these preformed IgM antibodies specific for A or B antigens causes massive intravascular hemolysis, renal tubular damage, and disseminated intravascular coagulation.
CMI5 380, 386-387

18. (C) Mycophenolate mofetil (MMF), like azathioprine, inhibits the maturation and proliferation of T cells. MMF is metabolized to mycophenolic acid, which blocks a lymphocyte-specific form of an enzyme required for the de novo synthesis of guanine nucleotides.
CMI5 381-383; BI2 190

19. (B) Cyclosporine is a cyclic fungal peptide that inhibits calcium-dependent calcineurin and thus prevents the dephosphorylation of NFAT. NFAT is an essential transcription factor for numerous T cell cytokine genes, including interleukin-2.
CMI5 381-383; BI2 190

20. (I) Corticosteroids are potent anti-inflammatory agents that are thought to block the synthesis and secretion of cytokines, primarily tumor necrosis factor and interleukin-1, by macrophages. Inhibition of these cytokines results in reduced graft endothelial cell activation and inflammatory cell recruitment. Corticosteroids are also thought to block other effector functions of macrophages, such as the production of reactive oxygen intermediates and nitric oxide.
CMI5 381-383; BI2 190

21. (D) Rapamycin is an antibiotic that binds to FK506 binding protein (FKBP) and inhibits T cell proliferation. The rapamycin-FKBP complex does this by binding another cellular protein, the mammalian target of rapamycin (MTOR), which has been observed to regulate cell cycle progression by modulating the expression of certain cyclins. Note that FK506, another immunosuppressive drug, also binds FKBP, and the complex binds and inhibits calcineurin, as does cyclosporine.
CMI5 381-383; BI2 190

22. (G) CTLA4-Ig is a fusion protein that binds to B7-1 and B7-2 and therefore blocks B7 binding to CD28. This is a method of blocking costimulation. If, at the time of transplantation, alloantigens provide signal 1 to alloreactive T cells, while signal 2 is blocked by CTLA4-Ig, the alloreactive T cells may become anergic.
CMI5 381-383; BI2 190

23. (E) A newly developed mass and a history of recent weight loss in a patient on long-term immunosuppressant therapy suggests malignancy. Immunocompromised patients are susceptible to viral infections, some of which can malignantly transform cells if not checked by the host's immune system. Two common malignant tumors found in transplantation patients are B cell lymphomas associated with Epstein-Barr virus and squamous cell carcinomas associated with human papillomavirus. Cyclosporine has not been shown to be carcinogenic. The lack of fevers or elevated white blood cell count in this patient does not point to an acute bacterial infection. An anti-cytomegalovirus response would not cause a massive replacement of lymph node by B cells. The sheets of B cells found on a biopsy specimen would not be seen in an immune response to infection in this immunosuppressed patient and, instead, are due to malignancy.
CMI5 383

24. (D) Karyotyping is a genetic test used to analyze chromosomal number and overt structural abnormalities. Karyotyping is not used for compatibility testing in transplantation. ABO blood type and HLA matching are performed in compatibility testing, as is screening for preformed antibodies to HLA antigens. Crossmatching is also a compatibility test performed in which a potential donor has already been identified and a screen is performed

to detect preformed antibodies to specific donor cells.
CMI5 383-385; BI2 190-191

25. (A) This patient's rash is due to acute graft-versus-host disease (GVHD). The histopathology includes sparse lymphocyte infiltration and damage to the epithelial layer, including apoptosis of keratinocytes. Acute GVHD also commonly affects biliary epithelial cells in the liver and mucosal epithelial cells in the gastrointestinal tract, with symptoms of jaundice, diarrhea, and gastrointestinal bleeding. The disease is caused by grafted mature T cells or natural killer (NK) cells in the bone marrow transplant that recognize the host cells as foreign. GVHD does occur when there is perfect MHC matching, and therefore minor histocompatibility antigens may be involved. Viral infection is not a cause of GVHD. Rarely, GVHD occurs after solid organ transplantation because these organs may carry mature T cells and NK cells.
CMI5 388; BI2 191

Chapter 17

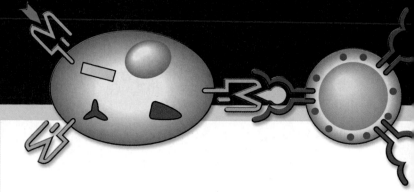

Immunity to Tumors

Cellular and Molecular Immunology, 5/E: Chapter 17—Immunity to Tumors

Basic Immunology, 2/E: Chapter 10—Immune Responses Against Tumors and Transplants

1. All of the following statements about immune responses to tumors are true EXCEPT:

   A. T cells specific for tumor antigens can be found in many human tumor patients.
   B. Antibodies specific for tumor antigens can be found in many human tumor patients.
   C. The presence of lymphocytic infiltrates in certain tumors is associated with a better prognosis than lymphocyte-poor tumors of the same histologic type.
   D. Immunodeficient individuals are more likely to develop the most common forms of cancer than are immunocompetent individuals.
   E. The host immune response is usually incapable of eradicating tumors once they are established.

2. The first experiments that demonstrated protective adaptive immune responses to tumors involved transplantation of chemical carcinogen-induced tumors between rodents. Which of the following facts was learned from these experiments?

   A. There are only a limited number of antigens that can evoke a protective anti-tumor response.
   B. Transplanted sarcomas can evoke protective cytolytic T lymphocyte responses.
   C. Carcinomas express tumor antigens that are recognized by T lymphocytes.
   D. Protective immune responses against tumors are largely mediated by antibodies.
   E. Spontaneously arising tumors are often eradicated by cytolytic T lymphocytes.

Questions 3-7

For each particular tumor antigen listed in questions 3-7, choose the class of tumor antigen (A-G) to which it belongs.

   A. Product of a cellular oncogene
   B. Overexpressed unmutated cellular proteins
   C. Product of unmutated genes normally silent in most tissues
   D. Overexpressed surface glycolipid
   E. Oncofetal antigen
   F. Tissue differentiation antigen
   G. Product of an oncogenic virus

3. Prostate-specific antigen ( )

4. E6 antigen ( )

5. Cancer testis antigens ( )

6. Carcinoembryonic antigen (CEA) ( )

7. Ras ( )

Questions 8-12

For each description in questions 8-12, choose the tumor antigen or gene (A-J) that is the best match.

   A. AFP
   B. *Bcr/Abl*
   C. CA-125
   D. CD20
   E. CEA
   F. EBNA
   G. MAGE
   H. *p53*
   I. PSA
   J. Ras

8. Differentiation antigen for B cells ( )

9. A patient presenting with jaundice and a recent 11-kg (20 lb) weight loss who has a history of hepatitis B infection will most likely have elevated levels of this glycoprotein ( )

10. Mutations in both allelic copies of this gene are required for malignant transformation ( )

11. A protein that is expressed only in immunologically privileged tissue ( )

12. A mucin that is often elevated in ovarian carcinoma ( )

13. A 17-year-old girl from southern China has had a sore throat and fever for 1 week. On physical examination, generalized lymphadenopathy is noted. A rapid strep test for streptococcal infection is negative and a CBC shows 20% atypical lymphocytes. A Monospot test for the presence of heterophile antibodies is positive. This illness is associated with eventual development of which of the following malignancies?

   A. Kaposi's sarcoma
   B. Cervical carcinoma
   C. Follicular lymphoma
   D. Human T cell lymphoma
   E. Nasopharyngeal carcinoma

14. Patients with which of the following disorders would be LEAST likely to develop Epstein-Barr virus–associated Burkitt's lymphoma?

   A. AIDS
   B. Bruton's disease
   C. DiGeorge syndrome (congenital absence of the thymus)
   D. Malarial infection
   E. Immunosuppressive therapy for renal allograft

15. Which of the following molecules is involved in the principal mechanism by which the immune system kills tumor cells?

   A. Perforin
   B. Complement C3
   C. IgG
   D. TGF-β
   E. Interleukin-2

16. Class I MHC-restricted T cell responses to tumors can be demonstrated in patients with various types of tumors, yet most of these tumors do not express costimulatory molecules. Which mechanism most likely explains how naive CD8⁺ T cells specific for antigens expressed by these tumors are stimulated to differentiate into cytolytic T lymphocytes?

   A. Malignant transformation of CD8⁺ T cells
   B. Tumor secretion of T cell–activating cytokines
   C. Cross reaction of microbe-specific CD8⁺ T cells with tumor antigens
   D. Cross priming
   E. Antigenic modulation

17. Which of the following is NOT a mechanism by which tumors evade immune responses?

   A. Decreased synthesis of TAP
   B. Increased expression of glycocalyx
   C. Lack of costimulatory molecule expression
   D. Increased expression of TGF-β
   E. Increased expression of Fas

18. A 56-year-old woman sees her primary care physician complaining of flank pain and hematuria and is found to have a hematocrit of 56%. She is subsequently diagnosed with advanced renal cell carcinoma. Part of the patient's management involves systemic cytokine therapy; however, the patient develops severe pulmonary edema as a result of the treatment. Which of the following cytokines was most likely used in this patient's therapy?

   A. Interleukin (IL)-2
   B. IL-6
   C. IL-12
   D. GM-CSF (granulocyte-macrophage colony-stimulating factor)
   E. TNF (tumor necrosis factor)

19. Injections of the mycobacterium Bacillus Calmette-Guérin (BCG) at the sites of tumor growth helps to activate which of the following effector immune cells?

A. B cells
B. Cytolytic T lymphocytes
C. Natural killer cells
D. Macrophages
E. Neutrophils

20. A 47-year-old woman had a mastectomy because she had breast carcinoma that was previously diagnosed by biopsy. Pathologic examination revealed that several axillary lymph nodes contained metastatic tumors. A test was performed on tumor cells extracted from the mastectomy specimen, which indicated that the tumor cells overexpressed a certain cellular proto-oncogene. On the basis of this test result, the patient was treated with an FDA-approved monoclonal antibody specific for the protein encoded by that gene. Which of the following was most likely the protein target of this antibody therapy?

A. p53
B. H-Ras
C. HPV E7
D. Rb
E. Her2

Questions 21-23

For each of the descriptions in questions 21-23, select the tumor immunotherapy strategy (A-J) that is best match.

A. Killed tumor vaccine
B. DNA vaccines
C. Interleukin (IL)-2
D. IL-4
E. GM-CSF (granulocyte-macrophage colony-stimulating factor)
F. Anti-CD3 antibodies
G. Lymphokine-activated killer cells
H. Anti-Her2/neu antibodies
I. Anti-idiotypic antibodies
J. Dendritic cell vaccine

21. Component of adoptive cellular immunotherapy used with IL-2 and/or chemotherapeutic drugs ( )

22. Tumor cells transfected with the gene encoding this protein have been used as a vaccine that promotes dendritic cell presentation of tumor antigens ( )

23. Therapy that targets an antigen that is not essential to the malignant phenotype of the tumor; antigen-loss variants can emerge during therapy ( )

Answers

1. (D) The most common tumors are carcinomas, originating from epithelial cells of organs such as the lung, colon, breast, and prostate. These tumors do not occur more frequently in immunocompromised hosts than in the general population. The types of tumors that do occur more frequently in immunocompromised hosts, such as AIDS patients or allograft recipients receiving chronic immuno-suppressive therapy, are those with a clear viral etiology. Examples include Epstein-Barr virus–associated lymphomas and human papillomavirus–associated cervical and skin carcinomas. It is true that T cells and antibodies specific for molecules expressed exclusively or abundantly on tumor cells can be found in tumor patients and that lymphocytic infiltrates are a histologic indication of better prognosis for a limited number of tumors. Nonetheless, the naturally occurring immune responses that occur against tumor antigens are usually not capable of eliminating tumors.
CMI5 391-392; BI2 177-178

2. (B) The chemical carcinogen used in many of the rodent tumor immunology experiments was methylcholanthrene (MCA), which causes tumors derived from mesenchymal cells of the skin, called sarcomas. When transplanted into naive mice, these MCA-induced sarcomas would evoke protective immune responses. Adoptive transfer studies showed that cytolytic T lymphocytes, and not antibodies, were mediating the protective effect. Interestingly, the T cells specific for one MCA-induced sarcoma usually could not recognize another MCA-induced sarcoma, indicating that there are innumerable potential T cell antigens expressed by these tumors. Most of these antigens are now known to be different, randomly mutated cellular proteins, which are presented by the class I MHC pathway on the surface of the tumor cells. These chemical carcinogen-induced sarcoma studies do not provide any information about antigens on carcinomas, nor do they prove that there are protective immune responses to spontaneously arising tumors in people.
CMI5 392, 393-396; BI2 177-179

3. (F) Prostate-specific antigen (PSA) is a glycoprotein that is expressed by both normal prostate epithelial cells and prostate cancer cells. The protein is secreted into the circulation, and the high degree of tissue specificity of PSA expression allows for the use of PSA as a specific marker for prostate cancer. Clinical trials have been performed using virally expressed PSA as a tumor vaccine.
CMI5 397

4. (G) Human papillomavirus (HPV) is the causative agent of cervical carcinoma, some skin cancers, and benign warts. HPV *E6* and *E7* are oncogenes whose protein products target and interfere with the function of the tumor suppressor genes p53 and Rb. HPV *E6* and *E7* are expressed by HPV-transformed tumor cells and stimulate host immune responses. These proteins have been used in experimental tumor vaccine protocols against cervical carcinoma.
CMI5 397; BI2 178-179

5. (C) The cancer testis antigens, including MAGE, BAGE, and GAGE, are proteins expressed in melanomas and many carcinomas, and they evoke

specific T cell responses. These proteins are normally found only in the testis and placenta.
CMI5 397

6. (E) Carcinoembryonic antigen (CEA, CD66e) is a glycoprotein adhesion molecule whose expression is usually limited to the gastrointestinal tract during the first two trimesters of gestation, but it is frequently expressed by carcinomas of the colon, pancreas, stomach, and breast. Serum levels of CEA are used to monitor the persistence or recurrence of treated tumors.
CMI5 399

7. (A) *Ras* genes with point mutations are oncogenes that promote malignant transformation of cells and are found in many different tumors. Patients with tumors often have circulating CD4$^+$ or CD8$^+$ T cells specific for Ras peptides containing the point mutations.
CMI5 393; BI2 178-179

8. (D) Differentiation antigens are molecules expressed on the normal cells from which the tumor was derived and are specific for particular cell differentiation stages or lineages. They are important in identifying the tissue of origin of tumors. CD20 is a differentiation antigen for B cell lymphomas, and PSA is a differentiation antigen for prostate carcinomas.
CMI5 400

9. (A) AFP (α-fetoprotein) is a circulating glycoprotein that normally is secreted during fetal life by the yolk sac and liver but is present only at low levels in adults. However, elevated levels of AFP are often detected in patients with hepatocellular carcinoma or germ cell tumors. The presenting signs of hepatocellular carcinoma can include jaundice, weight loss, and right upper quadrant abdominal pain. Previous infection with hepatitis B increases an individual's risk of developing this malignancy.
CMI5 399-400

10. (H) Tumor suppressor genes such as *p53* require loss-of-function mutations in both allelic copies for malignant transformation to occur. This is because one normal copy of the gene is sufficient to mediate antiproliferative effects. On the other hand, proto-oncogenes such as *Ras* and *Bcr/Abl* require only one activating mutation for malignant transformation to occur, because the mutant allele will act in a dominant fashion to activate cell proliferation.
CMI5 396-397

11. (G) Some tumor antigens are derived from genes that are silent in most tissues. The proteins encoded by many of these genes are not mutated and are not required for malignant transformation. However, they do act as tumor antigens and can elicit immune responses. Melanoma antigen (MAGE) is a cellular protein antigen recognized by tumor-specific cytolytic T lymphocyte clones derived not only from melanomas but also from carcinomas of the bladder, breast, skin, lung, and prostate. However, among normal tissues, MAGE expression is restricted to the testis, an immunologically privileged site that prevents the development of immune tolerance to this protein.
CMI5 397

12. (C) Mucins are high-molecular-weight glycoproteins containing numerous carbohydrate linkages on a core polypeptide. Many tumors have unregulated expression of enzymes that synthesize these carbohydrate side chains, thus leading to foreign carbohydrate epitopes. CA-125 and CA-19-9 are two mucins that are expressed in many ovarian carcinomas.
CMI5 400

13. (E) The clinical manifestations described are classic for infectious mononucleosis secondary to Epstein-Barr virus (EBV) infection. These include sore throat, fever, fatigue, and generalized lymphadenopathy. The differential diagnosis for sore throat includes streptococcal infection; however, the rapid strep test for streptococcal infection is negative in this patient. In addition, the peripheral blood smear of patients with mononucleosis often contains abundant numbers of large morphologically atypical lymphocytes. EBV infection is one of the etiologic factors associated with malignant tumors, including nasopharyngeal carcinoma in Chinese populations, Burkitt's lymphoma in equatorial African populations, and other B cell lymphomas in immunosuppressed populations.
CMI5 398

14. (B) Epstein-Barr virus (EBV) is a double-stranded DNA virus of the herpesvirus family that infects nasopharyngeal epithelial cells as well as B cells. The virus establishes a latent infection in these cells, and T cell–mediated immunity is required for control of EBV infections and, in particular, for killing of EBV-infected B cells. It has been demonstrated that loss of normal T cell function allows latently infected B cells to progress toward malignant transformation. Thus, patients with disorders that cause T cell immunodeficiencies (e.g., AIDS, DiGeorge syndrome, malarial infection, and transplantation patients taking immunosuppressive therapies) are at increased risk of developing Burkitt's lymphoma. Bruton's disease is an isolated B cell deficiency due to mutation of Btk, a tyrosine kinase required for the maturation of B cells in the bone marrow. Therefore, patients with Bruton's disease are not likely to develop B cell lymphomas.
CMI5 398-399

15. (A) Cytolytic T lymphocyte (CTL) killing of tumor cells is the principal known mechanism for tumor immunity in vivo. This requires class I MHC expression by the tumor cells. In addition, natural killer cells (NK cells) can kill tumor cells that lack class I MHC. CTL and NK cells employ the same mechanism to kill tumor cells, which depends on perforin and granzyme B release from cytoplasmic granules. Although antibodies (e.g., IgG) and complement can kill tumor cells in vitro and tumor-specific anti-

bodies can be detected in patients, it is not known if Ig or complement plays a significant role in tumor immunity in vivo. TGF-β (transforming growth factor-β) is an immunoregulatory cytokine produced by T cells and other cell types. TGF-β does not kill tumor cells. Interleukin-2 has been used in protocols to treat certain tumors, but its effect is indirect and it does not directly kill tumor cells.
CMI5 400-402; BI2 180-181

16. (D) Tumor cells, or the protein antigens they produce, may be taken up by professional antigen-presenting cells (APCs), especially dendritic cells, and the antigens may then be delivered into the cytoplasm to gain access to the class I MHC pathway of antigen presentation. In this way, naive T cells specific for the tumor antigens can be activated by the APCs; i.e., through cross-presentation. Once differentiated into cytolytic T lymphocytes (CTLs), the T cells can then be activated by and kill the tumor cells, which present the same antigen, even in the absence of costimulation. There is no reason why malignant transformation of the T cells should occur. There is no evidence for cross reactivity between microbes and tumor antigens, nor of tumors secreting T cell–activating cytokines. Antigenic modulation is a mechanism by which tumors evade T cells, not activate them.
CMI5 401; BI2 180

17. (E) Many tumor cells will up-regulate expression of Fas-ligand, not Fas, to signal for apoptosis in Fas-expressing leukocytes recruited to the site of the tumor. Other mechanisms of tumor evasion include down-regulation of MHC I molecules as well as the components of the antigen-processing machinery needed for MHC I presentation, such as proteasome subunits and the TAP transporter. Some tumors can also down-regulate costimulatory molecules such as B7. Tumors can also up-regulate expression of immunosuppressive cytokines, such as TGF-β, as well as increase production of glycocalyx polysaccharides that hide or "mask" tumor surface antigens from the immune system.
CMI5 402-403; BI2 181

18. (A) The classic clinical findings of renal cell carcinoma include flank pain and hematuria. These patients commonly have elevated hematocrits secondary to the overproduction of erythropoietin, which increases red blood cell production in the bone marrow. Of the systemic cytokine therapies used in cancer therapy, only interleukin (IL)-2 and IL-6 have been used frequently for renal cancer. Whereas IL-6 has not demonstrated any clinical benefit in these patients, IL-2 has been effective in inducing measurable tumor regression responses in a small percentage of patients (<15%). IL-2

therapy is highly toxic and can induce fever, pulmonary edema, and vascular shock.
CMI5 406-407

19. (D) Mycobacterial bacillus Calmette-Guérin (BCG) injections have been used for nonspecific immune stimulation at the sites of tumors and work by inducing a delayed-type hypersensitivity (DTH) reaction. The effector cells of a DTH response are macrophages.
CMI5 407

20. (E) Her2 is encoded by the *Her-2/neu* oncogene. It is a cell surface, transmembrane glycoprotein with intracellular tyrosine kinase activity. Presumably, *HER-2/neu* generates signals that regulate epithelial cell growth and differentiation. Twenty to 40 percent of breast cancers show amplification of the *Her2/neu* oncogene and overexpression of the product. A monoclonal antibody specific for the Her2 protein inhibits tumor growth and may have some clinical efficacy. H-Ras and HPV-E7 are oncogene products, but they are intracellular and inaccessible to monoclonal antibody treatment. p53 and Rb are intracellular tumor suppressor gene products, and there is no antibody-mediated therapy directed at these proteins.
CMI5 408-409; BI2 181

21. (G) Lymphokine activated killer (LAK) cells are activated natural killer cells derived from peripheral blood leukocytes of tumor patients by in vitro high-dose interleukin (IL)-2 treatment. LAK cells have been used in adoptive cellular immunotherapy protocols for certain cancers, such as melanoma and renal cell carcinoma, usually in conjunction with IL-2 and/or chemotherapeutic drugs.
CMI5 408

22. (E) Granulocyte-macrophage colony-stimulating factor (GM-CSF) is a hematopoietic cytokine that promotes dendritic cell maturation and cross-presentation of tumor antigens. Tumor cells transfected with the GM-CSF gene have been used in human tumor vaccine trials and induce long-lived memory responses to tumor antigens in mice.
CMI5 406-407

23. (I) Malignant tumors of B lymphocytes often express a membrane Ig; because they are clonal, all the tumor cells express the same Ig with the same idiotype. Therefore, the idiotype on these tumors is a very specific tumor antigen. Antiidiotypic antibodies have been used to treat these tumors, but often, the therapy "selects" for cells that no longer express the idiotype. Because the idiotype is not necessary for the malignant phenotype, the antigen-loss variants will continue to grow.
CMI5 409

Chapter 18

Diseases Caused by Immune Responses: Hypersensitivity and Autoimmunity

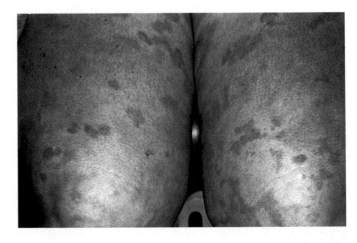

Cellular and Molecular Immunology, 5/E: Chapter 18—Diseases Caused by Immune Responses: Hypersensitivity and Autoimmunity

Basic Immunology, 2/E: Chapter 11—Hypersensitivity Diseases

1. Which of the following is a common cause of hypersensitivity diseases?

    A. Failure of lymphocyte maturation
    B. Treatment with corticosteroids
    C. Disseminated cancer
    D. Failure of self-tolerance
    E. Malnutrition

2. A 15-year-old girl experiences flushing, pruritus, and urticaria (see figure above), which began during a class field trip to the local botanical gardens. She is restless and uncomfortable and describes a sensation of "burning" and "pulling" in his skin. Which of the following best characterizes his condition?

A. Superantigen activation of CD4⁺ T cells

    A. Superantigen activation of CD4$^+$ T cells
    B. CD8$^+$ T cell-mediated cytolysis of keratinocytes in the skin
    C. CD4$^+$ T cell-mediated delayed-type hypersensitivity to poison ivy
    D. Complement activation by antibody-antigen immune complexes in the skin
    E. Activation of IgE-coated mast cells leading to histamine release

3. All of the following are effector mechanisms of antibody-mediated disease EXCEPT:

    A. Opsonization and phagocytosis of cells
    B. Fas-dependent apoptosis of cells
    C. Complement- and Fc receptor–mediated inflammation and tissue injury
    D. Antibody stimulation of cell surface receptors in the absence of the physiologic ligands
    E. FcεR crosslinking

4. A 43-year-old woman sees her physician with complaints of anxiety, heat intolerance, arm weakness, tremors, and fatigue. Physical examination reveals tachycardia, diffuse thyroid enlargement, and exophthalmos (see figure below). Laboratory tests indicate high serum thyroxine (T_4) and triiodothyronine (T_3) concentrations, with a high serum T_3 to T_4 ratio. The patient is treated with propylthiouracil and responded favorably. Which of the following is the underlying mechanism for the patient's condition?

    A. Autoantibody blockade of acetylcholine binding to acetylcholine receptors (AChR) in the neuromuscular junction
    B. Autoantibody specific for thyroid-stimulating hormone (TSH) that blocks TSH binding to the TSH receptor
    C. Autoantibody stimulation of TSH receptors
    D. Autoantibody stimulation of thyroid hormone receptors
    E. Autoreactive T cell–mediated damage to thyroid hormone–producing cells

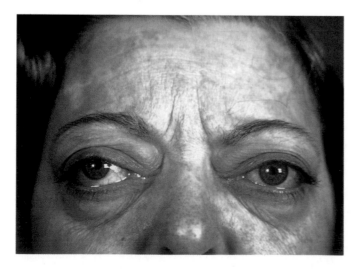

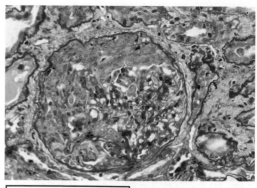

Light microscopy

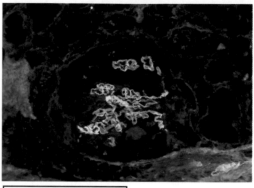

Immunofluorescence

5. The figure above shows routine histologic and immunofluorescence images of a kidney biopsy specimen taken from a 53-year-old man with acute-onset renal failure and hemoptysis (coughing up blood). The histologic section is notable for glomerular inflammation in a crescentic distribution. Staining, using fluorescently tagged anti-IgG antibody, shows linear deposits of IgG along the glomerular basement membrane. Urinalysis is positive for moderate proteinuria and red cell casts. A chest radiograph shows pulmonary infiltrates. Which of the following is the most likely diagnosis?

    A. Systemic lupus erythematosus
    B. Graves' disease
    C. Chronic allograft rejection
    D. Goodpasture's syndrome
    E. Poststreptococcal glomerulonephritis

6. Which type of hypersensitivity disease is caused by deposition of antigen-antibody complexes in blood vessel walls?

    A. Type I
    B. Type II
    C. Type III
    D. Type IV
    E. Type V

7. Which of the following statements about immune complex–mediated diseases is NOT true?

A. Immune complexes may contain antibodies bound to either self or foreign antigens.

B. Immune complex–mediated diseases generally show systemic manifestations.

C. Pathologic features of immune complex diseases are determined by the cellular source of the antigen.

D. Small complexes are deposited in vessels more than large complexes, which are usually efficiently phagocytosed.

E. Complexes containing cationic antigens are more likely to produce severe, long-lasting injury by depositing in blood vessels and renal glomeruli.

8. In which of the following disorders is the underlying pathogenic mechanism NOT due to antibody-mediated damage to cells or tissues?

A. Pernicious anemia
B. Autoimmune hemolytic anemia
C. Pemphigus vulgaris
D. Acute rheumatic fever
E. Hyperacute allograft rejection

9. A 26-year-old African-American woman visits her physician because of a prominent rash over her nose and cheeks, which she first noticed following her return from a vacation in Jamaica. She also complains of fever, fatigue, weight loss, and joint pain over the last several months. Serologic tests are conclusive for systemic lupus erythematosus (SLE), an autoimmune disease that can manifest clinically with rashes, arthritis, glomerulonephritis, hemolytic anemia, thrombocytopenia (low platelet count), and central nervous system involvement. The principal diagnostic test result specific for this condition is a high titer of autoantibodies against which of the following?

A. Glomerular basement membrane
B. Rh blood group antigen
C. Myelin
D. Double-stranded DNA
E. IgG

10. Which of the following is NOT associated with increased relative risk of developing systemic lupus erythematosus?

A. Female gender
B. Deficiency in complement protein C2
C. African-American ethnicity
D. Presence of HLA-DR3
E. Defect in B cell maturation

11. Which of the following conditions is NOT associated with immune complex deposition?

A. Arthus reaction
B. Autoimmune hemolytic anemia
C. Serum sickness
D. Systemic lupus erythematosus
E. Poststreptococcal glomerulonephritis

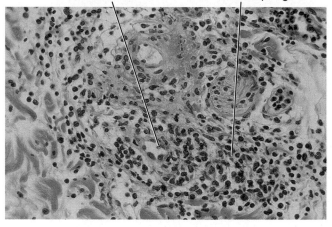

Vessel with activated endothelial cells

Activated lymphocytes and macrophages

12. A 22-year-old man who recently emigrated from South Africa received a PPD skin test for tuberculosis as part of the health screening requirements for a new job in a hospital. Within 48 hours there was an erythematous, indurated lesion 15 mm in diameter at the site on the forearm where the PPD was administered. A histologic section of this type of reaction is shown in the figure above. Which type of immunologic reaction has occurred at this site?

A. Immediate hypersensitivity
B. Anaphylaxis
C. Antibody-dependent cellular cytotoxicity (ADCC)
D. Autoimmune
E. Delayed-type hypersensitivity (DTH)

13. Individuals with the class I HLA-B27 allele have a 90-fold greater chance of developing which of the following inflammatory diseases, relative to HLA-B27-negative individuals?

A. Rheumatoid arthritis
B. Ankylosing spondylitis
C. Pemphigus vulgaris
D. Diabetes mellitus type 1 (insulin dependent)
E. Multiple sclerosis

14. An 8-year-old boy from the intermountain region of the United States is brought to the pediatrician with fever, rash, and pain in his knees and ankles. Pericarditis is evident on auscultation, and echocardiography confirms mitral valve regurgitation. Three weeks before this episode, the patient had experienced a sore throat but had not received medical attention. High titers of antistreptococcal antibodies are present in the serum. This child's disease is a result of which one of the following phenomena?

A. Clonal anergy
B. Peripheral tolerance
C. Epitope spreading
D. Central tolerance
E. Molecular mimicry

Questions 15 and 16

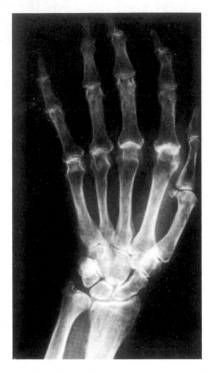

A 68-year-old woman displays symmetrical swelling of the proximal phalangeal joints. There are also small subcutaneous nodules over the extensor surfaces of her arms. A radiograph of her hand, shown in the figure above, shows loss of articular cartilage, narrowing of joint spaces, and ulnar deviation of the fingers. She reports that the hand pain and stiffness are most pronounced on arising in the morning.

15. Which of the following laboratory test results is typical of this patient's disease?

    A. Positive rheumatoid factor (IgG antibodies against the Fc region of autologous IgG)
    B. Cytolytic T lymphocyte activity in the blood specific for β cells of the islets of Langerhans
    C. Serum IgM specific for streptococcal antigens
    D. T_H1 cells in joint fluid specific for myelin basic protein
    E. IgA antibodies in blood specific for the acetylcholine receptor

16. Which of the following reagents is a newly developed therapy for the disease described in question 15?

    A. Anti-interleukin (IL)-10 monoclonal antibody
    B. RANK agonist
    C. Soluble tumor necrosis factor (TNF)-α receptor
    D. Recombinant IL-1 protein
    E. Rheumatoid factor

17. Experimental autoimmune encephalomyelitis (EAE) is a mouse model of a human organ-specific autoimmune disease mediated by T lymphocytes. In EAE, rodents are immunized with proteins found in the myelin sheath of central nervous system neurons. EAE is a model for which of the following human diseases?

    A. Rheumatoid arthritis
    B. Autoimmune myocarditis
    C. Systemic lupus erythematosus
    D. Diabetes mellitus type 1 (insulin-dependent)
    E. Multiple sclerosis

18. Which one of the following statements concerning autoimmune disease is true?

    A. Autoimmunity manifests as organ-specific, not systemic, disease.
    B. Infectious microorganisms are frequently present in autoimmune lesions.
    C. Effector mechanisms in autoimmunity include circulating autoantibodies, immune complexes, and autoreactive T lymphocytes.
    D. Among the genes associated with autoimmunity, associations are particularly prevalent with class I MHC genes.
    E. Many autoimmune diseases show higher incidence in males than in females.

19. Which of the following would NOT be a likely therapy for treating autoimmune diseases?

    A. Corticosteroids
    B. Small molecule inhibitor of VLA-4
    C. Cyclosporine
    D. CTLA-4 antagonist
    E. Plasmapheresis

Questions 20-23

For each of the clinical scenarios in questions 20-23, choose the hypersensitivity type (A-D) that best matches the associated immunologic disease. (Answers may be used more than once.)

    A. Type I hypersensitivity
    B. Type II hypersensitivity
    C. Type III hypersensitivity
    D. Type IV hypersensitivity

20. A 5-year-old girl is taken to the emergency department with lethargy, confusion, vomiting, abdominal pain, and flushed skin that is warm to the touch. Respirations are fast and shallow (Kussmaul) and emanate a strong, fruity odor. The mother notes that the child has been excessively thirsty over the past week and that she began wetting her bed during naps. Urine dipstick testing reveals markedly elevated levels of glucose and ketones. (   )

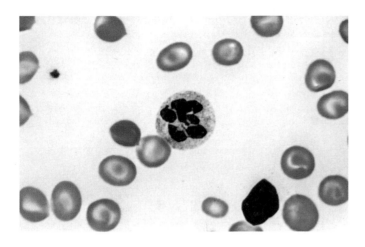

21. A 60-year-old man is evaluated for shortness of breath, lightheadedness, diarrhea, abdominal pain, and tingling in his fingers and toes. A blood smear from the patient is shown in the figure above. Antibodies to intrinsic factor are detected in his serum. (   )

22. A 29-year-old woman gives birth to an infant who is lethargic, jaundiced, and severely anemic and has an enlarged liver and spleen. The mother is RhD negative and the father is homozygous RhD positive. This is their second child. (   )

23. A 23-year-old medical student is taken to the emergency department because of diffuse facial erythema (redness), tightness of the chest, and difficulty breathing. He reports that the symptoms began shortly after he ate a shellfish dinner at a nearby Thai restaurant. On physical examination, he appears to be in acute distress with elevated heart rate and respiratory rate and a dangerously low blood pressure. He is treated with epinephrine. (   )

24. A 37-year-old homeless man is taken to a physician because of malaise, muscle aches, low-grade fever, and weight loss. He also complains of abdominal pain and melena (bloody stool). On physical examination, he is found to be hypertensive. Laboratory results show deteriorating renal function. His

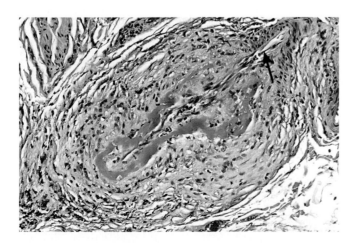

serum is positive for hepatitis B virus (HBV) surface antigen. Antinuclear antibody (ANA) tests are negative. A kidney biopsy is performed. A blood vessel from the biopsy specimen is shown at the bottom of the previous column. Which one of the following best describes the pathogenesis of this disease?

A. Antielastin autoantibodies bind to the media of small arteries in several organs, initiating arteritis.
B. CD4$^+$ T cells specific for vascular smooth muscle cell antigens are activated in the media of small arteries in several organs and initiate arteritis.
C. Immune complexes composed of DNA and anti-DNA antibodies have deposited in the glomerular basement membranes, causing glomerulonephritis.
D. Immune complexes composed of HBV antigens and antibodies specific for these antigens have deposited in medium-sized artery walls in various organs, causing arteritis.
E. HBV-specific cytolytic T lymphocytes lyse virally infected cells in the media of small arteries in several organs, causing damage to the vessel walls.

25. A 14-year-old boy is brought to the pediatrician's office in mid summer because of an itchy, blistering rash on his calves and forearms. The rash developed 24 hours after he returned from a weekend Boy Scout camping trip. The pediatrician suspects the lesion is caused by poison ivy. If the doctor is correct, which one of the following is NOT a prominent component in the immunologic mechanisms causing the skin lesions?

A. T cells
B. IgE-coated mast cells
C. Interferon-γ
D. Endothelial adhesion molecules
E. Chemokines

Answers

1. (D) Hypersensitivity diseases are caused by immune responses. A common underlying condition leading to hypersensitivity diseases is failure of self-tolerance, with subsequent immune responses directed against self antigens (autoimmune diseases). Hypersensitivity diseases may also result from uncontrolled or excessive responses against foreign antigens, including microbes and environmental substances. Failure of lymphocyte maturation, corticosteroid therapy, and malnutrition are associated with immunodeficiency.
CMI5 411; BI2 193-194

2. (E) This patient is experiencing an immediate (type I) hypersensitivity reaction to environmental allergens, such as pollen proteins, to which she has been previously exposed. This reaction begins rapidly, within minutes of antigen challenge, and is mediated by preformed IgE antibodies bound to Fc

receptors on mast cells. When these antibodies and associated Fc receptors are cross-linked by the antigen, the cells are activated to rapidly release various mediators that cause increased vascular permeability, vasodilation, bronchial and visceral smooth muscle contraction, and local inflammation. These effects manifest as the flushing, itching, hives, and discomfort experienced by the patient. Immediate hypersensitivity reactions are T_H2-dependent and may also involve basophils and eosinophils.
CMI5 412; BI2 194-199

3. (B) Fas-dependent apoptosis is a regulatory mechanism in T cell–mediated responses and may be involved in T cell–mediated damage to other cells, but the Fas pathway is not stimulated by antibodies. Antibody-mediated (types I to III) hypersensitivity diseases involve four main effector mechanisms: (1) IgE coats mast cells and links the presence of allergens with mast cell activation and release of inflammatory mediators; (2) antibody-mediated opsonization of cells and activation of complement promotes phagocytosis of cells through phagocyte Fc or C3 receptors; (3) antibody binding to tissues can promote recruitment of leukocytes via binding to Fc receptors on leukocytes or by activation of complement with release of chemotactic byproducts; and (4) autoantibodies specific for cell surface receptors either stimulate receptor activity in the absence of the physiologic ligand or inhibit binding of physiologic ligands to their receptors.
CMI5 413-414; BI2 194-204

4. (C) This patient's presentation is typical of Graves' disease, a hypersensitivity disease caused by autoantibodies that bind to and stimulate a physiologic receptor. In Graves' disease, there is hyperthyroidism due to autoantibodies specific for the thyroid-stimulating hormone (TSH) receptor on thyroid epithelial cells. The antibodies act as agonists, stimulating dysregulated production of thyroid hormones, T_3 (triiodothyronine) and T_4 (thyroxine). Exophthalmus in Graves' disease is due to orbital inflammation, edema, and accumulated glycosaminoglycans, likely due to autoimmune recognition of local antigens. Anti-acetylcholine receptor antibodies are involved in myasthenia gravis but not Graves' disease. Autoantibodies specific for TSH or T cell–mediated damage to thyroid-producing cells would be expected to cause symptoms of hypothyroidism, not hyperthyroidism. Autoantibodies specific for thyroid hormone receptors would not be expected to cause elevated thyroid hormone levels.
CMI5 414; BI2 202-204

5. (D) Goodpasture's syndrome is a type II hypersensitivity disease in which IgG antibodies against the glomerular basement membrane (GBM) of the kidney deposit in a linear distribution, causing complement- and Fc receptor–mediated inflammation and subsequent nephritis. These anti-GBM antibodies cross-react with pulmonary alveolar basement membranes to produce the typical clinical scenario of pulmonary hemorrhages associated with renal failure. Note that the pathology here contrasts to that seen in glomerulonephritis caused by type III hypersensitivity diseases (e.g., systemic lupus erythematosus, poststreptococcal glomerulonephritis) in that deposits are linear and smooth (antibody) versus granular and coarse (antigen-antibody immune complex). Chronic allograft rejection more closely resembles a type IV hypersensitivity reaction. Graves' disease does not directly involve the kidney.
CMI5 415-417; BI2 205

6. (C) Hypersensitivity diseases are often categorized by numerical designation. Type III is immune complex disease. Type I is immediate hypersensitivity (allergic) disease. Type II is disease caused by antibodies binding to antigens in tissues. Type IV is T cell–mediated disease. There is no type V hypersensitivity.
CMI5 411-412; BI2 194-195

7. (C) A hallmark of immune complex–mediated disease is that pathologic features reflect the site of immune complex deposition and are not determined by the cellular source of the antigen. As such, immune complex–mediated diseases tend to be systemic, with little or no specificity for particular tissues. Immune complexes that cause disease may be composed of either self antigens or foreign antigens with bound antibodies. These complexes are produced during normal immune responses, but they cause disease only when they are produced in excessive amounts or are not efficiently cleared so that they become deposited in tissues. Small complexes are often not phagocytosed and tend to be deposited in vessels more readily than large complexes, which are usually cleared by phagocytes. Complexes containing cationic antigens bind tightly to negatively charged components of basement membranes of blood vessels and kidney glomeruli, typically producing long-lasting injury.
CMI5 414-417; BI2 201-202

8. (A) Pernicious anemia is caused by neutralizing autoantibodies specific for intrinsic factor, which is a secreted protein required for absorption of vitamin B_{12} in the gastrointestinal tract. The lack of vitamin B_{12} absorption leads to decreased erythropoiesis, with subsequent anemia. Autoimmune hemolytic anemia is caused by opsonizing antibodies specific for erythrocyte membrane antigens, leading to their destruction by phagocytes. Pemphigus vulgaris occurs when autoantibodies specific for epidermal cell intracellular junctions cause inflammatory disruption of the skin, leading to formation of skin vesicles. Acute rheumatic fever is caused by antistreptococcal cell wall antibodies that cross-react with myocardial antigens, leading to inflammation and damage to myocardium. Hyperacute allograft rejection is caused by antibodies specific for alloantigens on graft endothelial cells, leading to blood vessel wall damage and thrombosis.
CMI5 415; BI2 205

9. (D) The most specific diagnostic test for systemic lupus erythematosus (SLE) is the detection of antibodies against double-stranded DNA. Nevertheless, many different autoantibodies are found in patients with SLE, including other "antinuclear" antibodies. These include autoantibodies against ribonucleoproteins, histones, and nucleolar antigens. Other autoantibodies found in SLE bind erythrocytes and platelets. Antibodies specific for the glomerular basement membrane are typical of Goodpasture's syndrome, and anti-IgG antibodies, called "rheumatoid factor," are found in several autoimmune diseases, including rheumatoid arthritis.
CMI5 418; BI2 205-206

10. (E) Systemic lupus erythematosus (SLE) is a chronic, remitting and relapsing, multisystem disease that affects predominantly women, with an incidence of 1 in 700 in women between the ages of 20 and 60 years. Incidence increases to about 1 in 250 in African-American women. The female-to-male ratio is 10:1. Deficiencies of classical complement proteins, especially C2 or C4, are seen in about 10% of patients with SLE; abnormal complement levels may result in defective clearance of immune complexes. Individuals with the class II DR2 or DR3 HLA allele have a five-fold higher probability of developing SLE. In contrast, patients with defects in B cell maturation would typically have impaired antibody synthesis; thus it is unlikely that these patients would develop an autoimmune disease characterized by the production of autoantibodies.
CMI5 418; BI2 206

11. (B) Autoimmune hemolytic anemia is a type II hypersensitivity disease caused by autoantibodies against erythrocyte membrane proteins, such as Rh blood group antigens. Antibody-mediated opsonization and phagocytosis of erythrocytes leads to hemolysis and subsequent anemia. All other choices listed (poststreptococcal glomerulonephritis, the Arthus reaction, serum sickness, and systemic lupus erythematosus) are examples of immune complex–mediated, or type III hypersensitivity, diseases.
CMI5 413; BI2 203-205

12. (E) This individual developed a typical positive PPD skin test, which is a form of delayed-type hypersensitivity (DTH). DTH reactions are CD4$^+$ T cell–mediated immune responses to protein antigens, with subsequent tissue damage. The positive test implies a previous exposure to *Mycobacterium tuberculosis*, or perhaps prior vaccination with bacille Calmette-Guérin (BCG), which shares antigens with *Mycobacterium tuberculosis*. The previous exposure resulted in generation of circulating memory T cells specific for PPG antigens, which migrate into the dermal site of the PPD injection, become activated, and induce an inflammatory response. Anaphylaxis is a systemic form of immediate hypersensitivity in which mast cells with pre-bound IgE become activated by an allergen. Skin lesions of immediate hypersensitivity are usually hives (loose edema) that typically develop within minutes after exposure to the allergen. PPD is a foreign antigen preparation; thus the reaction to it that develops is not autoimmune. In antibody-dependent cellular cytotoxicity (ADCC), natural killer cells bind via Fc receptors to IgG-opsonized target cells, causing their lysis. ADCC is not typically induced by PPD skin tests.
CMI5 419-423; BI2 204-207

13. (B) Individuals who are positive for the class I HLA-B27 allele have a 90- to 100-fold greater chance of developing ankylosing spondylitis than do individuals lacking B27. This constitutes the strongest HLA disease association thus far described. Ankylosing spondylitis is an autoimmune disease affecting vertebral joints. Rheumatoid arthritis, pemphigus vulgaris, diabetes mellitus, and multiple sclerosis are more likely to develop in individuals with certain class II MHC alleles, but these carry much lower relative risks (between 4 and 25).
CMI5 426-427; BI2 172-174

14. (E) This boy has acute rheumatic fever (ARF), which is caused by an immune response initially specific for streptococcal antigens, but that cross-reacts with heart antigens. Molecular mimicry refers to the postulated mechanism whereby immune responses to a microbe containing antigens that cross-react with self antigens may trigger an autoimmune response. This autoimmune response may then persist, even in the absence of the inciting microbe. In ARF, antistreptococcal antibodies cross-react with myocardial proteins. Molecular sequencing has revealed numerous short stretches of homologies between streptococcal protein and myocardial proteins. The incidence of ARF has declined dramatically in the United States because of widespread use of antibiotics in the treatment of streptococcal infections before antibody responses can fully develop. Clonal anergy, peripheral tolerance, and central tolerance are mechanisms that would prevent immune responses to self antigens, and thus do not explain this patient's disease. Epitope spreading occurs when autoimmune reactions develop against several different epitopes of self-molecules during the evolution of an autoimmune disease; these epitopes are different from the initial targets of autoreactive lymphocytes at the outset of the disease. Epitope spreading is due to the release of self antigens from damaged tissue and from activation of tissue-based antigen-presenting cells by the local inflammatory response.
CMI5 429; BI2 205

15. (A) Rheumatoid factors are circulating antibodies, which may be IgM or IgG, that are reactive to the Fc portions of a patient's own IgG molecules. The presence of these autoantibodies is used as a diagnostic test for rheumatoid arthritis, a disease characterized by inflammation of the synovium and destruction of cartilage, particularly in the small joints of

the extremities. Both cell-mediated and humoral immune responses may contribute to the development of synovitis, although the nature of the antigen or antibodies involved is not known. Rheumatoid factors may participate in the formation of immune complexes, but their pathogenic role has not been established. Adaptive immune responses specific for pancreatic beta cells, streptococcal antigens, myelin basic protein, or acetylcholine receptors are typical of diabetes mellitus, acute rheumatic fever, multiple sclerosis, and myasthenia gravis, respectively, but not rheumatoid arthritis.
CMI5 423; BI2 204-207

16. (C) In rheumatoid arthritis, proinflammatory cytokines (interleukin [IL]-1, IL-8, tumor necrosis factor [TNF], interferon-[IFN]-γ) present in the synovium are thought to activate proteolytic enzymes, which mediate joint tissue destruction. Antagonists of TNF have proven beneficial for patients. Soluble TNF receptor and anti-TNF antibody, which bind free TNF, are now approved for treatment of the disease. In contrast, depleting IL-10 levels with a monoclonal antibody, activating RANK (a TNF receptor family member), increasing IL-1 levels, and increasing rheumatoid factor autoantibody levels are likely to exacerbate inflammation in the setting of rheumatoid arthritis.
CMI5 423; BI2 204-207

17. (E) Experimental autoimmune encephalomyelitis (EAE) is an animal model for multiple sclerosis, a central nervous system (CNS) demyelinating disease with an autoimmune etiology. EAE is induced by immunizing mice with antigens normally present in CNS myelin, in conjunction with adjuvant, which is necessary to stimulate the innate immune system. One to 2 weeks after immunization, animals develop an encephalomyelitis, characterized by perivascular infiltrates composed of lymphocytes and macrophages in the CNS white matter, followed by demyelination. Neurologic lesions can be mild and self-limited or chronic and relapsing, depending on the animal species and strain and antigen-adjuvant preparation used.
CMI5 422; BI2 207

18. (C) Various effector mechanisms are responsible for tissue injury in different autoimmune diseases. These include circulating autoantibodies, immune complexes, and autoreactive T lymphocytes. Autoimmune diseases may be either systemic (i.e., systemic lupus erythematosus) or organ specific (i.e., type 1 diabetes mellitus, multiple sclerosis). Among the genes associated with autoimmunity, the strongest associations are with MHC genes and usually with class II MHC genes (ankylosing spondylitis is an exception). In most cases of autoimmunity, infectious microorganisms are neither present in lesions nor detectable in patients when autoimmunity develops; this suggests that lesions in autoimmunity result not from the infectious agent directly but from host immune

responses that may be triggered by microbes. Finally, many autoimmune diseases show higher incidence in females than in males, although the reasons for this are not well understood.
CMI5 424-430; BI2 172-176

19. (D) The mainstay therapy for hypersensitivity diseases is anti-inflammatory drugs, particularly corticosteroids. In contrast, blocking CTLA-4, a negative regulator of T cell responses, is likely to exacerbate preexisting conditions of hypersensitivity. (The CTLA-4 knockout mouse displays a lymphoproliferative phenotype.) An inhibitor of VLA-4 would be effective in blocking leukocyte transmigration into tissues, thus exerting an anti-inflammatory effect. Cyclosporine is a potent immunosuppressive drug used to block T cell activation. Plasmapheresis has been used during exacerbations of antibody-mediated diseases to reduce circulating levels of antibodies or immune complexes.
CMI5 430; BI2 204-205

20. (D) This patient is in diabetic ketoacidosis, a serious complication of her previously undiagnosed insulin-dependent diabetes mellitus (type 1). Her insulin deficiency results from destruction of the insulin-producing beta cells of the islets of Langerhans in the pancreas. Several mechanisms may contribute to beta cell destruction. Prominent among these mechanisms are type IV (delayed-type) hypersensitivity reactions mediated by $CD4^+$ T_H1 cells reactive with islet antigens, and cytotoxic T-lymphocyte (CTL)-mediated lysis of islet cells.
CMI5 421; BI2 207

21. (B) This patient has pernicious anemia, a type II hypersensitivity disease in which autoantibodies against intrinsic factor of gastric parietal cells lead to neutralization of intrinsic factor, which is required for intestinal absorption of vitamin B_{12}. Deficiency in vitamin B_{12} leads to abnormal erythropoiesis with macrocytic anemia and hypersegmented neutrophils (as shown in the figure).
CMI5 415; BI2 202-205

22. (B) This condition, called erythroblastosis fetalis, is a severe form of hemolytic disease of the newborn that occurs when an Rh-negative mother gives birth to an infant who is Rh positive (since the father is homozygous Rh positive). In this disease, the mother produces IgG antibodies against Rh-positive cells to which she has been previously exposed (i.e., during the delivery of her first Rh-positive child). Because the mother's immune system recognizes Rh antigen as "foreign," she produced large amounts of anti-Rh antibody when she encountered the antigen during the second pregnancy. This antibody crossed the placenta and mediated cellular injury in the second infant. Therefore, this is an example of type II hypersensitivity. Note that the most commonly involved antigen in erythroblastosis fetalis is RhD.
CMI5 413

23. (A) This young man is in anaphylactic shock, secondary to systemic exposure to shellfish antigens, to which he produced IgE antibodies when he was previously exposed. This is a classic example of type I (immediate) hypersensitivity.
CMI5 412, 448; BI2 198-200

24. (D) This patient's clinical presentation is consistent with polyarteritis nodosa, a systemic immune complex–mediated disease that leads to vasculitis of small or medium-sized arteries, often in the kidney. The figure shows fibrinoid necrosis of a small artery, which results from immune complex–dependent complement activation and neutrophil recruitment. Polyarteritis nodosa is frequently associated with chronic hepatitis virus B (HBV) infection and deposition of HBV surface antigen–containing immune complexes. Although DNA and anti-DNA immune complexes do deposit in vessel walls and cause vasculitis in systemic lupus erythematosus (SLE), the negative antinuclear antibody test in this patient suggests that he does not have SLE. Neither anti-elastin antibody deposition nor CD4$^+$ T cell infiltration is typical of the polyarteritis nodosa syndrome. HBV does not infect cells in the vessel wall, only hepatocytes.
CMI5 417; BI2 206

25. (B) Poison ivy rash is a form of contact dermatitis in which there is a delayed-type hypersensitivity (DTH) reaction. The patient's vesicular dermatitis was evoked by his repeated exposure to urushiol, the antigenic component of poison ivy. Endothelial adhesion molecules and chemokines mediate the recruitment of previously sensitized CD4$^+$ T cells of the T_H1 subset and CD8$^+$ T cells, which secrete cytokines such as interferon-γ and activate macrophages. Activated macrophages release enzymes and reactive oxygen intermediates that damage cellular tissue. IgE-coated mast cells are involved in immediate hypersensitivity reactions, not DTH reactions.
CMI5 419, 420; BI2 204-206

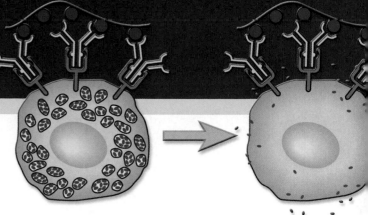

Chapter 19

Immediate Hypersensitivity

Cellular and Molecular Immunology, 5/E: Chapter 19—Immediate Hypersensitivity

Basic Immunology, 2/E: Chapter 11—Hypersensitivity Diseases

1. Which of the following is the most common disorder of immunity that affects 20% of all individuals in the United States?

   A. Atopy
   B. Diabetes mellitus
   C. Leukemia
   D. IgA deficiency
   E. Latent tuberculosis infection

2. All of the following are key mediators of immediate hypersensitivity reactions EXCEPT:

   A. Mast cells
   B. Basophils
   C. IgE
   D. Macrophages
   E. T_H2 cells

3. Immediate hypersensitivity differs from delayed-type hypersensitivity in which one of the following ways?

   A. Immediate hypersensitivity is a CD4⁺ T cell–mediated disease.
   B. Immediate hypersensitivity does not require previous exposure to an antigen.
   C. Immediate hypersensitivity does not involve inflammation.
   D. Immediate hypersensitivity is driven by cytokines such as interleukin (IL)-4, IL-5, and IL-13.
   E. Immediate hypersensitivity typically leads to granuloma formation.

4. Which of the following is required for the sensitization of mast cells?

A. Stimulation of IgD class switching in B cells
B. Multiple, repeated exposures to an allergen
C. Binding of antibody to high-affinity Fc receptors
D. Release of histamine and proteases
E. Antigen activation of T_H1 cells

5. Which one of the following is a property of mast cells but not of basophils?

   A. Mature in connective tissues, not in the bone marrow
   B. Express high levels of surface FcεRI receptors
   C. Have cytoplasmic granules containing histamine
   D. Cannot proliferate as mature cells
   E. Are recruited into tissues from the circulation

6. Which of the following favors the development of immediate hypersensitivity?

   A. T_H1 responses to antigens
   B. Infrequent exposure to antigens
   C. Strong innate immune responses to the antigens
   D. Production of interleukin-4 in response to antigens
   E. Nonprotein antigens

Questions 7-13

Match the definitions in questions 7-13 with the mast cell mediator (A-G) that most closely matches it.

   A. Histamine
   B. Tryptase
   C. Prostaglandin D_2
   D. Leukotriene C_4
   E. Platelet-activating factor
   F. Interleukin-5
   G. Tumor necrosis factor-α

7. Lipoxygenase-pathway product of arachidonic acid metabolism that causes prolonged bronchoconstriction, mucus secretion, and increased vascular permeability ( )

8. Soluble factor that promotes eosinophil maturation and activation ( )

9. Biogenic amine that transiently increases vascular permeability and smooth muscle contraction ( )

10. Cyclooxygenase-pathway product of arachidonic acid metabolism that causes vascular dilatation, smooth muscle contraction, and neutrophil chemotaxis ( )

11. Protein constituent of granules that contributes to tissue damage in immediate hypersensitivity reactions ( )

12. Soluble factor that promotes inflammation and late-phase reaction and activates endothelial expression of adhesion molecules critical for sequential neutrophilic infiltrate ( )

13. Membrane phospholipid derivative that causes bronchoconstriction, retraction of endothelial cells, and relaxation of vascular smooth muscle ( )

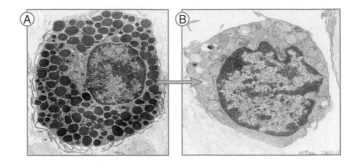

14. The figure above shows electron micrographs of a mast cell before (A) and after (B) activation by allergen. Which of the following statements most accurately describes the change in appearance of the mast cell and the mechanisms underlying the change?

   A. Many new cytoplasmic vacuoles are formed after activation, reflecting FcγR receptor-mediated enhancement of phagocytic activity.
   B. Secretory granules are depleted of their contents due to FcεR-crosslinking and generation of signals promoting granule exocytosis.
   C. There is an increase in rough endoplasmic reticulum after activation, reflecting enhanced production of IgE.
   D. There is accumulation of lipid-filled vacuoles, indicating uptake of oxidized lipoproteins.
   E. Lysosomes become depleted of their contents owing to the action of proteolytic enzymes induced by signaling from cross-linked FcεR.

15. A robust eosinophilic response is likely to be most protective in which of the following clinical scenarios?

   A. A 4-year-old Brazilian child with hookworm infection
   B. A 32-year-old florist with allergic rhinitis
   C. A 76-year-old Chinese man with latent tuberculosis
   D. A 13-year-old native of New York City with chronic asthma
   E. A 58-year-old woman with community-acquired lobar pneumonia

Questions 16 and 17

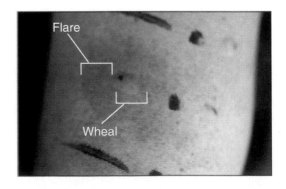

A 7-year-old girl with a history of chronic rhinitis visits an allergist's office for skin testing. She is given a series of intradermal injections and within 15 minutes develops a wheal and flare reaction (see figure at the bottom of the previous page) at the site of injection for *Dermatophagoides pteronyssinus* (house dust mite) allergen.

16. The wheal and flare reaction is characterized by all of the following EXCEPT:

    A. Cross-linking of IgE by antigen on sensitized mast cells
    B. Mast cell degranulation and release of histamine
    C. Vasodilation and vascular congestion
    D. Vascular leak and tissue edema
    E. Accumulation of inflammatory leukocytes

17. The patient has an older sister with eczema and an older brother with asthma. Which one of the following statements about these siblings is most likely true?

    A. Only the sister with rhinitis has a true allergy, as manifest by increased numbers of interleukin-4–secreting T cells in her circulation.
    B. Only the brother with asthma has an elevated eosinophil count.
    C. All three siblings will show higher than average plasma IgE levels.
    D. All three siblings have an autosomal dominant mutation for atopic disease.
    E. All three siblings should be treated with antihistamines.

18. The allergen associated with house dust mites is a cysteine protease. To act as an allergen, a molecule must be:

    A. A protein or hapten-protein conjugate
    B. An enzyme
    C. A polysaccharide
    D. A T cell–independent antigen
    E. A plant product

19. Which one of the following manifestations of atopy is due to repeated late phase-reactions to allergens?

    A. Hay fever
    B. Hives after eating shellfish
    C. Eczema
    D. Abdominal cramps and diarrhea after eating peanuts
    E. Anaphylaxis

Questions 20-22

An 18-year-old college student with a history of ragweed pollen allergy is brought to the university health care services complaining of shortness of breath, wheezing, angioedema, and red, itchy skin featuring prominent hives. An area on the back of his neck where he was stung by a bee 30 minutes ago while walking through campus, is warm, indurated, and tender. His breathing is now severely labored, and he is becoming cyanotic.

20. Which of the following does NOT accurately describe this patient's condition?

    A. Decrease in vascular tone
    B. Rise in blood pressure
    C. Laryngeal edema

D. Bronchoconstriction
E. Anaphylaxis

21. Based on the history and clinical presentation of this patient, which of the following statements is most likely true?

    A. The patient was at high risk for anaphylaxis because his mast cells were already coated with IgE specific for ragweed pollen allergens.
    B. The patient has a selective IgE deficiency.
    C. The patient was at high risk for an anaphylactic reaction to a bee sting because he had never been stung previously and therefore had not developed immunity to bee venom.
    D. The patient was previously stung by bees on several occasions but did not require medical attention.
    E. The patient had undergone chronic desensitization therapy throughout childhood.

22. Which of the following is the "gold standard" for acutely treating this patient?

    A. Intravenous corticosteroids
    B. High-dose oral antihistamines
    C. Parenteral epinephrine
    D. Intravenous anti-IgE antibody
    E. Inhaled sodium cromolyn

Questions 23 and 24

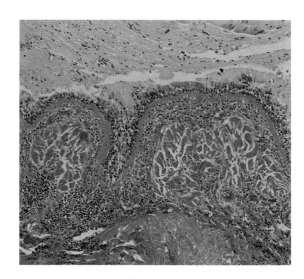

During a visit to the botanical gardens, a 26-year-old woman begins coughing, wheezing, and feeling short of breath. She has experienced similar episodes intermittently in the past, noting that they seem to recur more frequently when she is outside in the early morning. The image shown above is characteristic of chronic changes associated with her disease.

23. All of the following are prominent pathologic features of this tissue EXCEPT:

    A. Excess production of thick mucus
    B. Enlargement of air spaces distal to terminal bronchioles

C. Bronchial smooth muscle cell hypertrophy
D. Submucosal inflammatory infiltrate with eosinophils
E. Thickened basement membrane

24. Which of the following would be LEAST useful in treating this patient?

A. Oral antihistamines
B. Inhaled corticosteroids
C. Epinephrine
D. Inhaled sodium cromolyn
E. Inhaled theophylline

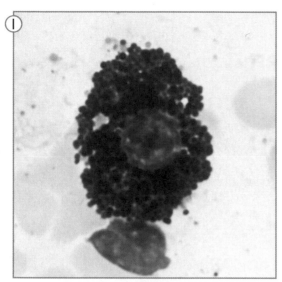

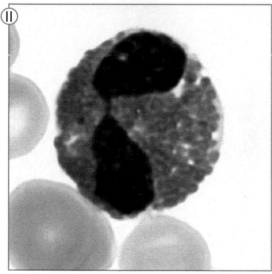

25. The figure above shows two blood cell types, labeled I and II, that play prominent roles in immediate hypersensitivity diseases. Which of the following statements about each of these cell types is most accurate?

A. I, granules contain major basic protein; II, granules contain histamine
B. I, activated by interleukin-5; II, resident in normal tissues

C. I, granules contain histamine; II, granules contain major basic protein
D. I, circulates in blood; II, cells proliferate when activated
E. I, resident in normal tissues; II, development stimulated by stem cell factor

Answers

1. **(A)** Atopy, or allergy, is the most common disorder of immunity and affects 20% of all individuals in the United States. Within this category, allergic rhinitis is perhaps the most common allergic disease and is a consequence of immediate hypersensitivity reactions to common allergens, such as plant pollen or house dust mites, localized to the upper respiratory tract by inhalation. Selective IgA deficiency is the most common known primary immunodeficiency.
CMI5 432; BI2 194

2. **(D)** The main cellular mediators of immediate hypersensitivity reactions are mast cells, basophils, and eosinophils. IgE antibody plays a major role in sensitizing these cellular mediators for subsequent activation. Activation of T_H2 cells is required for appropriate release of cytokines, such as interleukin (IL)-4 and IL-13, which stimulate IgE class switching in B cells. In contrast, macrophages are effector cells in delayed-type hypersensitivity reactions.
CMI5 432-434; BI2 196

3. **(D)** In contrast to delayed-type hypersensitivity (DTH), which is a T_H1-mediated disorder, immediate hypersensitivity is driven by cytokines, such as interleukin (IL)-4, IL-5, and IL-13, and is therefore a T_H2-mediated disorder. Note that both types of hypersensitivity reactions involve $CD4^+$ T cells (T_H1 vs. T_H2), although DTH also involves $CD8^+$ T cells. Importantly, both types of hypersensitivity reactions occur only after prior exposure to an antigen, and they are both characterized by inflammation. Granuloma formation, as a chronic response to persistent microbes, is a pathologic feature more typical of DTH than immediate hypersensitivity.
CMI5 434; BI2 197

4. **(C)** Sensitization of mast cells refers to the coating of mast cells with IgE (i.e., secreted IgE binding to FcεRI receptors on the surface of mast cells). In this way, mast cells are poised for immediate activation on subsequent antigen encounter. The sequence of events in immediate hypersensitivity reactions occurs as follows: (1) first exposure to allergen; (2) antigen activation of T_H2 cells and stimulation of IgE class switching in B cells; (3) production of IgE; (4) binding of IgE to FcεRI on mast cells; (5) repeated exposure to allergen; and (6) activation of mast cell with release of mediators, such as vasoactive amines and lipid mediators in the acute phase and cytokines in the late phase.
CMI5 433; BI2 196-198

5. (A) Mast cells differ from basophils in that they mature in connective tissues and do not circulate in blood. Mast cell progenitors in the bone marrow migrate to peripheral tissues as immature cells and undergo differentiation in situ. Mature mast cells are found throughout the body, predominantly near blood vessels and nerves and beneath epithelia; they are also present in lymphoid organs. Basophils can be thought of as the circulating counterpart of mast cells. Both mast cells and basophils express high surface levels of FcεRI, bind IgE, and can be triggered by antigen binding to the IgE. They both contain granules with histamine and protease mediators. In contrast to mature basophils, mature mast cells retain the ability to proliferate. Only basophils are recruited into tissues from blood circulation.
CMI5 437; BI2 198

6. (D) Interleukin (IL)-4 is an isotype switch factor for IgE synthesis by B cells, and IgE is essential for mast cell activation in allergic reactions. Therefore, the tendency to produce IL-4 in response to antigens, a hallmark of T_H2-type responses, favors development of immediate hypersensitivity disease. T_H1 responses, which are promoted by strong innate immune responses to microbial antigens, do not favor and may actually suppress the development of immediate hypersensitivity. Allergens must be protein antigens or haptenated-protein antigens, because IgE is a T cell–dependent antibody. In most cases, allergens are environmental antigens to which a person is repetitively and frequently exposed.
CMI5 434-435; BI2 194-196

7. (D) Leukotriene C_4 (LTC_4) is rapidly synthesized by the lipoxygenase pathway of arachidonic acid metabolism in activated mast cells. It is one component of a so-called slow-reacting substance of anaphylaxis, which also includes LTD_4 and LTE_4. These leukotrienes are major mediators of bronchoconstriction in allergic asthma.
CMI5 443-444; BI2 199

8. (F) Interleukin-5 is a cytokine synthesized by activated mast cells (as well as T_H2 cells) and promotes eosinophilia and eosinophilic inflammation, which are characteristic of chronic immediate hypersensitivity conditions.
CMI5 443-444; BI2 199

9. (A) Histamine, one of several biogenic amines in mast cell granules, is partly responsible for the rapid increases in vascular permeability causing wheals (or hives) and for the smooth muscle contraction in bronchi and intestines, causing some of the pulmonary and gastrointestinal symptoms of immediate hypersensitivity reactions.
CMI5 443; BI2 199

10. (C) Prostaglandin D_2 (PGD_2) is the major arachidonic acid product of the cyclooxygenase pathway in mast cells. PGD_2 causes vasodilation and bronchoconstriction, which contribute to the early signs and symptoms of immediate hypersensitivity reactions. It also is a chemoattractant for neutrophils, which accumulate in tissues as part of the late-phase inflammatory response to allergens.
CMI5 441; BI2 199

11. (B) Tryptase is a neutral serine protease stored in mast cell granules. When released into the extracellular matrix, this enzyme cleaves fibrinogen and activates collagenases, contributing to tissue damage.
CMI5 443-444; BI2 199

12. (G) When tumor necrosis factor-α is released during IgE-mediated mast cell activation, it activates endothelial expression of the adhesion molecules, accounting for subsequent infiltration of neutrophils. As such, it is critical for inflammation and the late-phase allergic reaction.
CMI5 444

13. (E) Platelet-activating factor (PAF) is synthesized after mast cell activation by acylation of a membrane phospholipid derivative; it acts on bronchial smooth muscle cells and endothelial cells. Genetic deficiency of an enzyme that inactivates PAF is associated with asthma.
CMI5 444

14. (B) The numerous dark, circular structures in the cytoplasm of the mast cell before activation are secretory granules, which are filled with histamine, proteoglycans, and enzymes. The contents of these granules are rapidly released after FcεR cross-linking by allergen, leaving empty membrane-bound vesicles. Mast cells are not phagocytic, do not synthesize IgE, and do not accumulate oxidized lipids. Although there are some proteolytic enzymes in the mast cell granules, these enzymes are not active until they are released from the cell.
CMI5 438-441; BI2 197-198

15 (A) Eosinophil-mediated killing of IgE-coated helminths by the process of antibody-dependent cell-mediated cytotoxicity (ADCC) is an effective defense against these organisms. Thus, the activities of interleukin (IL)-4, IL-5, and IL-13 in IgE production and eosinophil activation would contribute to a coordinated defense against hookworm infection. It has also been speculated that IgE-dependent mast cell activation in the gastrointestinal tract promotes the expulsion of parasites by increasing peristalsis and mucus secretion.
CMI5 444, 451

16. (E) The wheal and flare reaction that occurs in response to intradermal injection of an allergen is a manifestation of the early vascular changes that occur during immediate hypersensitivity reactions. It is caused by cross-linking of IgE by antigen on sensitized mast cells, mast cell degranulation and release of vasoactive mediators, vasodilation and vascular congestion, and vascular leak and tissue edema. In contrast, accumulation of leukocytic

infiltrate rich in eosinophils, neutrophils, and T cells occurs in the late-phase reaction, in response to chemotactic agents and cytokines released at the site of antigen.
CMI5 445-446; BI2 198

17. (C) Abnormally high levels of IgE and associated atopy often are found in families. Although family studies have shown clear autosomal transmission of atopy, the full inheritance pattern is probably multigenic. Although the target organ of atopic disease can vary within a family so that hay fever, asthma, and eczema can be present to various degrees in different family members, all atopic individuals within that family are likely to manifest higher than average plasma IgE levels. Similarly, all atopic individuals tend to have increased levels of interleukin (IL)-4–secreting T cells, and eosinophilia is associated with late-phase reactions of allergic responses. Because asthma and eczema have prominent late-phase inflammatory reactions, antihistamines are not indicated in the treatment of these diseases, whereas they are commonly used to treat rhinitis.
CMI5 447, 450-451; BI2 194

18. (A) An allergen is defined as an antigen that elicits an immediate hypersensitivity reaction. Because such reactions are dependent on T cells, allergens must be proteins, or chemicals bound to proteins, that induce IgE antibody responses in atopic individuals. Therefore, T cell–independent antigens, such as polysaccharides, are not allergens unless they form hapten-carrier conjugates (i.e., a small molecule drug conjugated to the amino acid residues of a self protein). Although many allergens, such as the cysteine protease of the house dust mite, are enzymes, the importance of enzymatic activity in triggering immediate hypersensitivity reactions is not known. Allergenic proteins are produced by animals, plants, and molds.
CMI5 434; BI2 194, 197

19. (C) Eczema and bronchial asthma are diseases in which there is chronic inflammation with accumulation of eosinophils and T_H2 cells without the vascular changes that are characteristic of the early-phase wheal and flare response. In these disorders, the cytokines that induced the chronic late-phase reaction are likely derived from T_H2 cells. Rhinitis, hives, and acute gastrointestinal symptoms are due to the rapid release of mast cell mediators, and anaphylaxis is an extreme systemic reaction to large quantities of these mediators.
CMI5 447

20. (B) This patient is experiencing anaphylactic shock, which refers to the dramatic drop in blood pressure that is occurring in the setting of a systemic, immediate, hypersensitivity reaction. The severe hypotension occurs secondary to decreased vascular tone and leakage of plasma caused by mast cell mediators in response to systemic presence of antigen (i.e., as introduced into the blood via a bee sting or absorption from the intestines). Cardiovas-cular collapse is accompanied by airway obstruction due to laryngeal edema and bronchoconstriction with outpouring of mucus.
CMI5 448; BI2 200

21. (D) Immediate hypersensitivity reactions occur only in the setting of previous exposure to an antigen. The most dramatic examples of the importance of repeated exposure to antigen in allergic disease are seen in cases of bee stings. Whereas protein toxins in insect venoms usually are not of concern on the first encounter (because an atopic individual has no preexisting specific IgE antibodies), an IgE response may occur after a single encounter with antigen so that a second sting by an insect of the same species may induce fatal anaphylaxis. Although an individual may be allergic to many different allergens, IgE specific for one allergen does not usually cross-react with another allergen. Thus, pollen-specific IgE will not contribute to the reaction against bee venom. Neither a patient with selective IgE deficiency nor a patient with chronic desensitization therapy (for bee venom) would be expected to mount such a robust immediate hypersensitivity reaction.
CMI5 434-435; BI2 194

22. (C) Epinephrine is the drug of choice for treating anaphylaxis because, when delivered systemically, it can rapidly reverse the bronchoconstrictive and vasodilatory effects of mast cell mediators. Patients presenting with severe bronchospasm and hypotension should receive intravenous epinephrine, whereas those with mild to moderate symptoms may be managed with intramuscular epinephrine. Epinephrine also improves cardiac output, further aiding survival from threatened circulatory collapse. Although antihistamines may also be beneficial as adjunct therapy in anaphylaxis, fatality rates are highest in patients in whom treatment with epinephrine is delayed. Inhaled sodium cromolyn and corticosteroids are used as a prophylactic therapy for allergic diseases such as asthma, but not as a treatment for acute allergic reactions.
CMI5 448; BI2 200

23. (B) This patient's clinical presentation is consistent with atopic bronchial asthma, which results from repeated immediate hypersensitivity reactions in the lungs with chronic late-phase reactions. The image shown is a cross-section of a bronchus from a patient with asthma. The diseased tissue shows excessive secretion of thick mucus, hypertrophied bronchial smooth muscle cells, prominent submucosal inflammatory infiltrate with eosinophils, and a thickened basement membrane. All of these changes contribute to bronchial obstruction and respiratory difficulties. In contrast, enlargement of air spaces distal to terminal bronchioles occurs in emphysema.
CMI5 448-449; BI2 200

24. (A) Current therapy for asthma has two major targets: (1) prevention and reversal of inflamma-

tion and (2) relaxation of airway smooth muscle. Corticosteroids inhibit the production of inflammatory cytokines. Sodium cromolyn is thought to antagonize IgE-induced release of mediators (i.e., mast cell degranulation). Epinephrine and theophylline promote bronchial smooth muscle cell relaxation, the former by activating adenylate cyclase and the latter by inhibiting the phosphodiesterase enzymes that degrade cyclic adenosine monophosphate (cAMP). By raising cAMP levels in mast cells, theophylline also acts to inhibit mast cell degranulation. In contrast, because histamine has little role in airway constriction, antihistamines are not useful in the treatment of asthma. Rather, because many antihistamines are also anticholinergics, these drugs may worsen airway obstruction by causing thickening of mucus secretions and should therefore be avoided in patients with asthma.

CMI5 449-450; BI2 200

25. (C) The two cells are a basophil (I) and an eosinophil (II). Basophils, which are stained dark purple in many histologic preparations, contain granules with similar contents to mast cell granules, including histamine and other mediators, but not major basic protein (MBP). Eosinophil granules, which appear red in most histologic preparations, do not contain histamine, but do contain MBP, a cationic protein toxic to helminths and capable of tissue damage. Basophils develop in the bone marrow, circulate in the blood, unlike mast cells, and are recruited in some sites of inflammation. Basophils are not resident in normal tissues. Eosinophils develop in the bone marrow in response to interleukin-5, circulate in the blood, and are recruited to inflammatory sites in tissues and release granule contents upon activation. Stem cell factor promotes mast cell development, but not basophil or eosinophil development.

CMI5 439-445; BI2 197-198

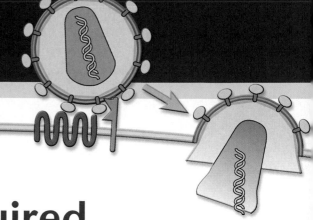

Chapter 20

Congenital and Acquired Immunodeficiencies

Cellular and Molecular Immunology, 5/E: Chapter 20—Congenital and Acquired Immunodeficiencies

Basic Immunology, 2/E: Chapter 12—Congenital and Acquired Immunodeficiencies

1. All of the following may result in an acquired immunodeficiency EXCEPT:

   A. Malnutrition
   B. Treatment with corticosteroids
   C. Disseminated cancer
   D. Inherited defect in B cell maturation
   E. Infection with human immunodeficiency virus (HIV)

2. Which one of the following is typically NOT associated with T cell immunodeficiencies?

   A. Cancer
   B. Viral infection
   C. Autoimmunity
   D. Infection with intracellular microbes
   E. Infection with pyogenic bacteria

Questions 3 and 4

3. In which of the following conditions would you be LEAST likely to see a robust delayed-type hypersensitivity (DTH) response to a *Candida* antigen skin challenge?

   A. X-linked agammaglobulinemia
   B. DiGeorge syndrome
   C. Selective IgA deficiency
   D. Common variable immunodeficiency
   E. Chronic granulomatous disease

4. A generalized deficiency in the ability to mount delayed-type hypersensitivity (DTH) responses, as described in question 3, is called:

   A. Clinical atopy
   B. Clonal ignorance

C. Clinical anergy

D. Clonal deletion

E. Seroconversion

Questions 5-9

A 7-month-old boy is evaluated in the clinic for recurrent bacterial infections. His tonsils are not visible on physical examination. Serum immunoglobulin A (IgA) and IgG levels are markedly decreased, and serum IgM levels are slightly below normal.

5. Based on the findings described, which one of the following should be excluded from the differential diagnosis?

   A. X-linked agammaglobulinemia

   B. X-linked severe combined immunodeficiency disease (X-linked SCID)

   C. Common variable immunodeficiency

   D. X-linked hyper-IgM syndrome

   E. Adenosine deaminase deficiency (ADA)

6. Careful examination of this infant reveals white plaques along the buccal mucosa, palate, and tongue, consistent with oral candidiasis (thrush). Analysis of blood cells reveals normal numbers of B cells and very few CD3+ cells. In addition, maternally-derived T cells, as determined by HLA typing, are detectable. The infant's mother reports that two of her three brothers died of infection as young children. Collectively, this presentation and history are most consistent with which of the following disorders?

   A. X-linked agammaglobulinemia

   B. X-linked severe combined immunodeficiency disease (X-linked SCID)

   C. Common variable immunodeficiency

   D. X-linked hyper-IgM syndrome

   E. Adenosine deaminase deficiency (ADA)

7. Based on this family's history and clinical presentation, a mutation in which of the following genes is most likely to be found in this patient?

   A. *JAK3* kinase

   B. Adenosine deaminase

   C. Common cytokine receptor γ chain

   D. *RAG2*

   E. Purine nucleoside phosphorylase

8. The gene identified in this patient plays a critical role in receptor binding to all of the following ligands EXCEPT:

   A. Interleukin (IL)-2

   B. IL-4

   C. IL-7

   D. IL-12

   E. IL-15

9 This infant should NOT be given the measles-mumps-rubella (MMR) vaccination because:

   A. The vaccine would have no effect because he is not susceptible to infection with measles, mumps, or rubella.

   B. The vaccine would have no effect because he cannot mount an appropriate humoral response.

   C. The vaccine could be dangerous because he is predisposed to develop a type I hypersensitivity response to the MMR vaccine.

   D. The vaccine could be dangerous because vaccination with MMR would put him at risk for developing a fatal infection.

   E. Vaccination with MMR is not contraindicated in his case and should be performed to prevent future infection.

10. A lymph node biopsy from a young boy with X-linked agammaglobulinemia is expected to show which of the following histologic features?

    A. Marked perivascular lymphocytic infiltrate

    B. Abundant polymorphonuclear inflammation

    C. Reduced follicles and germinal centers

    D. Nearly absent parafollicular cortical regions

    E. Enlarged follicles

11. Which of the following is the most common known primary immunodeficiency with a prevalence of 1 in 700 white individuals?

    A. X-linked agammaglobulinemia

    B. Selective IgA deficiency

    C. Common variable immunodeficiency

    D. Chronic granulomatous disease

    E. Chédiak-Higashi syndrome

Questions 12-16

Match each of the following descriptions in questions 12-16 with the appropriate disease (A-G).

   A. X-linked agammaglobulinemia

   B. X-linked hyper-IgM syndrome

   C. X-linked lymphoproliferative syndrome

   D. Bare lymphocyte syndrome

   E. Chronic granulomatous disease (CGD)

   F. Leukocyte adhesion deficiency-1 (LAD-1)

   G. Leukocyte adhesion deficiency-2 (LAD-2)

12. Impaired CD4+ T cell development and activation due to lack of class II MHC expression, resulting in defective cell-mediated immunity and impaired T cell–dependent humoral immunity (   )

13. Defect in leukocyte adhesion-dependent functions, resulting from mutations in the gene encoding the CD18 integrin β chain, and leading to recurrent bacterial and fungal infections (   )

14. Defect in lymphocyte activation due to mutations in the gene encoding the SAP adapter protein required for inhibition of signaling by the SLAM molecule. Lack of SAP results in uncontrolled B cell proliferation, hypogammaglobulinemia, and B cell lymphoma in the setting of Epstein-Barr virus (EBV) infection. (   )

15. Defect in B cell maturation at the pre-B cell stage caused by mutations in the gene encoding the B cell tyrosine kinase (Btk), resulting in undetectable levels of serum Ig (   )

16. Defect in phagocyte microbicidal activity as a result of defective production of reactive oxygen intermediates, most commonly from a mutation in the gene encoding cytochrome b_{558} (   )

17. An 18-month-old girl is brought to the pediatrician because of recurrent upper respiratory tract infections. She has a fever, labored breathing, and a dry cough. Diagnostic tests confirm infection with *Pneumocystis jaroveci*. Serum studies are remarkable for negligible levels of IgG and IgA in the presence of high concentrations of IgM. The family history is unremarkable; in particular, the patient's three older brothers are in excellent health. This patient most likely carries a mutation in which of the following molecules?

    A. CD18
    B. CD40L
    C. ZAP-70
    D. B7
    E. CD40

Questions 18 and 19

A 3-year-old boy is taken to the pediatrician because of a nosebleed (epistaxis). He has a history of severe, recurrent sinopulmonary infection. Physical examination is remarkable for dry, red patches of skin (eczema) and multiple petechiae (tiny hemorrhagic spots). Laboratory findings include thrombocytopenia and reduced IgM levels. The boy's maternal uncle died of bleeding complications after an emergency appendectomy.

18. Which of the following is the most likely diagnosis?

    A. Reticular dysgenesis
    B. Wiskott-Aldrich syndrome (WAS)
    C. Chédiak-Higashi syndrome
    D. Ataxia-telangiectasia
    E. DiGeorge syndrome

19. Which of the following represents a curative therapy currently available for this patient?

    A. Passive immunization with gamma globulin
    B. Bone marrow transplantation
    C. Treatment with corticosteroids
    D. Enzyme replacement
    E. Gene therapy

20. Which of the following patients is particularly susceptible to infection with *Streptococcus pneumoniae*, an encapsulated bacterium?

    A. A 23-year-old man with malaise, rash, and diffuse lymphadenopathy consistent with early infection with human immunodeficiency virus
    B. A 54-year-old woman receiving local corticosteroid injections for knee pain
    C. A 35-year-old man with Hodgkin's disease and a deficient delayed-type hypersensitivity (DTH) response to *Candida* antigen
    D. A 6-year-old boy with sickle cell anemia who had a splenectomy
    E. A 77-year-old woman on chronic renal dialysis and a strict low-protein diet

21. Human immunodeficiency virus (HIV) is NOT a:

    A. Herpesvirus
    B. RNA virus
    C. Enveloped virus
    D. Retrovirus
    E. Lentivirus

22. All of the following have a direct role in mediating human immunodeficiency virus (HIV) entry into susceptible cells EXCEPT:

    A. CD4
    B. MHC class I
    C. CCR5
    D. CXCR4
    E. Env

Questions 23-26

Match the descriptions in questions 23-26 with the associated HIV gene (A-G).

    A. *env*
    B. *gag*
    C. *nef*
    D. *pol*
    E. *rev*
    F. *tat*
    G. *vif*

23. Late gene product; encodes reverse transcriptase, integrase, protease (   )

24. Early gene product; required for elongation of viral transcripts (   )

25. Late gene product; encodes coat proteins gp120 and gp41 (   )

26. Late gene product; encodes nucleocapsid core and matrix proteins (   )

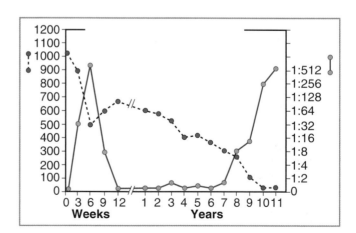

27. The purple (I) and yellow (II) lines in the chart above represent two different parameters measured in the blood of an individual infected with human immunodeficiency virus (HIV) over time. Which of the following properly identifies these parameters?

A. I, anti-p24 antibody concentration; II, CD4:CD8 T cell ratio

B. I, virion titer; II, CD4⁺ T cell count

C. I, CD4⁺ T cell count; II, virion titer

D. I, CD8⁺ T cell count; II, CD4:CD8 T cell ratio

E. I, virions/μL; II, CD8:CD4 T cell ratio

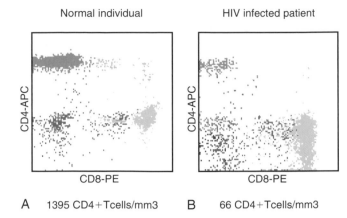

Questions 28 and 29

28. A 36-year-old man with a history of a positive anti-HIV antibody test comes to the clinic with fever, sore throat, nonproductive cough, and weight loss. The patient has a high serum viral load, quantified by reverse transcriptase polymerase chain reaction (RT-PCR). This patient is LEAST likely to suffer from which of the following?

A. Kaposi's sarcoma
B. *Pneumocystis jaroveci* pneumonia
C. Encephalopathy
D. Cachexia
E. T cell lymphoma

29. This patient has had a partner for 8 years with whom he has frequently engaged in unprotected sexual intercourse. The partner is a healthy 29-year-old man who is HIV negative. The partner's relative "resistance" to HIV infection may be due to a loss-of-function mutation in which of the following proteins?

A. CD4
B. CD8
C. CCR5
D. Tumor necrosis factor (TNF)
E. NF-κB

30. Which of the following strategies would be expected to be LEAST effective in the prevention and/or treatment of AIDS?

A. Abstinence from intravenous drug use and unprotected sexual intercourse
B. Vaccination with recombinant gp120 protein to elicit antibodies against HIV
C. Chronic administration of a single non-nucleoside reverse transcriptase inhibitor
D. Chronic administration of highly active anti-retroviral therapy (HAART)
E. Short-term administration of a nucleoside reverse transcriptase inhibitor to HIV-positive pregnant women during labor and the months preceding delivery

31. A 28-year-old man with a history of intravenous drug abuse and a positive test for anti-HIV antibodies 7 years ago comes to the emergency department complaining of shortness of breath. A chest radiograph shows bilateral pulmonary air space infiltrates, and a sputum sample is positive for *Pneumocystis jaroveci*. A blood sample is taken and analyzed for CD4⁺ and CD8⁺ T cells by flow cytometry. The results are shown in the figure above. Based on the flow cytometry data and the clinical history, which of the following statements about this patient is most likely true?

A. After treatment of the current respiratory problem, the patient may remain relatively healthy for several more years before developing AIDS.
B. The patient is likely to successfully control the current pulmonary infection because of a strong CD8⁺ T cell response.
C. The patient is unlikely to have any detectable HIV virions in his blood.
D. The patient's HIV infection has been successfully controlled by therapy until now.
E. The patient is now at risk for multiple opportunistic infections, neoplasia, and wasting, even if the current infection responds to therapy.

Answers

1. (D) An inherited defect in B cell maturation is, by definition, a primary immunodeficiency, not an acquired immunodeficiency. In particular, abnormalities in B lymphocyte development and function result in deficient antibody production and increased susceptibility to infection by extracellular microbes. In contrast, malnutrition, treatment with corticosteroids, disseminated cancer, and infection with human immunodeficiency virus (HIV) would all result in acquired, or secondary, immunodeficiencies. Administration of corticosteroids to intentionally create an immunosuppressive state, such as in the treatment of inflammatory diseases or the prevention of tissue allograft rejection, is referred to as iatrogenic immunosuppression.
CMI5 453; BI2 209, 216

2. (E) B cell, not T cell, immunodeficiencies are associated with increased incidence of infection with pyogenic bacteria. In contrast, increased incidence of cancer is most often seen in T cell immunodeficiencies, because T cells are critical for surveillance against oncogenic viruses and the tumors they cause. Defects in cell-mediated immunity lead to infection by viruses and other intracellular microbes. Interestingly, certain immunodeficiencies are associated with increased incidence of autoimmunity; the mechanism for this phenomenon may reflect a deficiency of regulatory T cells that normally serve to maintain self-tolerance.
CMI5 453-454

3. (B) A delayed-type hypersensitivity (DTH) response is an immune reaction in which T cell–dependent macrophage activation and inflammation cause tissue injury. The severity of the reaction to the subcutaneous injection of antigen is used as an assay for cell-mediated immunity. A deficient cutaneous DTH response to common microbial antigens, such as *Candida* antigens, suggests a T cell immunodeficiency. DiGeorge syndrome is a selective T cell deficiency caused by a congenital malformation that results in defective development of the thymus and other embryologically associated structures. In contrast, X-linked agammaglobulinemia, selective IgA deficiency, and common variable immunodeficiency are B cell immunodeficiencies. Chronic granulomatous disease is a congenital disorder in which phagocytes cannot generate free radicals and kill ingested microbes.
CMI5 308, 454; BI2 210, 213

4. (C) A generalized deficiency in delayed-type hypersensitivity (DTH) responses is called clinical anergy. Note that clonal (or lymphocyte) anergy refers to the failure of clones of T or B cells to react to antigen. Anergy may be a mechanism of maintaining immunologic tolerance to self. Atopy refers to allergic disease. Clonal ignorance and clonal deletion are mechanisms of tolerance to antigens. Seroconversion refers to the appearance in the serum of antibodies specific for a particular antigen after infection or immunization.
CMI5 463

5. (D) The infant's presentation suggests an underlying congenital immunodeficiency. X-linked hyper-IgM syndrome is characterized by failure of the B cell heavy chain to undergo switching from the IgM isotype, excess levels of IgM antibody (hyper-IgM) are often detectable in sera from patients. Thus, these patients are predisposed to both pyogenic and protozoal infections. X-linked severe combined immunodeficiency disease (SCID) and adenosine deaminase (ADA) deficiency are both forms of SCID and will present as very low levels of T cell–dependent Ig isotypes (IgG and IgA), as well as defects in cell-mediated immunity. X-linked agammaglobulinemia is a defect in B cell maturation and will present as very low levels of all antibody isotypes. Common variable immunodeficiency includes a number of defects in B cell differentiation into antibody-secreting cells and may present as pan-Ig deficiency.
CMI5 454-460; BI2 213

6. (B) Oral candidiasis suggests impaired cell-mediated immunity, and a low number of CD3+ cells implies a defect in T cell maturation. The persistence of transplacentally-derived maternal T cells also implies a lack of cell-mediated immunity in the child, because these T cells will express MHC alleles not inherited by the child and should therefore be recognized and eliminated by him. The information presented in Question 5 indicates that the infant also exhibits signs and symptoms consistent with humoral immunodeficiency. This pattern of severe combined immunodeficiency (SCID) can be caused by both X-linked SCID and by adenosine deaminase (ADA) deficiency, which is an autosomal recessive disease. The patient's family history is highly suggestive of an X-linked recessive pattern of inheritance: the infant is male, and two of his maternal uncles died in childhood of possible infections. His clinical picture is therefore most consistent with X-linked SCID, the predominant cause of severe combined immunodeficiency, occurring in approximately 50% of cases.
CMI5 455-456; BI2 211

7. (C) X-linked severe combined immunodeficiency disease (SCID) results from mutations in the gene encoding the cytokine receptor common γ chain. Mutations in any of the other genes listed (*JAK3* kinase, adenosine deaminase, *RAG2*, or purine nucleoside phosphorylase) cause severe combined immunodeficiency syndrome with autosomal recessive patterns of inheritance.
CMI5 455-457; BI2 211

8. (D) The common γ chain protein is shared by receptors for the interleukins (IL)-2, IL-4, IL-7, IL-9, and IL-15.
CMI5 455; BI2 211

9. (D) The measles-mumps-rubella (MMR) preparation is a live, attenuated viral vaccine. The great advantage of this type of vaccine is that it elicits all the innate and adaptive immune responses that would naturally arise as a result of infection with the pathogenic viruses. As such, it is the ideal way of inducing protective immunity. Nevertheless, whereas the viruses in the vaccine have been manipulated in the laboratory to become nonpathogenic in individuals with intact immune systems, they can potentially cause disease in vulnerable patients, such as those with congenital immunodeficiencies. As such, administration of the MMR vaccine is contraindicated in an infant with X-linked severe combined immunodeficiency disease (SCID), because vaccination would place him at risk of developing fatal infection.
CMI5 363, 455-456; BI2 159

10. (C) X-linked agammaglobulinemia, or Bruton's agammaglobulinemia, is an immunodeficiency disease characterized by a block in early B cell maturation and absence of serum Ig. As in other B cell deficiencies, morphology of lymphoid tissues is most remarkable for absent or reduced follicles and germinal centers (i.e., the B cell zones). In contrast, T cell deficiencies usually do not affect follicle size, but follicles will lack germinal centers and there may be reduced parafollicular cortical regions (i.e., the T cell zones).
CMI5 454; BI2 210, 213

11. (B) Selective IgA deficiency is the most common (known) primary immunodeficiency and is believed to affect approximately 1 in 700 white individuals. Most cases occur sporadically. Whereas many patients show no clinical symptoms, others experience occasional respiratory infections and diarrhea. In rare cases, patients present with severe, recurrent infections that lead to permanent intestinal and airway damage, with other associated autoimmune disorders.
CMI5 458; BI2 213

12. (D) Bare lymphocyte syndrome is a form of severe combined immunodeficiency disease (SCID) caused by inherited mutations in genes encoding factors required for class II MHC transcription. The absence of class II MHC in the thymus results in a lack of positive selection and maturation of CD4$^+$ T cells.
CMI5 460; BI2 215

13. (F) LAD-1 is a rare disorder in which integrins with the CD18 chain, such as LFA-1, are not expressed. Migration and function of neutrophils, monocytes, and lymphocytes are all impaired.
CMI5 462; BI2 215

14. (C) X-linked lymphoproliferative syndrome is characterized by a severe CD8$^+$ T cell response to Epstein-Barr virus (EBV), the virus that causes infectious mononucleosis. In a way, this is an example of a lethal exaggerated response to an infection, rather than a true immunodeficiency.
CMI5 460

15. (A) Btk is required for pre-B cell receptor signaling and maturation from pre-B to immature B cells. In females carrying the mutated Btk gene on one X chromosome, the B cells that do mature have all inactivated the X chromosome carrying the mutant allele; thus, these individuals do not show a clinical phenotype. This disease is effectively controlled by injections of pooled gamma globulin.
CMI5 457; BI2 213

16. (E) Chronic granulomatous disease (CGD) is a disorder of the innate immune system. The failure to generate reactive oxygen intermediates (free radicals) leads to persistent intracellular bacterial infections, with chronic T cell stimulation of macrophages and development of granulomas.
CMI5 461-462; BI2 215

17. (E) The patient's clinical presentation is consistent with hyper-IgM syndrome, which is associated with defective switching of B cells to the IgG and IgA isotypes. Whereas IgG and IgA levels may be undetectable in blood, IgM titers are often concomitantly increased. The molecular defect arises from impaired interaction between CD40L on T cells and CD40 on B cells; thus T cells cannot provide B cells with the stimulatory signals required for heavy chain isotype switching. Patients also show defects in cell-mediated immunity, since CD40 ligand-receptor interactions are important for T cell–dependent activation of macrophages. These patients therefore are particularly susceptible to infection by the opportunistic intracellular microbe *Pneumocystis jaroveci*. Because this patient is a girl with healthy brothers and maternal uncles, she is unlikely to have X-linked hyper-IgM syndrome, which is caused by mutations in CD40L (expressed on T cells). Rather, she is more likely to carry a rare mutation in CD40 (expressed on B cells), which results in hyper-IgM syndrome with an autosomal recessive pattern of inheritance.
CMI5 459; BI2 213

18. (B) This patient most likely has Wiskott-Aldrich syndrome (WAS), an X-linked immunodeficiency disease involving multiple organ systems. It is characterized by eczema, a low platelet count (thrombocytopenia), and susceptibility to bacterial infection. Patients with WAS have a mutation in a gene that encodes a cytoplasmic protein expressed exclusively in bone marrow–derived cells. This protein interacts both with adapter molecules, such as Grb-2, and with small G proteins of the Rho family that regulate the actin cytoskeleton. Expression of many cell surface glycoproteins on lymphocytes, macrophages, neutrophils, and platelets is also reduced. All of these changes likely interfere with trafficking of leukocytes to sites of inflammation.
CMI5 461; BI2 215

19. (B) Bone marrow transplantation, in which the immunodeficient patient's marrow is reconstituted with functional immune cell precursors, is the only curative therapy currently available for Wiskott-

Aldrich syndrome (WAS) or severe combined immunodeficiency disease (SCID). In particular, bone marrow transplantation from HLA-matched sibling donors have had very high success rates. Passive immunization with gamma globulin only prevents or minimizes future infections. Corticosteroids, which exhibit immunosuppressive effects, are contraindicated in already immunodeficient patients. Enzyme replacement therapy has shown transient benefit in patients with well-characterized enzyme deficiencies, including adenosine deaminase (ADA) and purine nucleoside phosphorylase (PNP) deficiencies. Gene therapy to restore the affected *WASP* gene in WAS syndrome, although potentially curable, remains a distant clinical goal.
CMI5 462-463

20. (D) A patient who has undergone splenectomy, or surgical removal of the spleen, is particularly susceptible to infection with encapsulated bacteria such as *Streptococcus pneumoniae*. This occurs because the spleen is a major site for production of antibodies specific for T cell–independent polysaccharide antigens found in bacterial capsules. In addition, the spleen is important for the phagocytic clearance of opsonized blood-borne microbes.
CMI5 464; BI2 216-217

21. (A) Human immunodeficiency virus (HIV) is a member of the Lentivirus family of retroviruses. Retroviruses are all enveloped RNA viruses. Herpesviruses are a family of DNA viruses, many of which cause human diseases, including Epstein-Barr virus, cytomegalovirus, herpes simplex virus, and varicella.
CMI5 464; BI2 217

22. (B) Human immunodeficiency virus (HIV) entry into host cells occurs when gp120, a glycoprotein expressed on the HIV envelope, binds to CD4 expressed on host T cells. This induces a conformational change in gp120, promoting its binding to a chemokine coreceptor, such as CCR5 or CXCR4, on host cells. A conformational change in gp41, another glycoprotein expressed on the HIV envelope, exposes a fusion peptide, which inserts into the T cell membrane, allowing fusion of viral and cell membranes and subsequent infection of the host cell. Thus, CD4, CCR5, and CXCR4 are host proteins that are directly involved in mediating HIV entry into susceptible T cells, macrophages, and dendritic cells. Env, the HIV envelope glycoprotein that includes gp120 and gp41, is also directly involved in mediating HIV entry into host cells. In contrast, MHC class I molecules do not have a direct role in this process.
CMI5 465-467; BI2 217-219

23. (D) The *pol* (polymerase) gene encodes the enzymes required for viral genome integration into the host cell genome (reverse transcriptase, integrase, protease, ribonuclease). Integrase is critical for processing viral proteins.
CMI5 465, 468; BI2 218

24. (F) *tat* is essential for HIV gene expression and serves to enhance the formation of full length RNA transcripts from the proviral DNA.
CMI5 465, 468; BI2 218

25. (A) The *env* gene encodes a precursor polypeptide that is cleaved to form the gp120 and gp41 glycoproteins found in the HIV envelope; gp120 and gp41 are involved in CD4 binding and membrane fusion, respectively.
CMI5 465, 468; BI2 218

26. (B) The *gag* gene encodes the p24 (capsid) and p17 (matrix) proteins required for packaging the human immunodeficiency virus (HIV) genome. Antibodies against these proteins are used as diagnostic markers of HIV infection.
CMI5 465, 468; BI2 218

27. (C) Plasma virion concentration rises and falls rapidly during the first few weeks of infection with human immunodeficiency virus (HIV) and then remains very low for several years, detectable only with sensitive reverse transcriptase polymerase chain reaction (RT-PCR) analysis. During this clinical latency period, there is active viral replication in lymphoid tissues. Eventually, when the immune system is severely damaged, the viral titer rises again to very high levels. (The virion concentration is indicated by a dilution titer.) The CD4+ T cell count may drop slightly early after infection, but then there is a gradual decline over many years, reflecting the chronic destruction of lymphoid tissues by viral infection. Opportunistic infections begin to occur when the CD4+ count drops below 200 cells/mm^3.
CMI5 465, 470, 473; BI2 221

28. (E) Based on this patient's severe clinical presentation, his human immunodeficiency virus (HIV) disease has already progressed to AIDS. This final, almost invariably lethal phase is characterized by essentially complete destruction of peripheral lymphoid tissue, such that the blood CD4+ T cell count drops below 200 cells/mm^3 and HIV viremia increases dramatically as viral replication proceeds unchecked. As a result, patients with AIDS often suffer from (1) multiple opportunistic infections, including *Pneumocystis jaroveci* pneumonia and oral candidiasis; (2) tumors such as Kaposi's sarcoma; (3) central nervous system degeneration (encephalopathy); (4) kidney failure (nephropathy); and (5) generalized wasting (cachexia). Although AIDS patients are at risk for B cell lymphomas, T cell lymphomas are not a typical complication. HIV does not act as an oncovirus.
CMI5 465, 468; BI2 220, 222

29. (C) CCR5 is one of the coreceptors required for human immunodeficiency virus (HIV) infection in vivo. Individuals who do not express the normal CCR5 chemokine receptor because of genetic mutations are resistant to HIV infection despite repeated exposure. This finding underscores the importance of CCR5 as a cofactor in mediating HIV viral fusion with the host cell membrane. Interest-

ingly, many HIV-infected individuals transition from the production of virus that uses CCR5 (macrophage-tropic virus), early in the disease to virus that binds to CXCR4, another chemokine receptor (T cell line tropic virus) late in the disease. A loss-of-function mutation in CD4 would also "protect" an individual from HIV infection, but because this individual would also lack CD4$^+$ T cells, he would not present as a healthy 29-year-old man. **CMI5 465, 468**

30. **(B)** Vaccination with an HIV envelope-derived protein would induce a largely humoral response, but this has been shown to be ineffective in preventing disease. In particular, antibody responses to a variety of HIV antigens are detectable within 6 to 9 weeks in the natural course of HIV infection, but there is little evidence that these antibodies have any beneficial effect in controlling infection. Rather, it is likely that an effective vaccine will have to stimulate both humoral and cell-mediated responses to viral antigens critical for the life cycle. In the future, this may be safely accomplished with the use of live recombinant non-HIV viral vectors carrying HIV genes. Protection from contact with HIV through abstinence from risky behavior is the most effective means of preventing infection. Chronic administration of HAART (highly active antiretroviral therapy), a triple-drug therapy combining a protease inhibitor with two non-nucleoside reverse transcriptase inhibitors, has proven to be remarkably effective in reducing plasma viral RNA to undetectable levels in treated patients for several years. Note that single drug therapy against HIV is less effective than HAART because the virus has an extremely high mutation rate and can more readily develop resistance to the drug. Also, even short-term administration of a nucleoside reverse transcriptase inhibitor, such as zidovudine (AZT), to HIV-positive pregnant women has been shown to remarkably decrease rates of transmission to newborns. **CMI5 465, 468; BI2 222-223**

31. **(E)** The flow cytometry finding of a CD4$^+$ T cell count well below 200 cells/mm^3 and the current infection with *Pneumocystis jaroveci* indicate that the patient has frank AIDS and will be at a high risk of acquiring other infections, neoplasia (e.g., Kaposi's sarcoma or B cell lymphoma), cachexia, and AIDS encephalopathy. Treatment of the current pneumonia with antibiotics will not prevent these other complications from arising in the near future. The flow cytometry data show a high CD8$^+$:CD4$^+$ ratio, but this does not mean there is an effective CD8$^+$ T cell response to *Pneumocystis jaroveci*. In contrast, it reflects a low CD4$^+$ cell count, and the CD8$^+$ T cell response may be impaired because of lack of adequate help. Human immunodeficiency virus (HIV) viremia rises sharply when the CD4$^+$ T cell count drops as low as this patient's, because lymphoid tissues are severely damaged and cannot maintain a reservoir of unreleased virus. The advanced stage of this patient's HIV disease implies antiviral therapy has not been successful. **CMI5 468-471; BI2 220-222, 298-299**

Glossary

αβ T cell receptor (αβ TCR). The most common form of TCR, expressed on both CD4$^+$ and CD8$^+$ T cells. The αβ TCR recognizes peptide antigen bound to an MHC molecule. Both α and β chains contain highly variable (V) regions that together form the antigen-binding site as well as constant (C) regions. TCR V and C regions are structurally homologous to the V and C regions of Ig molecules.

ABO blood group antigens. Glycosphingolipid antigens present on many cell types, including red blood cells. These antigens differ between different individuals, depending on inherited alleles encoding the enzymes required for synthesis of the antigens. The ABO antigens act as alloantigens responsible for blood transfusion reactions and hyperacute rejection of allografts.

Accessory molecule. A lymphocyte cell surface molecule distinct from the antigen receptor complex that mediates adhesive or signaling functions important for activation or migration of the lymphocyte.

Acquired immunodeficiency. A deficiency in the immune system that is acquired after birth, usually because of infection (e.g., AIDS), and that is not related to a genetic defect.

Acquired immunodeficiency syndrome (AIDS). A disease caused by human immunodeficiency virus (HIV) infection that is characterized by depletion of CD4$^+$ T cells leading to a profound defect in cell-mediated immunity. Clinically, AIDS includes opportunistic infections, malignant tumors, wasting, and encephalopathy.

Activation protein-1 (AP-1). A family of DNA-binding transcription factors composed of dimers of two proteins that bind to one another through a shared structural motif called a leucine zipper. The best characterized AP-1 factor is composed of the proteins Fos and Jun. AP-1 is involved in transcriptional regulation of many different genes important in the immune system, such as cytokine genes.

Active immunity. The form of adaptive immunity that is induced by exposure to a foreign antigen and activation of lymphocytes and in which the immunized individual plays an active role in responding to the antigen. This type contrasts with passive immunity, in which an individual receives antibodies or lymphocytes from another individual who was previously actively immunized.

Acute-phase reactants. Proteins, mostly synthesized in the liver, whose plasma concentrations increase shortly after infection as part of the systemic inflammatory response syndrome. Examples include C-reactive protein, fibrinogen, and serum amyloid A protein. Hepatic synthesis of these molecules is upregulated by inflammatory cytokines, especially IL-6 and TNF. The acute-phase reactants play various roles in the innate immune response to microbes.

Acute-phase response. The increase in plasma concentrations of several proteins, called acute-phase reactants, that occurs as part of the early innate immune response to infections.

Acute rejection. A form of graft rejection involving vascular and parenchymal injury mediated by T cells, macrophages, and antibodies that usually begins after the first week of transplantation. Differentiation of effector T cells and production of antibodies that mediate acute rejection occur in response to the graft, thus the delay in onset.

Adapter protein. Proteins involved in lymphocyte signal transduction pathways by serving as bridge molecules or scaffolds for the recruitment of other signaling molecules. During lymphocyte activation, adapter molecules may be phosphorylated on tyrosine residues to enable them to bind other proteins containing Src homology 2 (SH2) domains. Adapter molecules involved in T cell activation include LAT, SLP-76, and Grb-2.

Adaptive immunity. The form of immunity that is mediated by lymphocytes and stimulated by exposure to infectious agents. In contrast to innate immunity, adaptive immunity is characterized by exquisite specificity for distinct macromolecules and memory, which is the ability to respond more vigorously to repeated exposure to the same microbe. Adaptive immunity is also called specific immunity.

Addressin. Molecules expressed on endothelial cells in different anatomic sites that bind to counter-receptors on lymphocytes called homing receptors and that direct organ-specific lymphocyte homing. Mucosal addressin cell adhesion molecule-1 (MadCAM-1) is an example of an addressin expressed in Peyer's patch in the intestinal wall that binds to the integrin α$_4$β$_7$ on gut-homing T cells.

Adhesion molecule. A cell surface molecule whose function is to promote adhesive interactions with other cells or the extracellular matrix. Leukocytes express various types of adhesion molecules, such as selectins, integrins, and members of the Ig superfamily, and these molecules play crucial roles in cell migration and cellular activation in innate and adaptive immune responses.

Adjuvant. A substance, distinct from antigen, that enhances T cell activation by promoting the accumulation and activation of other leukocytes, called accessory cells, at a site of antigen exposure. Adjuvants enhance

149

accessory cell expression of T cell–activating costimulators and cytokines and may also prolong the expression of peptide-MHC complexes on the surface of APCs.

Adoptive transfer. The process of transferring lymphocytes from one, usually immunized, individual into another individual. Adoptive transfer is used in research to define the role of a particular cell population (e.g., CD4+ T cells) in an immune response. Clinically, adoptive transfer of tumor-reactive T lymphocytes is used in experimental cancer therapy.

Affinity. The strength of the binding between a single binding site of a molecule (e.g., an antibody) and a ligand (e.g., an antigen). The affinity of a molecule X for a ligand Y is represented by the dissociation constant (K_d), which is the concentration of Y that is required to occupy the combining sites of half the X molecules present in a solution. A smaller K_d indicates a stronger or higher affinity interaction, and a lower concentration of ligand is needed to occupy the sites.

Affinity chromatography. A technique used to purify an antigen from a solution by passing it through a column packed with antibody that binds the antigen and is attached to a solid support such as agarose beads.

Affinity maturation. The process that leads to increased affinity of antibodies for a particular protein antigen as a humoral response progresses. Affinity maturation is the result of somatic mutation of Ig genes, followed by selective survival of the B cells producing the highest affinity antibodies.

Allele. One of different forms of a gene present at a particular chromosomal locus. An individual who is heterozygous at a locus has two different alleles, each on a different member of a pair of chromosomes, one inherited from the mother and one from the father. If a particular gene in a population has many different alleles, the gene or locus is said to be polymorphic. The MHC locus is extremely polymorphic.

Allelic exclusion. The exclusive expression of only one of two inherited alleles encoding Ig heavy and light chains and TCR β chains. Allelic exclusion occurs when the protein product of one productively recombined antigen receptor locus on one chromosome blocks rearrangement of the corresponding locus on the other chromosome. This property ensures that all the antigen receptors expressed by one clone of lymphocytes will have the identical antigen specificities. Because the TCR α chain locus does not show allelic exclusion, some T cells do express two different types of TCR.

Allergen. An antigen that elicits an immediate hypersensitivity (allergic) reaction. Allergens are proteins or chemicals bound to proteins that induce IgE antibody responses in atopic individuals.

Allergy. A form of atopy or immediate hypersensitivity disease, often referring to the type of antigen that elicits the disease, such as food allergy, bee sting allergy, and penicillin allergy. All these conditions are related to antigen-induced mast cell or basophil activation.

Alloantibody. An antibody specific for an alloantigen (i.e., an antigen present in some individuals of a species but not in others).

Alloantigen. A cell or tissue antigen that is present in some members of a species and not in others and that is recognized as foreign on an allograft. Alloantigens are usually products of polymorphic genes.

Alloantiserum. The alloantibody-containing serum of an individual who has previously been exposed to one or more alloantigens.

Allogeneic graft. An organ or tissue graft from a donor who is of the same species but genetically nonidentical to the recipient (also called an allograft).

Alloreactive. Reactive to alloantigens; describes T cells or antibodies from one individual that will recognize antigens on cells or tissues of another genetically nonidentical individual.

Allotype. The property of a group of antibody molecules defined by their sharing a particular allotope; that is, antibodies that share a particular allotope belong to the same allotype. Allotype is also often used synonymously with allotope, which refers to an antigenic determinant found on the antibodies of some individuals but not others.

Altered peptide ligands (APLs). Peptides with altered TCR contact residues that elicit responses different from the responses to native peptide ligands. Altered peptide ligands may be important in the regulation of T cell activation in physiologic, pathologic, or therapeutic situations.

Alternative pathway of complement activation. An antibody-independent pathway of activation of the complement system that occurs when the C3b protein binds to microbial cell surfaces. The alternative pathway is a component of the innate immune system and mediates inflammatory responses to infection as well as direct lysis of microbes.

Anaphylactic shock. Cardiovascular collapse occurring in the setting of a systemic immediate hypersensitivity reaction.

Anaphylatoxins. The C5a, C4a, and C3a complement fragments that are generated during complement activation. The anaphylatoxins bind specific cell surface receptors and promote acute inflammation by stimulating neutrophil chemotaxis and activating mast cells. At high concentrations, anaphylatoxins activate enough mast cells to mimic anaphylaxis.

Anaphylaxis. An extreme systemic form of immediate hypersensitivity in which mast cell or basophil mediators cause bronchial constriction, massive tissue edema, and cardiovascular collapse.

Anchor residues. The amino acid residues of a peptide whose side chains fit into pockets in the peptide-binding cleft of an MHC molecule. The side chains bind to complementary amino acids in the MHC molecule and therefore serve to anchor the peptide in the cleft of the MHC molecule.

Anergy. A state of unresponsiveness to antigenic stimulation. Clinically, anergy describes the lack of T cell–dependent cutaneous delayed-type hypersensitivity reactions to common antigens. Lymphocyte anergy (also called clonal anergy) is the failure of clones of T or B cells to react to antigen and may be a mechanism of maintaining immunologic tolerance to self.

Angiogenesis. New blood vessel formation regulated by a variety of protein factors elaborated by cells of the innate and adaptive immune systems and often accompanying chronic inflammation.

Antagonist peptide. Variant peptide ligands of a TCR in which one or two TCR contact residues have been changed and in which negative signals are delivered to specific T cells that inhibit responses to native peptides.

Antibody. A type of glycoprotein molecule, also called immunoglobulin (Ig), produced by B lymphocytes that binds antigens, often with a high degree of specificity and affinity. The basic structural unit of an antibody is composed of two identical heavy chains and two identical light chains. N-terminal variable regions of the heavy and light chains form the antigen-binding sites, whereas the C-terminal constant regions of the heavy chains functionally interact with other molecules in the immune system. Every individual has millions of different antibodies, each with a unique antigen-binding site. Secreted antibodies perform various effector functions, including neutralizing antigens, activating complement, and promoting leukocyte-dependent destruction of microbes.

Antibody-dependent cell-mediated cytotoxicity (ADCC). A process by which NK cells are targeted to IgG-coated cells, resulting in lysis of the antibody-coated cells. A specific receptor for the constant region of IgG, called FcγRIII (CD16), is expressed on the NK cell membrane and mediates binding to the IgG.

Antibody feedback. The down-regulation of antibody production by secreted IgG antibodies that occurs when antigen-antibody complexes simultaneously engage B cell membrane Ig and Fcγ receptors (FcγRII). Under these conditions, the cytoplasmic tails of the Fcγ receptors transduce inhibitory signals inside the B cell.

Antibody repertoire. The collection of different antibody specificities expressed in an individual.

Antibody-secreting cell. A B lymphocyte that has undergone differentiation and produces the secretory form of Ig. Antibody-secreting cells are produced in response to antigen and reside in the spleen and lymph nodes as well as in the bone marrow.

Antigen. A molecule that binds to an antibody or a TCR. Antigens that bind to antibodies include all classes of molecules. TCRs bind only peptide fragments of proteins complexed with MHC molecules; both the peptide ligand and the native protein from which it is derived are called T cell antigens.

Antigen presentation. The display of peptides bound by MHC molecules on the surface of an APC that permits specific recognition by TCRs and activation of T cells.

Antigen processing. The intracellular conversion of protein antigens derived from the extracellular space or the cytosol into peptides and loading of these peptides onto MHC molecules for display to T lymphocytes.

Antigen-presenting cell (APC). A cell that displays peptide fragments of protein antigens, in association with MHC molecules, on its surface and activates antigen-specific T cells. In addition to displaying peptide-MHC complexes, APCs must also express costimulatory molecules to activate T lymphocytes optimally.

Antiserum. Serum from an individual previously immunized against an antigen that contains antibody specific for that antigen.

Apoptosis. A process of cell death characterized by DNA cleavage, nuclear condensation and fragmentation, and plasma membrane blebbing that leads to phagocytosis of the cell without inducing an inflammatory response. This type of cell death is important in lymphocyte development, regulation of lymphocyte responses to foreign antigens, and maintenance of tolerance to self antigens.

Arthus reaction. A localized form of experimental immune complex–mediated vasculitis induced by injection of an antigen subcutaneously into a previously immunized animal or into an animal that has been given intravenous antibody specific for the antigen. Circulating antibodies bind to the injected antigen and form immune complexes that are deposited in the walls of small arteries at the injection site and give rise to a local cutaneous vasculitis with necrosis.

Atopy. The propensity of an individual to produce IgE antibodies in response to various environmental antigens and to develop strong immediate hypersensitivity (allergic) responses. People who have allergies to environmental antigens, such as pollen or house dust, are said to be atopic.

Autoantibody. An antibody produced in an individual that is specific for a self antigen. Autoantibodies can cause damage to cells and tissues and are produced in excess in systemic autoimmune diseases, such as systemic lupus erythematosus.

Autocrine factor. A molecule that acts on the same cell that produces the factor. For example, IL-2 is an autocrine T cell growth factor that stimulates mitotic activity of the T cell that produces it.

Autoimmune disease. A disease caused by a breakdown of self-tolerance such that the adaptive immune system responds to self antigens and mediates cell and tissue damage. Autoimmune diseases can be organ specific (e.g., thyroiditis or diabetes) or systemic (e.g., systemic lupus erythematosus).

Autoimmunity. The state of adaptive immune system responsiveness to self antigens that occurs when mechanisms of self-tolerance fail.

Autologous graft. A tissue or organ graft in which the donor and recipient are the same individual. Autologous bone marrow and skin grafts are commonly performed in clinical medicine.

Avidity. The overall strength of interaction between two molecules, such as an antibody and antigen. Avidity depends on both the affinity and the valency of interactions. Therefore, the avidity of a pentameric IgM antibody, with 10 antigen-binding sites, for a multivalent antigen may be much greater than the avidity of a dimeric IgG molecule for the same antigen. Avidity can be used to describe the strength of cell-cell interactions, which are mediated by many binding interactions between cell surface molecules.

B cell tyrosine kinase (Btk). A tyrosine kinase of the Src family that plays an essential role in B cell maturation. Mutations in the gene encoding Btk cause X-linked agammaglobulinemia, a disease characterized by failure of B cells to mature beyond the pre-B cell stage.

B lymphocyte. The only cell type capable of producing antibody molecules and therefore the central cellular component of humoral immune responses. B lymphocytes, or B cells, develop in the bone marrow, and mature B cells are found mainly in lymphoid follicles in secondary lymphoid tissues, in bone marrow, and in low numbers in the circulation.

B lymphocyte antigen receptor (BCR) complex. A multiprotein complex expressed on the surface of B lymphocytes that recognizes antigen and transduces activating signals into the cell. The BCR includes membrane Ig, which is responsible for binding antigen, and Igα and Igβ proteins, which initiate signaling events.

Bare lymphocyte syndrome. An immunodeficiency disease characterized by a lack of class II MHC molecule expression that leads to defects in antigen presentation and cell-mediated immunity. The disease is caused by mutations in genes encoding factors that regulate class II MHC gene transcription.

Basophil. A type of bone marrow–derived, circulating granulocyte with structural and functional similarities to mast cells that has granules containing many of the same inflammatory mediators as mast cells and expresses a high-affinity Fc receptor for IgE. Basophils that are recruited into tissue sites where antigen is present may contribute to immediate hypersensitivity reactions.

Biogenic amines. Low molecular weight, nonlipid compounds, such as histamine, that share the structural feature of an amine group, are stored in and released from the cytoplasmic granules of mast cells, and mediate many of the biologic effects of immediate hypersensitivity (allergic) reactions. (Biogenic amines are sometimes called vasoactive amines.)

Biologic response modifiers. Molecules, such as cytokines, used clinically as modulators of inflammation, immunity, and hematopoiesis.

Bone marrow. The central cavity of bone that is the site of generation of all circulating blood cells in adults, including immature lymphocytes, and the site of B cell maturation.

Bone marrow transplantation. The transplantation of bone marrow, including stem cells that give rise to all mature blood cells and lymphocytes; it is performed clinically to treat hematopoietic or lymphopoietic disorders and malignant diseases and is also used in various immunologic experiments in animals.

Bronchial asthma. An inflammatory disease usually caused by repeated immediate hypersensitivity reactions in the lung that leads to intermittent and reversible airway obstruction, chronic bronchial inflammation with eosinophils, and bronchial smooth muscle cell hypertrophy and hyperreactivity.

Burkitt's lymphoma. A malignant B cell tumor that is defined by histologic features but almost always carries a reciprocal chromosomal translocation involving Ig gene loci and the cellular *myc* gene on chromosome 8. Many cases of Burkitt's lymphoma are associated with Epstein-Barr virus infection.

C (constant region) gene segments. The DNA sequences in the Ig and TCR gene loci that encode the nonvariable portions of Ig heavy and light chains and TCR α, β, γ, and δ chains.

C1. A serum complement system protein composed of several polypeptide chains that initiates the classical pathway of complement activation by attaching to the Fc portions of IgG or IgM antibody that has bound antigen.

C1 inhibitor (C1 INH). A plasma protein inhibitor of the classical pathway of complement activation. C1 INH is a serine protease inhibitor (serpin) that mimics the normal substrates of the C1r and C1s components of C1. A genetic deficiency in C1 INH causes the disease hereditary angioneurotic edema.

C3. The central and most abundant complement system protein; it is involved in both the classical and alternative pathway cascades. C3 is proteolytically cleaved during complement activation to generate a C3b fragment, which covalently attaches to cell or microbial surfaces, and a C3a fragment, which has various proinflammatory activities.

C3 convertase. A multiprotein enzyme complex generated by the early steps of either the classical or alternative pathway of complement activation. C3 convertase cleaves C3, which gives rise to two proteolytic products called C3a and C3b.

C5 convertase. A multiprotein enzyme complex generated by C3b binding to C3 convertase. C5 convertase cleaves C5 and initiates the late steps of complement activation leading to formation of the membrane attack complex and lysis of cells.

Calcineurin. A cytoplasmic serine/threonine phosphatase that dephosphorylates and thereby activates the transcription factor NFAT. Calcineurin is activated by calcium signals generated through TCR signaling in response to antigen recognition, and the immunosuppressive drugs cyclosporine and FK-506 work by blocking calcineurin activity.

Carcinoembryonic antigen (CEA, CD66). A highly glycosylated membrane protein; increased expression of CEA in many carcinomas of the colon, pancreas, stomach, and breast results in a rise in serum levels. The level of serum CEA is used to monitor the persistence or recurrence of metastatic carcinoma after treatment. Because CEA expression is normally high in many tissues during fetal life but is suppressed in adults except in tumor cells, it is called an oncofetal tumor antigen.

Caspases. Intracellular proteases with cysteines in their active sites that cleave substrates at the C-terminal sides of aspartic acid residues and are components of enzymatic cascades that cause apoptotic death of cells. Lymphocyte caspases may be activated by two pathways; one is associated with mitochondrial permeability changes in growth factor–deprived cells, and the other is associated with signals from death receptors in the plasma membrane.

Cathepsins. Thiol and aspartyl proteases with broad substrate specificities. The most abundant proteases of endosomes in APCs, cathepsins probably play an important role in generating peptide fragments from exogenous protein antigens that bind to class II MHC molecules.

CD molecules. Cell surface molecules expressed on various cell types in the immune system that are designated by the "cluster of differentiation" or CD number. See Appendix II for a list of CD molecules.

Cell-mediated immunity (CMI). The form of adaptive immunity that is mediated by T lymphocytes and serves as the defense mechanism against microbes that survive within phagocytes or infect nonphagocytic cells. CMI responses include CD4$^+$ T cell–mediated activation of macrophages that have phagocytosed microbes and CD8$^+$ CTL killing of infected cells.

Central tolerance. A form of self-tolerance induced in generative (central) lymphoid organs as a consequence of immature self-reactive lymphocytes recognizing self antigens and subsequently leading to their death or inactivation. Central tolerance prevents the emergence of lymphocytes with high-affinity receptors for the ubiquitous self antigens that are likely to be present in the bone marrow or thymus.

Chédiak-Higashi syndrome. A rare autosomal recessive immunodeficiency disease caused by a defect in the cytoplasmic granules of various cell types that affects the lysosomes of neutrophils and macrophages as well as the granules of CTLs and NK cells. Patients show reduced resistance to infection with pyogenic bacteria.

Chemokine receptors. Cell surface receptors for chemokines that transduce signals stimulating the migration of leukocytes. These receptors are members of the seven-transmembrane α-helical, G protein–linked family of receptors.

Chemokines. A large family of structurally homologous, low molecular weight cytokines that stimulate leukocyte movement and regulate the migration of leukocytes from the blood to tissues.

Chemotaxis. Movement of a cell directed by a chemical concentration gradient. The movement of lymphocytes, polymorphonuclear leukocytes, monocytes, and other leukocytes into various tissues is often directed by gradients of low molecular weight cytokines called chemokines.

Chromosomal translocation. A chromosomal abnormality in which a segment of one chromosome is transferred to another. Many malignant diseases of lymphocytes are associated with chromosomal translocations involving an Ig or TCR locus and a chromosomal segment containing a cellular oncogene.

Chronic granulomatous disease. A rare inherited immunodeficiency disease caused by a defect in the gene encoding a component of the phagocyte oxidase enzyme that is needed for microbial killing by polymorphonuclear leukocytes and macrophages. The disease is characterized by recurrent intracellular bacterial and fungal infections, often accompanied by chronic cell-mediated immune responses and the formation of granulomas.

Chronic rejection. A form of allograft rejection characterized by fibrosis with loss of normal organ structures occurring during a prolonged period. In many cases, the major pathologic event in chronic rejection is graft arterial occlusion, which is caused by proliferation of intimal smooth muscle cells and is called graft arteriosclerosis.

c-Kit ligand (stem cell factor). A protein required for hematopoiesis, early steps in T cell development in the thymus, and mast cell development. c-Kit ligand is produced in membrane-bound and soluble forms by stromal cells in the bone marrow and thymus and binds to the c-Kit tyrosine kinase membrane receptor on pluripotent stem cells.

Class I major histocompatibility complex (MHC) molecule. One of two forms of polymorphic, heterodimeric membrane proteins that bind and display peptide fragments of protein antigens on the surface of APCs for recognition by T lymphocytes. Class I MHC molecules usually display peptides derived from the cytoplasm of the cell.

Class II–associated invariant chain peptide (CLIP). A peptide remnant of the invariant chain that sits in the class II MHC peptide-binding cleft and is removed by action of the HLA-DM molecule before the cleft becomes accessible to peptides produced from extracellular protein antigens.

Class II major histocompatibility complex (MHC) molecule. One of two forms of polymorphic, heterodimeric membrane proteins that bind and display peptide fragments of protein antigens on the surface of APCs for recognition by T lymphocytes. Class II MHC molecules usually display peptides derived from extracellular proteins that are internalized into phagocytic or endocytic vesicles.

Class II vesicle (CIIV). A membrane-bound organelle identified in murine B cells that is important in the class II MHC pathway of antigen presentation. The CIIV is similar to the MHC class II compartment (MIIC) identified in other cells and contains all the components required for the formation of complexes of peptide antigens and class II MHC molecules, including the enzymes that degrade protein antigens, class II molecules, invariant chain, and HLA-DM.

Classical pathway of complement activation. The pathway of activation of the complement system that is initiated by binding of antigen-antibody complexes to the C1 molecule and induces a proteolytic cascade involving multiple other complement proteins. The classical pathway is an effector arm of the humoral immune system that generates inflammatory mediators, opsonins for phagocytosis of antigens, and lytic complexes that destroy cells.

Clonal anergy. A state of antigen unresponsiveness of a clone of T lymphocytes experimentally induced by recognition of antigen in the absence of additional signals (costimulatory signals) required for functional activation. Clonal anergy is considered a model for one mechanism of tolerance to self antigens and may be applicable to B lymphocytes as well.

Clonal deletion. A mechanism of lymphocyte tolerance in which an immature T cell in the thymus or an immature B cell in the bone marrow undergoes apoptotic death as a consequence of recognizing an abundant antigen in the generative organ.

Clonal expansion. The increase in number of lymphocytes specific for an antigen that results from antigen stimulation and proliferation of naive T cells. Clonal expansion occurs in lymphoid tissues and is required to generate enough antigen-specific effector lymphocytes from rare naive precursors to eradicate infections.

Clonal ignorance. A form of lymphocyte unresponsiveness in which self antigens are ignored by the immune system even though lymphocytes specific for those antigens remain viable and functional.

Clonal selection hypothesis. A fundamental tenet of the immune system (no longer a hypothesis) stating that every individual possesses numerous clonally derived lymphocytes, each clone having arisen from a single precursor and being capable of recognizing and responding to a distinct antigenic determinant. When an antigen enters, it selects a specific preexisting clone and activates it.

c-myc. A cellular proto-oncogene that encodes a nuclear factor involved in cell cycle regulation. Translocations of the c-myc gene into Ig gene loci are associated with B cell malignant neoplasms.

Collectins. A family of proteins, including mannose-binding lectin, that are characterized by a collagen-like domain and a lectin (i.e., carbohydrate-binding) domain. Collectins play a role in the innate immune system by acting as microbial pattern recognition receptors, and they may activate the complement system by binding to C1q.

Colony-stimulating factors (CSFs). Cytokines that promote the expansion and differentiation of bone marrow progenitor cells. CSFs are essential for the maturation of red blood cells, granulocytes, monocytes, and lymphocytes. Examples of CSFs are granulocyte-monocyte colony-stimulating factor (GM-CSF), c-Kit ligand, IL-3, and IL-7.

Combinatorial diversity. Combinatorial diversity describes the many different combinations of variable, diversity, and joining segments that are possible as a result of somatic recombination of DNA in the Ig and TCR loci during B cell or T cell development. Combinatorial diversity is one mechanism for the generation of large numbers of different antigen receptor genes from a limited number of DNA gene segments.

Complement. A system of serum and cell surface proteins that interact with one another and with other molecules of the immune system to generate important effectors of innate and adaptive immune responses. The classical and alternative pathways of the complement system are activated by antigen-antibody complexes or microbial surfaces, respectively, and consist of a cascade of proteolytic enzymes that generate inflammatory mediators and opsonins. Both pathways lead to the formation of a common terminal cell lytic complex that is inserted in cell membranes.

Complement receptor type 1 (CR1). A high-affinity receptor for the C3b and C4b fragments of complement. Phagocytes use CR1 to mediate internalization of C3b- or C4b-coated particles. CR1 on erythrocytes serves in the clearance of immune complexes from the circulation. CR1 is also a regulator of complement activation.

Complement receptor type 2 (CR2). A receptor expressed on B cells and follicular dendritic cells that binds proteolytic fragments of the C3 complement protein, including C3d, C3dg, and iC3b. CR2 functions to stimulate humoral immune responses by enhancing B cell activation by antigen and by promoting the trapping of antigen-antibody complexes in germinal centers. CR2 is also the receptor for Epstein-Barr virus.

Complementarity-determining region (CDR). Short segments of Ig and TCR proteins that contain most of the sequence differences among different antibodies or TCRs and that make contact with antigen. Three CDRs are present in the variable domain of each antigen receptor polypeptide chain and six CDRs in an intact Ig or TCR molecule. These hypervariable segments assume loop structures that together form a surface that is complementary to the three-dimensional structure of the bound antigen.

Congenic mouse strains. Inbred mouse strains that are identical to one another at every genetic locus except the one for which they are selected to differ; such strains are created by repetitive back-crossbreeding and selection for a particular trait. Congenic strains that differ from one another only at a particular MHC allele have been useful in defining the function of MHC molecules.

Constant (C) region. The portion of Ig or TCR polypeptide chains that does not vary in sequence among different clones and is not involved in antigen binding.

Contact sensitivity. The propensity for a T cell–mediated, delayed-type hypersensitivity reaction to develop in the skin on contact with a particular chemical agent. Chemicals that elicit contact hypersensitivity bind to and modify self proteins or molecules on the surfaces of APCs, which are then recognized by CD4$^+$ or CD8$^+$ T cells.

Coreceptor. A lymphocyte surface receptor that binds to an antigen complex at the same time that membrane Ig or TCR binds the antigen and delivers signals required for optimal lymphocyte activation. CD4 and CD8 are T cell coreceptors that bind nonpolymorphic parts of an MHC molecule concurrently with the TCR binding to polymorphic residues and the bound peptide. CR2 is a coreceptor on B cells that binds to complement-opsonized antigens at the same time that membrane Ig binds another part of the antigen.

Costimulator. A molecule on the surface of or secreted by an APC that provides a stimulus (or second signal) required for the activation of naive T cells, in addition to antigen. The best defined costimulators are the B7 molecules on professional APCs that bind to the CD28 molecule on T cells.

CpG nucleotides. Unmethylated cytidine-guanine sequences found in bacterial DNA that have adjuvant properties in the mammalian immune system and may be important to the efficacy of DNA vaccines.

C-reactive protein (CRP). A member of the pentraxin family of plasma proteins involved in innate immune responses to bacterial infections. CRP is an acute-phase reactant, and it binds to the capsule of pneumococcal bacteria. CRP also binds to C1q and may thereby activate complement or act as an opsonin by interacting with phagocyte C1q receptors.

Crossmatching. A screening test performed to minimize the chance of graft rejection in which a patient in need of an allograft is tested for the presence of preformed antibodies against donor cell surface antigens (usually MHC antigens). The test involves mixing the recipient serum with leukocytes from potential donors, adding complement, and observing whether cell lysis occurs.

Cross-priming. A mechanism by which a professional APC activates (or primes) a naive CD8+ CTL specific for the antigens of a third cell (e.g., a virus-infected or tumor cell). Cross-priming occurs, for example, when an infected (often apoptotic) cell is ingested by a professional APC and the microbial antigens are processed and presented in association with class I MHC molecules, just like any other phagocytosed antigen. The professional APC also provides costimulation for the T cells. Also called **cross-presentation**.

Cutaneous immune system. The components of the innate and adaptive immune system found in the skin that function together in a specialized way to detect and respond to environmental antigens. Components of the cutaneous immune system include keratinocytes, Langerhans cells, intraepithelial lymphocytes, and dermal lymphocytes.

Cyclosporine. An immunosuppressive drug used to prevent allograft rejection that functions by blocking T cell cytokine gene transcription. Cyclosporine (also called cyclosporin A) binds to a cytosolic protein called cyclophilin, and cyclosporine-cyclophilin complexes bind to and inhibit calcineurin, thereby inhibiting activation and nuclear translocation of the transcription factor NFAT.

Cytokines. Proteins produced by many different cell types that mediate inflammatory and immune reactions. Cytokines are principal mediators of communication between cells of the immune system.

Cytolytic (or cytotoxic) T lymphocyte (CTL). A type of T lymphocyte whose major effector function is to recognize and kill host cells infected with viruses or other intracellular microbes. CTLs usually express CD8 and recognize microbial peptides displayed by class I MHC molecules. CTL killing of infected cells involves the release of cytoplasmic granules whose contents include membrane pore-forming proteins and enzymes.

Cytopathic effect of viruses. Harmful effects of viruses on host cells that are caused by any of a variety of biochemical or molecular mechanisms and are independent of the host immune response to the virus. Some viruses have little cytopathic effect but still cause disease because the immune system recognizes and destroys the infected cells.

Defensins. Cysteine-rich peptides present in the skin and in neutrophil granules that act as broad-spectrum antibiotics to kill a wide variety of bacteria and fungi. The synthesis of defensins is increased in response to inflammatory cytokines such as IL-1 and TNF.

Delayed-type hypersensitivity (DTH). An immune reaction in which T cell–dependent macrophage activation and inflammation cause tissue injury. A DTH reaction to the subcutaneous injection of antigen is often used as an assay for cell-mediated immunity (e.g., the purified protein derivative skin test for immunity to *Mycobacterium tuberculosis*). DTH is a frequent accompaniment of protective cell-mediated immunity against microbes.

Delayed xenograft rejection. A frequent form of rejection of xenografts that occurs within 2 to 3 days of transplantation and is characterized by intravascular thrombosis and fibrinoid necrosis of vessel walls. Delayed xenograft rejection is likely to be caused by antibody- and cytokine-mediated endothelial activation and damage.

Dendritic cells. Bone marrow–derived immune accessory cells found in epithelial and lymphoid tissues that are morphologically characterized by thin membranous projections. Dendritic cells function as APCs for naive T lymphocytes and are important for initiation of adaptive immune responses to protein antigen.

Desensitization. A method of treating immediate hypersensitivity disease (allergies) that involves repetitive administration of low doses of an antigen to which individuals are allergic. This process often prevents severe allergic reactions on subsequent environmental exposure to the antigen, but the mechanisms are not well understood.

Determinant. The specific portion of a macromolecular antigen to which an antibody binds. In the case of a protein antigen recognized by a T cell, the determinant is the peptide portion that binds to an MHC molecule for recognition by the TCR. Synonymous with **epitope**.

Determinant selection model. A model to explain MHC-linked immune responses that was proposed before the demonstration of peptide-MHC molecule binding. The model states that the products of MHC genes in each individual select which determinants of protein antigens will be immunogenic in that individual.

Diacylglycerol (DAG). A membrane-bound signaling molecule generated by phospholipase C (PLCγ1)–mediated hydrolysis of the plasma membrane phospholipid phosphatidylinositol 4,5-bisphosphate (PIP$_2$) during antigen activation of lymphocytes. The main function of DAG is to activate an enzyme called protein kinase C that participates in the generation of active transcription factors.

DiGeorge syndrome. A selective T cell deficiency caused by a congenital malformation that results in defective development of the thymus, parathyroid glands, and other structures that arise from the third and fourth pharyngeal pouches.

Direct antigen presentation (or direct allorecognition). Presentation of cell surface allogeneic MHC molecules by graft cells to a graft recipient's T cells that leads to T cell activation, with no requirement for processing. Direct recognition of foreign MHC molecules is a cross-reaction in which a normal TCR that recognizes a self MHC molecule plus foreign peptide cross-reacts with an allogeneic MHC molecule plus peptide. Direct presentation is partly responsible for strong T cell responses to allografts.

Diversity. The existence of a large number of lymphocytes with different antigenic specificities in any individual (i.e., the lymphocyte repertoire is large and diverse). Diversity is a fundamental property of the adaptive immune system and is the result of variability in the structures of the antigen-binding sites of lymphocyte receptors for antigens (antibodies and TCRs).

Diversity (D) segments. Short coding sequences between the variable (V) and constant (C) gene segments in the Ig heavy chain and TCR β and γ loci that together with J segments are somatically recombined with V segments during lymphocyte development. The resulting recombined VDJ DNA codes for the carboxyl terminal ends of the antigen receptor V regions, including the third hypervariable (CDR) regions. Random use of D segments contributes to the diversity of the antigen receptor repertoire.

DNA vaccine. A vaccine composed of a bacterial plasmid containing a complementary DNA encoding a protein antigen. DNA vaccines presumably work because professional APCs are transfected *in vivo* by the plasmid and express immunogenic peptides that elicit specific responses. Furthermore, the plasmid DNA contains CpG nucleotides that act as potent adjuvants. DNA vaccines may elicit strong CTL responses.

Double-negative thymocyte. A subset of developing T cells (thymocytes) in the thymus that express neither CD4 nor CD8. Most double-negative thymocytes are at an early developmental stage and do not express antigen receptors. They will later express both CD4 and CD8 during the intermediate double-positive stage before further maturation to single-positive T cells expressing only CD4 or CD8.

Double-positive thymocyte. A subset of developing T cells (thymocytes) in the thymus at an intermediate developmental stage that express both CD4 and CD8. Double-positive thymocytes also express TCRs and are subject to selection processes, the survivors of which mature to single-positive T cells expressing only CD4 or CD8.

Ectoparasite. Parasites that live on the surface of an animal, such as ticks and mites. Both the innate and adaptive immune systems may play a role in protection against ectoparasites, often by destroying the larval stages of these organisms.

Effector cells. The cells that perform effector functions during an immune response, such as secreting cytokines (e.g., helper T cells), killing microbes (e.g., macrophages), killing microbe-infected host cells (e.g., CTLs), or secreting antibodies (e.g., differentiated B cells).

Effector phase. The phase of an immune response, after the recognition and activation phases, in which a foreign antigen is actually destroyed or inactivated. For example, in a humoral immune response, the effector phase may be characterized by antibody-dependent complement activation and phagocytosis of antibody- and complement-opsonized bacteria.

Endosome. An intracellular membrane-bound vesicle into which extracellular proteins are internalized during antigen processing. Endosomes have an acidic pH and contain proteolytic enzymes that degrade proteins into peptides that bind to class II MHC molecules. A subset of class II MHC–rich endosomes, called MIIC, play a special role in antigen processing and presentation by the class II pathway.

Endotoxin. A component of the cell wall of gram-negative bacteria, also called **lipopolysaccharide** (LPS), that is released from dying bacteria and stimulates many innate immune responses, including the secretion of cytokines, induction of microbicidal activities of macrophages, and expression of leukocyte adhesion molecules on endothelium. Endotoxin contains both lipid components and carbohydrate (polysaccharide) moieties.

Enhancer. A regulatory nucleotide sequence in a gene that is located either upstream or downstream of the promoter, binds transcription factors, and increases the activity of the promoter. In cells of the immune system, enhancers are responsible for integrating cell surface signals that lead to induced transcription of genes encoding many of the effector proteins of an immune response, such as cytokines.

Envelope glycoprotein (Env). A membrane glycoprotein encoded by a retrovirus that is expressed on the plasma membrane of infected cells and on the host cell–derived membrane coat of viral particles. Env proteins are often required for viral infectivity. The Env proteins of HIV include gp41 and gp120, which bind to CD4 and chemokine receptors, respectively, on human T cells and mediate fusion of the viral and T cell membranes.

Enzyme-linked immunosorbent assay (ELISA). A method of quantifying an antigen immobilized on a solid surface by use of a specific antibody with a covalently coupled enzyme. The amount of antibody that binds the antigen is proportional to the amount of antigen present and is determined by spectrophotometrically measuring the conversion of a clear substrate to a colored product by the coupled enzyme.

Eosinophil. A bone marrow–derived granulocyte that is abundant in the inflammatory infiltrates of immediate hypersensitivity late-phase reactions and that contributes to many of the pathologic processes in allergic diseases. Eosinophils are important in defense against extracellular parasites, including helminths.

Epitope. The specific portion of a macromolecular antigen to which an antibody binds. In the case of a protein antigen recognized by a T cell, an epitope is the peptide portion that binds to an MHC molecule for recognition by the TCR. Synonymous with **determinant**.

Epstein-Barr virus (EBV). A double-stranded DNA virus of the herpesvirus family that is the etiologic agent of infectious mononucleosis and is associated with some B cell malignant tumors and nasopharyngeal carcinoma. EBV infects B lymphocytes and some epithelial cells by specifically binding to CR2 (CD21).

Equilibrium dialysis. A method of determining the affinity of interaction between a macromolecule such as an antibody and a small ligand such as a hapten. A solution of the macromolecule, at a defined concentration, is confined within a semipermeable membrane and immersed in a solution containing the small ligand. The membrane does not permit the macromolecule to pass through, but the small ligand can pass across the membrane freely. The concentration of the small ligand in solution at equilibrium is used to calculate the affinity of binding to the macromolecule.

Experimental autoimmune encephalomyelitis. An animal model of autoimmune demyelinating disease of the central nervous system (e.g., multiple sclerosis) that is induced in rodents by immunization with components of the myelin sheath (e.g., myelin basic protein) of nerves, mixed with an adjuvant. The disease is mediated in large part by cytokine-secreting $CD4^+$ T cells specific for the myelin sheath proteins.

Extravasation. Escape of the fluid and cellular components of blood from a blood vessel into tissues.

Fab (fragment, antigen-binding). A proteolytic fragment of an IgG antibody molecule that includes one complete light chain paired with one heavy chain fragment containing the variable domain and only the first constant domain. Fab fragment retains the ability to monovalently bind an antigen but cannot interact with IgG Fc receptors on cells or with complement. Therefore, Fab preparations are used in research and therapeutic applications when antigen binding is desired without activation of effector functions. (Fab' fragment retains the hinge region of the heavy chain.)

F(ab')₂ fragment. A proteolytic fragment of an IgG molecule that includes two complete light chains but only the variable domain, first constant domain, and hinge region of the two heavy chains. F(ab')₂ fragments retain the entire bivalent antigen-binding region of an intact IgG molecule but cannot bind complement or IgG Fc receptors. They are used in research and therapeutic applications when antigen binding is desired without antibody effector functions.

Fas (CD95). A member of the TNF receptor family that is expressed on the surface of T cells and many other cell types and initiates a signaling cascade leading to apoptotic death of the cell. The death pathway is initiated when Fas binds to Fas ligand expressed on activated T cells. Fas-mediated killing of T cells, called activation-induced cell death, is important for the maintenance of self-tolerance. Mutations in the Fas gene cause systemic autoimmune disease.

Fas ligand (CD95 ligand). A membrane protein that is a member of the TNF family of proteins expressed on activated T cells. Fas ligand binds to Fas, thereby stimulating a signaling pathway leading to apoptotic cell death of the Fas-expressing cell. Mutations in the Fas ligand gene cause systemic autoimmune disease in mice.

Fc (fragment, crystalline). A proteolytic fragment of IgG that contains only the disulfide-linked carboxyl terminal regions of the two heavy chains. Fc is also used to describe the corresponding region of an intact Ig molecule that mediates effector functions by binding to cell surface receptors or the C1q complement protein. (Fc fragments are so named because they tend to crystallize out of solution.)

Fc receptor. A cell surface receptor specific for the carboxyl terminal constant region of an Ig molecule. Fc receptors are typically multichain protein complexes that include signaling components and Ig-binding components. Several types of Fc receptors exist, including those specific for different IgG isotypes, IgE, and IgA. Fc receptors mediate many of the cell-dependent effector functions of antibodies, including phagocytosis of antibody-bound antigens, antigen-induced activation of mast cells, and targeting and activation of NK cells.

FcεRI. A high-affinity receptor for the carboxyl terminal constant region of IgE molecules that is expressed on mast cells and basophils. FcεRI molecules on mast cells are usually occupied by IgE, and antigen-induced cross-linking of these IgE-FcεRI complexes activates the mast cell and initiates immediate hypersensitivity reactions.

Fcγ receptor (FcγR). A specific cell surface receptor for the carboxyl terminal constant region of IgG molecules. There are several different types of Fcγ receptors, including a high-affinity FcγRI that mediates phagocytosis by macrophages and neutrophils, a low-affinity FcγRIIB that transduces inhibitory signals in B cells, and a low-affinity FcγRIIIA that mediates targeting and activation of NK cells.

First-set rejection. Allograft rejection in an individual who has not previously received a graft or otherwise been exposed to tissue alloantigens from the same donor. First-set rejection usually takes about 7 to 10 days.

FK-506. An immunosuppressive drug used to prevent allograft rejection that functions by blocking T cell cytokine gene transcription, similar to cyclosporine. FK-506 binds to a cytosolic protein called FK-506–binding protein, and the resulting complex binds to calcineurin, thereby inhibiting activation and nuclear translocation of the transcription factor NFAT.

Flow cytometry. A method of analysis of the phenotype of cell populations requiring a specialized instrument (flow cytometer) that can detect fluorescence on individual cells in a suspension and thereby determine the number of cells expressing the molecule to which a fluorescent probe binds. Suspensions of cells are incubated with fluorescently labeled antibodies or other probes, and the amount of probe bound by each cell in the population is measured by passing the cells one at a time through a fluorimeter with a laser-generated incident beam.

Fluorescence-activated cell sorter (FACS). An adaptation of the flow cytometer that is used for the purification of cells from a mixed population according to which and how much fluorescent probe the cells bind.

Cells are first stained with fluorescently labeled probe, such as an antibody specific for a surface antigen of a cell population. The cells are then passed one at a time through a fluorimeter with a laser-generated incident beam and are differentially deflected by electromagnetic fields whose strength and direction are varied according to the measured intensity of the fluorescence signal.

Follicle. See **Lymphoid follicle.**

Follicular dendritic cells. Cells found in lymphoid follicles that express complement receptors, Fc receptors, and CD40 ligand and have long cytoplasmic processes that form a meshwork integral to the architecture of a lymphoid follicle. Follicular dendritic cells display antigens on their surface for B cell recognition and are involved in the activation and selection of B cells expressing high-affinity membrane Ig during the process of affinity maturation.

N-Formylmethionine. An amino acid that initiates all bacterial proteins and no mammalian proteins (except those synthesized within mitochondria) and serves as a signal to the innate immune system of infection. Specific receptors for N-formylmethionine–containing peptides are expressed on neutrophils and mediate activation of the neutrophils.

G protein–coupled receptor family. A diverse family of receptors for hormones, lipid inflammatory mediators, and chemokines that use associated trimeric G proteins for intracellular signaling.

G proteins. Proteins that bind guanyl nucleotides and act as exchange molecules by catalyzing the replacement of bound guanosine diphosphate (GDP) by guanosine triphosphate (GTP). G proteins with bound GTP can activate a variety of cellular enzymes in different signaling cascades. Trimeric GTP-binding proteins are associated with the cytoplasmic portions of many cell surface receptors, such as chemokine receptors. Other small soluble G proteins, such as Ras and Rac, are recruited into signaling pathways by adapter proteins.

γδ T cell receptor (γδ TCR). A form of TCR that is distinct from the more common αβ TCR and is expressed on a subset of T cells found mostly in epithelial barrier tissues. Although structurally similar to the αβ TCR, the forms of antigen recognized by γδ TCRs are poorly understood; they do not recognize peptide complexes bound to polymorphic MHC molecules.

Generative lymphoid organ. Organs in which lymphocytes develop from immature precursors. The bone marrow and thymus are the major generative lymphoid organs in which B cells and T cells develop, respectively.

Germinal center. A lightly staining region within a lymphoid follicle in spleen, lymph node, or mucosal lymphoid tissue that forms during T cell–dependent humoral immune responses and is the site of B cell affinity maturation.

Germline organization. The inherited arrangement of variable, diversity, joining, and constant region gene segments of the antigen receptor loci in nonlymphoid cells or in immature lymphocytes. In developing B or T lymphocytes, the germline organization is modified by somatic recombination to form functional Ig or TCR genes.

Glomerulonephritis. Inflammation of the renal glomeruli, often initiated by immunopathologic mechanisms such as deposition of circulating antigen-antibody complexes in the glomerular basement membrane or binding of antibodies to antigens expressed in the glomerulus. The antibodies can activate complement and phagocytes, and the resulting inflammatory response can lead to renal failure.

Graft. A tissue or organ that is removed from one site and placed in another site, usually in a different individual.

Graft arteriosclerosis. Occlusion of graft arteries caused by proliferation of intimal smooth muscle cells. This process is evident within 6 months to a year after transplantation and is responsible for chronic rejection of vascularized organ grafts. The mechanism is likely to be a result of a chronic immune response to vessel wall alloantigens. Graft arteriosclerosis is also called accelerated arteriosclerosis.

Graft rejection. A specific immune response to an organ or tissue graft that leads to inflammation, damage, and possibly graft failure.

Graft-versus-host disease. A disease occurring in bone marrow transplant recipients that is caused by the reaction of mature T cells in the marrow graft with alloantigens on host cells. The disease most often affects the skin, liver, and intestines.

Granulocyte colony-stimulating factor (G-CSF). A cytokine made by activated T cells, macrophages, and endothelial cells at sites of infection that acts on bone marrow to increase the production of and mobilize neutrophils to replace those consumed in inflammatory reactions.

Granulocyte-monocyte colony-stimulating factor (GM-CSF). A cytokine made by activated T cells, macrophages, endothelial cells, and stromal fibroblasts that acts on bone marrow to increase the production of neutrophils and monocytes. GM-CSF is also a macrophage-activating factor and promotes the differentiation of Langerhans cells into mature dendritic cells.

Granuloma. A nodule of inflammatory tissue composed of clusters of activated macrophages and T lymphocytes, often with associated necrosis and fibrosis. Granulomatous inflammation is a form of chronic delayed-type hypersensitivity, often in response to persistent microbes, such as *Mycobacterium tuberculosis* and some fungi, or in response to particulate antigens that are not readily phagocytosed.

Granzyme. A serine protease enzyme found in the granules of CTLs and NK cells that is released by exocytosis, enters target cells and proteolytically cleaves and activates caspases, which in turn cleave several substrates and induce target cell apoptosis.

H-2 molecule. An MHC molecule in the mouse. The mouse MHC was originally called the H-2 locus.

Haplotype. The set of MHC alleles inherited from one parent and therefore on one chromosome.

Hapten. A small chemical that can bind to an antibody but must be attached to a macromolecule (carrier) to stimulate an adaptive immune response specific for that chemical. For example, immunization with dinitrophenol (DNP) alone will not stimulate an anti-DNP antibody response, but immunization with a protein with covalently bonded DNP hapten will.

Heavy chain class (isotype) switching. The process by which a B lymphocyte changes the class, or isotype, of the antibodies that it produces, from IgM to IgG, IgE, or IgA, without changing the antigen specificity of the antibody. Heavy chain class switching is regulated by helper T cell cytokines and CD40 ligand and involves recombination of B cell VDJ segments with downstream heavy chain gene segments.

Helminth. A parasitic worm. Helminthic infections often elicit T_H2-regulated immune responses characterized by eosinophil-rich inflammatory infiltrates and IgE production.

Helper T cells. The functional subset of T lymphocytes whose main effector functions are to activate macrophages in cell-mediated immune responses and to promote B cell antibody production in humoral immune responses. These effector functions are mediated by secreted cytokines and by T cell CD40 ligand binding to macrophage or B cell CD40. Most helper T cells express the CD4 molecule.

Hematopoiesis. The development of mature blood cells, including erythrocytes, leukocytes, and platelets, from pluripotent stem cells in the bone marrow and fetal liver. Hematopoiesis is regulated by several different cytokine growth factors produced by bone marrow stromal cells, T cells, and other cell types.

Hematopoietic stem cell. An undifferentiated bone marrow cell that divides continuously and gives rise to additional stem cells and cells of multiple different lineages. A hematopoietic stem cell in the bone marrow will give rise to cells of the lymphoid, myeloid, and erythrocytic lineage.

High endothelial venule (HEV). Specialized venules that are the sites of lymphocyte extravasation from the blood into the stroma of a peripheral lymph node or mucosal lymphoid tissue. HEVs are lined by plump endothelial cells that protrude into the vessel lumen and express unique adhesion molecules involved in binding naive T cells.

Highly active antiretroviral therapy (HAART). Combination chemotherapy for HIV infection consisting of reverse transcriptase inhibitors and a viral protease inhibitor. HAART can reduce plasma virus titers to below detectable levels for more than 1 year and slow the progression of HIV disease.

Hinge region. A region of Ig heavy chains between the first two constant domains that can assume multiple conformations, thereby imparting flexibility in the orientation of the two antigen-binding sites. Because of the hinge region, an antibody molecule can simultaneously bind two epitopes that are anywhere within a range of distances from one another.

Histamine. A biogenic amine stored in the granules of mast cells that is one of the important mediators of immediate hypersensitivity. Histamine binds to specific receptors in various tissues and causes increased vascular permeability and contraction of bronchial and intestinal smooth muscle.

HLA. See **Human leukocyte antigens.**

HLA-DM. A peptide exchange molecule that plays a critical role in the class II MHC pathway of antigen presentation. HLA-DM is found in the specialized MIIC endosomal compartment and facilitates removal of the invariant chain–derived CLIP peptide and the binding of other peptides to class II MHC molecules. HLA-DM is encoded by a gene in the MHC and is structurally similar to class II MHC molecules, but it is not polymorphic.

Homeostasis. In the adaptive immune system, the maintenance of a constant number and diverse repertoire of lymphocytes, despite the emergence of new lymphocytes and tremendous expansion of individual clones that may occur during responses to immunogenic antigens. Homeostasis is achieved by several regulated pathways of lymphocyte death and inactivation.

Homing receptor. Adhesion molecules expressed on the surface of lymphocytes that are responsible for the different pathways of lymphocyte recirculation and tissue homing. Homing receptors bind to ligands (addressins) expressed on endothelial cells in particular vascular beds.

Human immunodeficiency virus (HIV). The etiologic agent of AIDS. HIV is a retrovirus that infects a variety of cell types, including CD4-expressing helper T cells, macrophages, and dendritic cells, and causes chronic progressive destruction of the immune system.

Human leukocyte antigens (HLA). MHC molecules expressed on the surface of human cells. Human MHC molecules were first identified as alloantigens on the surface of white blood cells (leukocytes) that bound serum antibodies from individuals previously exposed to other individuals' cells (e.g., mothers or transfusion recipients).

Humanized antibody. A monoclonal antibody encoded by a recombinant hybrid gene and composed of the antigen-binding sites from a murine monoclonal antibody and the constant region of a human antibody. Humanized antibodies are less likely than mouse monoclonal antibodies to induce an anti-antibody response in humans; they are used clinically in the treatment of tumors and transplant rejection.

Humoral immunity. The type of adaptive immune response mediated by antibodies produced by B lymphocytes. Humoral immunity is the principal defense mechanism against extracellular microbes and their toxins.

Hybridoma. A cell line derived by cell fusion, or somatic cell hybridization, between a normal lymphocyte and an immortalized lymphocyte tumor line. B cell hybridomas created by fusion of normal B cells of defined antigen specificity with a myeloma cell line are used to produce monoclonal antibodies. T cell hybridomas created by fusion of a normal T cell of defined specificity with a T cell tumor line are commonly used in research.

Hyperacute rejection. A form of allograft or xenograft rejection that begins within minutes to hours after transplantation and that is characterized by thrombotic occlusion of the graft vessels. Hyperacute rejection is mediated by preexisting antibodies in the host circulation that bind to donor endothelial antigens, such as blood group antigens or MHC molecules, and activate the complement system.

Hypersensitivity diseases. Disorders caused by immune responses. Hypersensitivity diseases include autoimmune diseases, in which immune responses are directed against self antigens, and diseases that result from uncontrolled or excessive responses against foreign antigens, such as microbes and allergens. The tissue damage that occurs in hypersensitivity diseases is due to the same effector mechanisms used by the immune system to protect against microbes.

Hypervariable loop (hypervariable region). Short segments of about 10 amino acid residues within the variable regions of antibody or TCR proteins that form loop structures that contact antigen. Three hypervariable loops, also called CDRs, are present in each antibody heavy chain and light chain and in each TCR chain. Most of the variability between different antibodies or TCRs is located within these loops.

Idiotype. The property of a group of antibodies or TCRs defined by their sharing a particular idiotope; that is, antibodies that share a particular idiotope belong to the same idiotype. Idiotype is also used to describe the collection of idiotopes expressed by an Ig molecule, and it is often used synonymously with idiotope.

Idiotypic network. A network of complementary interactions involving idiotypes and anti-idiotypic antibodies (or T cells) that, according to the network hypothesis, reach a steady state at which the immune system is at homeostasis. Theoretically, when one or a few clones of lymphocytes respond to a foreign antigen, their idiotypes are expanded and anti-idiotype responses are triggered that function to shut off the antigen-specific response.

Igα and Igβ. Proteins that are required for surface expression and signaling functions of membrane Ig on B cells. Igα and Igβ pairs are disulfide linked to one another, noncovalently associated with the cytoplasmic tail of membrane Ig, and form the BCR complex. The cytoplasmic domains of Igα and Igβ contain ITAMs that are involved in early signaling events during antigen-induced B cell activation.

IL-1 receptor antagonist (IL-1ra). A natural inhibitor of IL-1 produced by mononuclear phagocytes that is structurally homologous to IL-1 and binds to the same receptors but is biologically inactive. Attempts to use IL-1 inhibitors to reduce inflammation in diseases such as rheumatoid arthritis are ongoing.

Immature B lymphocyte. A membrane IgM$^+$, IgD$^-$ B cell, recently derived from marrow precursors, that does not proliferate or differentiate in response to antigens but rather may undergo apoptotic death or become functionally unresponsive. This property is important for the negative selection of B cells that are specific for self antigens present in the bone marrow.

Immediate hypersensitivity. The type of immune reaction responsible for allergic diseases and dependent on IgE plus antigen-mediated stimulation of tissue mast cells and basophils. The mast cells and basophils release mediators that cause increased vascular permeability, vasodilation, bronchial and visceral smooth muscle contraction, and local inflammation.

Immune complex. A multimolecular complex of antibody molecules with bound antigen. Because each antibody molecule has a minimum of two antigen-binding sites and many antigens are mutivalent, immune complexes can vary greatly in size. Immune complexes activate effector mechanisms of humoral immunity, such as the classical complement pathway and Fc receptor–mediated phagocyte activation. Deposition of circulating immune complexes in blood vessel walls or renal glomeruli can lead to inflammation and disease.

Immune complex disease. An inflammatory disease caused by the deposition of antigen-antibody complexes in blood vessel walls resulting in local complement activation and phagocyte recruitment. Immune complexes may form because of overproduction of antibodies to microbial antigens or as a result of autoantibody production in the setting of an autoimmune disease such as systemic lupus erythematosus. Immune complex deposition in the specialized capillary basement membranes of renal glomeruli can cause glomerulonephritis and impair renal function. Systemic deposition of immune complexes in arterial walls can cause thrombosis and ischemic damage to various organs.

Immune deviation. The conversion of a T cell response associated with one set of cytokines, such as T_H1 cytokines that stimulate cell-mediated immunity, to a response associated with other cytokines, such as T_H2 cytokines that stimulate the production of selected antibody isotypes.

Immune inflammation. Inflammation that is a result of an adaptive immune response to antigen. The cellular infiltrate at the inflammatory site may include cells of the innate immune system such as neutrophils and macrophages, which are recruited as a result of the actions of T cell cytokines.

Immune response. A collective and coordinated response to the introduction of foreign substances in an individual mediated by the cells and molecules of the immune system.

Immune response (Ir) genes. Originally defined as genes in inbred strains of rodents that were inherited in a dominant mendelian manner and that controlled the ability of the animals to make antibodies against simple synthetic polypeptides. We now know that Ir genes are polymorphic MHC genes that encode peptide-binding molecules required for the activation of T lymphocytes and are therefore also required for helper T cell–dependent B cell (antibody) responses to protein antigens.

Immune surveillance. The concept that a physiologic function of the immune system is to recognize and destroy clones of transformed cells before they grow into tumors and to kill tumors after they are formed. The term *immune surveillance* is sometimes used in a general sense to describe the function of T lymphocytes to detect and destroy any cell, not necessarily a tumor cell, that is expressing foreign (e.g., microbial) antigens.

Immune system. The molecules, cells, tissues, and organs that collectively function to provide immunity, or protection, against foreign organisms.

Immunity. Protection against disease, usually infectious disease, mediated by a collection of molecules, cells, and tissues collectively called the immune system. In a broader sense, immunity refers to the ability to respond to foreign substances, including microbes or molecules.

Immunoblot. An analytical technique in which antibodies are used to detect the presence of an antigen bound to (i.e., blotted on) a solid matrix such as filter paper (also known as a Western blot).

Immunodominant epitope. A linear amino acid sequence of a multideterminant protein antigen for which most of the responding T cells in any individual are specific. Immunodominant epitopes correspond to the peptides proteolytically generated within APCs that bind most avidly to MHC molecules and are most likely to stimulate T cells.

Immunofluorescence. A technique in which a molecule is detected by use of an antibody labeled with a fluorescent probe. For example, in immunofluorescence microscopy, cells that express a particular surface antigen can be stained with a fluorescein-conjugated antibody specific for the antigen and then visualized with a fluorescent microscope.

Immunogen. An antigen that induces an immune response. Not all antigens are immunogens. For example, small molecular weight compounds may not stimulate an immune response unless they are linked to macromolecules.

Immunoglobulin domain. A three-dimensional globular structural motif found in many proteins in the immune system, including Igs, TCRs, and MHC molecules. Ig domains are about 110 amino acid residues in length, include an internal disulfide bond, and contain two layers of β-pleated sheet, each layer composed of three to five strands of antiparallel polypeptide chain. Ig domains are classified as V-like or C-like on the basis of closest homology to either the Ig V or C domains.

Immunoglobulin superfamily. A large family of proteins that contain a globular structural motif called an Ig domain, or Ig fold, originally described in antibodies. Many proteins of importance in the immune system, including antibodies, TCRs, MHC molecules, CD4, and CD8, are members of this superfamily.

Immunoglobulin (Ig). Synonymous with antibody (see **Antibody**).

Immunoglobulin heavy chain. One of two types of polypeptide chains in an antibody molecule. The basic structural unit of an antibody includes two identical, disulfide-linked heavy chains and two identical light chains. Each heavy chain is composed of a variable (V) Ig domain and three or four constant (C) Ig domains. The different antibody isotypes, including IgM, IgD, IgG, IgA, and IgE, are distinguished by structural differences in their heavy chain constant regions. The heavy chain constant regions also mediate effector func-

tions, such as complement activation or engagement of phagocytes.

Immunoglobulin light chain. One of two types of polypeptide chains in an antibody molecule. The basic structural unit of an antibody includes two identical light chains, each disulfide linked to one of two identical heavy chains. Each light chain is composed of one variable (V) Ig domain and one constant (C) Ig domain. There are two light chain isotypes, called κ and λ, both functionally identical. About 60% of human antibodies have κ light chains and 40% have λ light chains.

Immunohistochemistry. A technique to detect the presence of an antigen in histologic tissue sections by use of an enzyme-coupled antibody that is specific for the antigen. The enzyme converts a colorless substrate to a colored insoluble substance that precipitates at the site where the antibody and thus the antigen are localized. The position of the colored precipitate, and therefore the antigen, in the tissue section is observed by conventional light microscopy. Immunohistochemistry is a routine technique in diagnostic pathology and various fields of research.

Immunologic tolerance. See **Tolerance.**

Immunologically privileged site. A site in the body that is inaccessible to or constitutively suppresses immune responses. The anterior chamber of the eye, the testes, and the brain are examples of immunologically privileged sites.

Immunoperoxidase technique. A common immunohistochemical technique in which a horseradish peroxidase–coupled antibody is used to identify the presence of an antigen in a tissue section. The peroxidase enzyme converts a colorless substrate to an insoluble brown product that is observable by light microscopy.

Immunoprecipitation. A technique for the isolation of a molecule from a solution by binding it to an antibody and then rendering the antigen-antibody complex insoluble, either by precipitation with a second antibody or by coupling the first antibody to an insoluble particle or bead.

Immunoreceptor tyrosine-based activation motif (ITAM). A conserved motif composed of two copies of the sequence tyrosine-X-X-leucine (where X is an unspecified amino acid) found in the cytoplasmic tails of various membrane proteins in the immune system that are involved in signal transduction. ITAMS are present in the ζ and CD3 proteins of the TCR complex, in Igα and Igβ proteins in the BCR complex, and in several Ig Fc receptors. When these receptors bind their ligands, the tyrosine residues of the ITAMs become phosphorylated and form docking sites for other molecules involved in propagating cell-activating signal transduction pathways.

Immunoreceptor tyrosine-based inhibition motif (ITIM). A six–amino acid (isoleucine-X-tyrosine-X-X-leucine) motif found in the cytoplasmic tails of various inhibitory receptors in the immune system, including FcγRIIB on B cells and killer cell Ig-like receptors (KIR) on NK cells. When these receptors bind their ligands, the ITIMs become phosphorylated on their tyrosine residue and form a docking site for protein tyrosine phosphatases, which in turn function to inhibit other signal transduction pathways.

Immunosuppression. Inhibition of one or more components of the adaptive or innate immune system as a result of an underlying disease or intentionally induced by drugs for the purpose of preventing or treating graft rejection or autoimmune disease. A commonly used immunosuppressive drug is cyclosporine, which blocks T cell cytokine production.

Immunotherapy. The treatment of a disease with therapeutic agents that promote or inhibit immune responses. Cancer immunotherapy, for example, involves promoting active immune responses to tumor antigens or administering anti-tumor antibodies or T cells to establish passive immunity.

Immunotoxins. Reagents that may be used in the treatment of cancer and consist of covalent conjugates of a potent cellular toxin, such as ricin or diphtheria toxin, with antibodies specific for antigens expressed on the surface of tumor cells. It is hoped that such reagents can specifically target and kill tumor cells without damaging normal cells, but safe and effective immunotoxins have yet to be developed.

Inbred mouse strain. A strain of mice created by repetitive mating of siblings that is characterized by homozygosity at every genetic locus. Every mouse of an inbred strain is genetically identical (syngeneic) to every other mouse of the same strain.

Indirect antigen presentation (or indirect allorecognition). In transplantation immunology, a pathway of presentation of donor (allogeneic) MHC molecules by recipient APCs that involves the same mechanisms used to present microbial proteins. The allogeneic MHC proteins are processed by recipient professional APCs, and peptides derived from the allogeneic MHC molecules are presented, in association with recipient (self) MHC molecules, to host T cells. In contrast to indirect antigen presentation, direct antigen presentation involves recipient T cell recognition of unprocessed allogeneic MHC molecules on the surface of graft cells.

Inflammation. A complex reaction of the innate immune system in vascularized tissues that involves the accumulation and activation of leukocytes and plasma proteins at a site of infection, toxin exposure, or cell injury. Inflammation is initiated by changes in blood vessels that promote leukocyte recruitment. Local adaptive immune responses can promote inflammation. Although inflammation serves a protective function in controlling infections and promoting tissue repair, it can also cause tissue damage and disease.

Inflammatory bowel disease (IBD). A group of disorders, including ulcerative colitis and Crohn's disease, characterized by chronic inflammation in the gastrointestinal tract. The etiology of IBD is not known, but some evidence indicates that immune mechanisms may be involved. IBD develops in gene knockout mice lacking IL-2, IL-10, or the TCR α chain.

Innate immunity. Protection against infection that relies on mechanisms that exist before infection, are capable of a rapid response to microbes, and react in essentially the same way to repeated infections. The innate immune system includes epithelial barriers, phagocytic cells (neutrophils, macrophages), NK cells, the complement system, and cytokines, largely made by mononuclear phagocytes, that regulate and coordinate many of the activities of the cells of innate immunity.

Inositol 1,4,5-triphosphate (IP₃). A cytoplasmic signaling molecule generated by phospholipase C (PLCγ1)–mediated hydrolysis of the plasma membrane phospholipid PIP₂ during antigen activation of lymphocytes. The main function of IP₃ is to stimulate the release of intracellular stores of calcium from membrane-bound compartments such as the endoplasmic reticulum.

Insulin-dependent diabetes mellitus. A disease characterized by a lack of insulin that leads to various metabolic and vascular abnormalities. The insulin deficiency results from autoimmune destruction of the insulin-producing β cells of the islets of Langerhans in the pancreas, usually during childhood. CD4⁺ and CD8⁺ T cells, antibodies, and cytokines have been implicated in the islet cell damage. Also called type 1 diabetes mellitus.

Integrins. Heterodimeric cell surface proteins whose major functions are to mediate the adhesion of leukocytes to other leukocytes, endothelial cells, and extracellular matrix proteins. Integrins are important for T cell interactions with APCs and for migration of leukocytes from blood into tissues. The ligand-binding affinity of the integrins can be regulated by various stimuli, and the cytoplasmic domains of integrins bind to the cytoskeleton. There are two main subfamilies of integrins; the members of each family express a conserved β chain (β₁, or CD29, and β₂, or CD18) associated with different α chains. VLA-4 (very late activation protein-4) is a β₁ integrin expressed on T cells, and LFA-1 (leukocyte function–associated antigen-1) is a β₂ integrin expressed on T cells and phagocytes.

Interferon-γ (IFN-γ). A cytokine produced by T lymphocytes and NK cells whose principal function is to activate macrophages in both innate immune responses and adaptive cell-mediated immune responses. (IFN-γ is also called immune or type II interferon.)

Interleukin (IL). Another name for a cytokine originally used to describe a cytokine made by leukocytes that acts on leukocytes. The term is now generally used with a numerical suffix to designate a structurally defined cytokine regardless of its source or target.

Interleukin-1 (IL-1). A cytokine produced mainly by activated mononuclear phagocytes whose principal function is to mediate host inflammatory responses in innate immunity. The two forms of IL-1 (α and β) bind to the same receptors and have identical biologic effects, including induction of endothelial cell adhesion molecules, stimulation of chemokine production by endothelial cells and macrophages, stimulation of the synthesis of acute-phase reactants by the liver, and fever.

Interleukin-2 (IL-2). A cytokine produced by antigen-activated T cells that acts in an autocrine manner to stimulate T cell proliferation and also potentiates the apoptotic cell death of antigen-activated T cells. Thus, IL-2 is required for both the induction and self-regulation of T cell–mediated immune responses.

IL-2 also stimulates the proliferation and effector functions of NK cells and B cells.

Interleukin-3 (IL-3). A cytokine produced by CD4$^+$ T cells that promotes the expansion of immature marrow progenitors of all known mature blood cell types. IL-3 is also known as multilineage colony-stimulating factor.

Interleukin-4 (IL-4). A cytokine produced mainly by the T$_H$2 subset of CD4$^+$ helper T cells whose functions include induction of differentiation of T$_H$2 cells from naive CD4$^+$ precursors, stimulation of IgE production by B cells, and suppression of IFN-γ–dependent macrophage functions.

Interleukin-5 (IL-5). A cytokine produced by CD4$^+$ T$_H$2 cells and activated mast cells that stimulates the growth and differentiation of eosinophils and activates mature eosinophils.

Interleukin-6 (IL-6). A cytokine produced by many cell types, including activated mononuclear phagocytes, endothelial cells, and fibroblasts, that functions in both innate and adaptive immunity. IL-6 stimulates the synthesis of acute-phase proteins by hepatocytes as well as the growth of antibody-producing B lymphocytes.

Interleukin-7 (IL-7). A cytokine secreted by bone marrow stromal cells that stimulates survival and expansion of immature, but lineage-committed, precursors of B and T lymphocytes.

Interleukin-10 (IL-10). A cytokine produced by activated macrophages and some helper T cells whose major function is to inhibit activated macrophages and therefore to maintain homeostatic control of innate and cell-mediated immune reactions.

Interleukin-12 (IL-12). A cytokine produced by mononuclear phagocytes and dendritic cells that serves as a mediator of the innate immune response to intracellular microbes and is a key inducer of cell-mediated immune responses to these microbes. IL-12 activates NK cells, promotes IFN-γ production by NK cells and T cells, enhances the cytolytic activity of NK cells and CTLs, and promotes the development of T$_H$1 cells.

Interleukin-15 (IL-15). A cytokine produced by mononuclear phagocytes and other cells in response to viral infections whose principal function is to stimulate the proliferation of NK cells. It is structurally similar to IL-2.

Interleukin-18 (IL-18). A cytokine produced by macrophages in response to LPS and other microbial products that functions together with IL-12 as an inducer of cell-mediated immunity. IL-18 synergizes with IL-12 in stimulating the production of IFN-γ by NK cells and T cells. IL-18 is structurally homologous to but functionally different from IL-1.

Intracellular bacterium. A bacterium that survives or replicates within cells, usually in endosomes. The principal defense against intracellular bacteria, such as *Mycobacterium tuberculosis,* is cell-mediated immunity.

Intraepidermal lymphocytes. T lymphocytes found within the epidermal layer of the skin. In the mouse, most of the intraepidermal T cells express the γδ form of TCR (see **Intraepithelial T lymphocytes**).

Intraepithelial T lymphocytes. T lymphocytes present in the epidermis of the skin and in mucosal epithelia that typically express a limited diversity of antigen receptors. Some of these lymphocytes may recognize microbial products, such as glycolipids, associated with nonpolymorphic class I MHC–like molecules. Intraepithelial T lymphocytes may be considered effector cells of innate immunity and function in host defense by secreting cytokines and activating phagocytes and by killing infected cells.

Invariant chain (I$_i$). A nonpolymorphic protein that binds to newly synthesized class II MHC molecules in the endoplasmic reticulum. The invariant chain prevents loading of the class II MHC peptide-binding cleft with peptides present in the endoplasmic reticulum, and such peptides are left to associate with class I molecules. The invariant chain also promotes folding and assembly of class II molecules and directs newly formed class II molecules to the specialized endosomal MIIC compartment, where peptide loading takes place.

Isotype. One of five types of antibodies, determined by which of five different forms of heavy chain are present. Antibody isotypes include IgM, IgD, IgG, IgA, and IgE, and each isotype performs a different set of effector functions. Additional structural variations characterize distinct subtypes of IgG and IgA.

J chain. A small polypeptide that is disulfide bonded to the tail pieces of multimeric IgM and IgA antibodies.

JAK/STAT signaling pathway. A signaling pathway initiated by cytokine binding to type I and type II cytokine receptors. This pathway sequentially involves activation of receptor-associated Janus kinase (JAK) tyrosine kinases, JAK-mediated tyrosine phosphorylation of the cytoplasmic tails of cytokine receptors, docking of signal transducers and activators of transcription (STATs) to the phosphorylated receptor chains, JAK-mediated tyrosine phosphorylation of the associated STATs, dimerization and nuclear translocation of the STATs, and STAT binding to regulatory regions of target genes causing transcriptional activation of those genes.

Janus kinases (JAK kinases). A family of tyrosine kinases that associate with the cytoplasmic tails of several different cytokine receptors, including the receptors for IL-2, IL-4, IFN-γ, IL-12, and others. In response to cytokine binding and receptor dimerization, JAKs phosphorylate the cytokine receptors to permit the binding of STATs, and then the JAKs phosphorylate and thereby activate the STATs. Different JAK kinases associate with different cytokine receptors.

Joining (J) segments. Short coding sequences, between the variable (V) and constant (C) gene segments in all the Ig and TCR loci, that together with D segments are somatically recombined with V segments during lymphocyte development. The resulting recombined VDJ DNA codes for the carboxyl terminal ends of the antigen receptor V regions, including the third hypervariable (CDR) regions. Random use of different J segments contributes to the diversity of the antigen receptor repertoire.

Junctional diversity. The diversity in antibody and TCR repertoires that is attributed to the random addition or removal of nucleotide sequences at junctions between V, D, and J gene segments.

Kaposi's sarcoma. A malignant tumor of vascular cells that frequently arises in patients with AIDS. Kaposi's sarcoma is associated with infection by the Kaposi's sarcoma–associated herpesvirus (human herpesvirus 8).

Killer Ig-like receptors (KIRs). Ig superfamily receptors expressed by NK cells that recognize different alleles of HLA-A, HLA-B, and HLA-C molecules. Some KIRs have signaling components with ITIMS in their cytoplasmic tails, and these deliver inhibitory signals to inactivate the NK cells. Some members of the KIR family have short cytoplasmic tails without ITIMs, and these function as activating receptors.

Knockout mouse. A mouse with a targeted disruption of one or more genes that is created by homologous recombination techniques. Knockout mice lacking functional genes encoding cytokines, cell surface receptors, signaling molecules, and transcription factors have provided extensive information about the roles of these molecules in the immune system.

Langerhans cells. Immature dendritic cells found as a continuous meshwork in the epidermal layer of the skin whose major function is to trap and transport protein antigens to draining lymph nodes. During their migration to the lymph nodes, Langerhans cells mature into lymph node dendritic cells, which can efficiently present antigen to naive T cells.

Large granular lymphocyte. Another name for an NK cell based on the morphologic appearance of this cell type in the blood.

Late-phase reaction. A component of the immediate hypersensitivity reaction that ensues 2 to 4 hours after mast cell and basophil degranulation and that is characterized by an inflammatory infiltrate of eosinophils, basophils, neutrophils, and lymphocytes. Repeated bouts of this late-phase inflammatory reaction can cause tissue damage.

Lck. An Src family nonreceptor tyrosine kinase that noncovalently associates with the cytoplasmic tails of CD4 and CD8 molecules in T cells and is involved in the early signaling events of antigen-induced T cell activation. Lck mediates tyrosine phosphorylation of the cytoplasmic tails of CD3 and ζ proteins of the TCR complex.

Lectin pathway of complement activation. A pathway of complement activation triggered, in the absence of antibody, by the binding of microbial polysaccharides to circulating lectins such as MBL. MBL is structurally similar to C1q and activates the C1r–C1s enzyme complex (like C1q) or activates another serine esterase, called mannose-binding protein–associated serine esterase. The remaining steps of the lectin pathway, beginning with cleavage of C4, are the same as the classical pathway.

Leishmania. An obligate intracellular protozoan parasite that infects macrophages and can cause a chronic inflammatory disease involving many tissues. *Leishmania* infection in mice has served as a model system for study of the effector functions of several cytokines and the helper T cell subsets that produce them. T_H1 responses to *Leishmania major* and associated IFN-γ production control infection, whereas T_H2 responses

with IL-4 production lead to disseminated lethal disease.

Lethal hit. A term used to describe the events that result in irreversible damage to a target cell when a CTL binds to it. The lethal hit includes CTL granule exocytosis, perforin polymerization in the target cell membrane, and entry of calcium ions and apoptosis-inducing enzymes (granzymes) into the target cell cytoplasm.

Leukemia. A malignant disease of bone marrow precursors of blood cells in which large numbers of leukemic cells usually occupy the bone marrow and often circulate in the blood stream. Lymphocytic leukemias are derived from B or T cell precursors, myelogenous leukemias are derived from granulocyte or monocyte precursors, and erythroid leukemias are derived from red blood cell precursors.

Leukocyte adhesion deficiency (LAD). One of a rare group of immunodeficiency diseases with infectious complications that is caused by defective expression of the leukocyte adhesion molecules required for tissue recruitment of phagocytes and lymphocytes. LAD-1 is due to mutations in the gene encoding the CD18 protein, which is part of β_2 integrins. LAD-2 is caused by mutations in a gene that encodes a fucose transporter involved in the synthesis of leukocyte ligands for endothelial selectins.

Leukotrienes. A class of arachidonic acid–derived lipid inflammatory mediators produced by the lipoxygenase pathway in many cell types. Mast cells make abundant leukotriene C_4 (LTC_4) and its degradation products LTD_4 and LTE_4, which bind to specific receptors on smooth muscle cells and cause prolonged bronchoconstriction. Leukotrienes contribute to the pathologic processes of bronchial asthma. Collectively, LTC_4, LTD_4, and LTE_4 constitute what was once called slow-reacting substance of anaphylaxis.

Lipopolysaccharide. Synonymous with **endotoxin**.

Live viral vaccine. A vaccine composed of a live but nonpathogenic (attenuated) form of a virus. Attenuated viruses carry mutations that interfere with the viral life cycle or pathogenesis. Because live virus vaccines actually infect the recipient cells, they can effectively stimulate immune responses, such as the CTL response, that are optimal for protecting against wild-type viral infection. A commonly used live virus vaccine is the Sabin poliovirus vaccine, and there is much interest in development of an attenuated live virus vaccine to protect against HIV infection.

LMP-2 and LMP-7. Two catalytic subunits of the proteasome, the organelle that degrades cytosolic proteins into peptides in the class I MHC pathway of antigen presentation. LMP-2 and LMP-7 are encoded by genes in the MHC, are up-regulated by IFN-γ, and are particularly important for generating class I MHC–binding peptides.

Lymph node. Small nodular, encapsulated aggregates of lymphocyte-rich tissue situated along lymphatic channels throughout the body where adaptive immune responses to lymph-borne antigens are initiated.

Lymphatic system. A system of vessels throughout the body that collects tissue fluid called lymph, originally derived from the blood, and returns it, through the thoracic duct, to the circulation. Lymph nodes are interspersed along these vessels and trap and retain antigens present in the lymph.

Lymphocyte homing. The directed migration of subsets of circulating lymphocytes into particular tissue sites. Lymphocyte homing is regulated by the selective expression of adhesion molecules, called homing receptors, on the lymphocytes and the tissue-specific expression of endothelial ligands for these homing receptors, called addressins, in different vascular beds. For example, some T lymphocytes preferentially home to intestinal lymphoid tissue (e.g., Peyer's patches), and this directed migration is regulated by binding of the VLA-4 integrin on the T cells to the MadCAM addressin on Peyer's patch endothelium.

Lymphocyte maturation. The process by which pluripotent bone marrow precursor cells develop into mature, antigen receptor–expressing naive B or T lymphocytes that populate peripheral lymphoid tissues. This process takes place in the specialized environments of the bone marrow (for B cells) and the thymus (for T cells).

Lymphocyte migration. The movement of lymphocytes from the blood stream into peripheral tissues.

Lymphocyte recirculation. The continuous movement of lymphocytes through the blood stream and lymphatics, between the lymph nodes or spleen, and, if activated, to peripheral inflammatory sites.

Lymphocyte repertoire. The complete collection of antigen receptors and therefore antigen specificities expressed by the B and T lymphocytes of an individual.

Lymphoid follicle. A B cell–rich region of a lymph node or the spleen that is the site of antigen-induced B cell proliferation and differentiation. In T cell–dependent B cell responses to protein antigens, a germinal center forms within the follicles.

Lymphokine. An old name for a cytokine (soluble protein mediator of immune responses) produced by lymphocytes.

Lymphokine-activated killer (LAK) cell. NK cells with enhanced cytolytic activity for tumor cells as a result of exposure to high doses of IL-2. LAK cells generated *in vitro* have been adoptively transferred back into patients with cancer to treat their tumors.

Lymphoma. A malignant tumor of B or T lymphocytes usually arising in and spreading between lymphoid tissues but that may spread to other tissues. Lymphomas often express phenotypic characteristics of the normal lymphocytes from which they were derived.

Lymphotoxin (LT, TNF-β). A cytokine produced by T cells that is homologous to and binds to the same receptors as TNF. Like TNF, LT has proinflammatory effects, including endothelial and neutrophil activation. LT is also critical for the normal development of lymphoid organs.

Lysosome. A membrane-bound, acidic organelle abundant in phagocytic cells that contains proteolytic enzymes that degrade proteins derived both from the extracellular environment and from within the cell. Lysosomes are involved in the class II MHC pathway of antigen processing.

M cells. Specialized epithelial cells overlying Peyer's patches in the gut that play a role in delivering antigens to Peyer's patches.

Macrophage. A tissue-based phagocytic cell derived from blood monocytes that plays important roles in innate and adaptive immune responses. Macrophages are activated by microbial products such as endotoxin and by T cell cytokines such as IFN-γ. Activated macrophages phagocytose and kill microorganisms, secrete proinflammatory cytokines, and present antigens to helper T cells. Macrophages may assume different morphologic forms in different tissues, including the microglia of the central nervous system, Kupffer cells in the liver, alveolar macrophages in the lung, and osteoclasts in bone.

Major histocompatibility complex (MHC). A large genetic locus (on human chromosome 6 and mouse chromosome 17) that includes the highly polymorphic genes encoding the peptide-binding molecules recognized by T lymphocytes. The MHC locus also includes genes encoding cytokines, molecules involved in antigen processing, and complement proteins.

Major histocompatibility complex (MHC) molecule. A heterodimeric membrane protein encoded in the MHC locus that serves as a peptide display molecule for recognition by T lymphocytes. Two structurally distinct types of MHC molecules exist. Class I MHC molecules are present on most nucleated cells, bind peptides derived from cytosolic proteins, and are recognized by CD8+ T cells. Class II MHC molecules are restricted largely to professional APCs, bind peptides derived from endocytosed proteins, and are recognized by CD4+ T cells.

Mannose receptor. A carbohydrate-binding receptor (lectin) expressed by macrophages that binds mannose and fucose residues on microbial cell walls and mediates phagocytosis of the organisms.

Mannose-binding lectin (MBL). A plasma protein that binds to mannose residues on bacterial cell walls and acts as an opsonin by promoting phagocytosis of the bacterium by macrophages. Macrophages express a surface receptor for C1q that can also bind MBL and mediate uptake of the opsonized organisms.

Marginal zone. A peripheral region of splenic lymphoid follicles containing macrophages that are particularly efficient at trapping polysaccharide antigens. Such antigens may persist for prolonged periods on the surfaces of marginal zone macrophages, where they are recognized by specific B cells, or they may be transported into follicles.

Mast cell. The major effector cell of immediate hypersensitivity (allergic) reactions. Mast cells are derived from the marrow, reside in most tissues adjacent to blood vessels, express a high-affinity Fc receptor for IgE, and contain numerous mediator-filled granules. Antigen-induced cross-linking of IgE bound to the mast cell Fc receptors causes release of their granule contents as well as new synthesis and secretion of other mediators, leading to an immediate hypersensitivity reaction.

Mature B cell. IgM- and IgD-expressing, functionally competent naive B cells that represent the final stage of

B cell maturation in the bone marrow and that populate peripheral lymphoid organs.

Membrane attack complex (MAC). A lytic complex of the terminal components of the complement cascade, including multiple copies of C9, that forms in the membranes of target cells. The MAC causes lethal ionic and osmotic changes in cells.

Memory. The property of the adaptive immune system to respond more rapidly, with greater magnitude, and more effectively to a repeated exposure to an antigen, compared with the response to the first exposure.

Memory lymphocytes. B or T lymphocytes that mediate rapid and enhanced (i.e., memory or recall) responses to second and subsequent exposures to antigens. Memory B and T cells are produced by antigen stimulation of naive lymphocytes and survive in a functionally quiescent state for many years after the antigen is eliminated.

MHC class II (MIIC) compartment. A subset of endosomes (membrane-bound vesicles involved in cell trafficking pathways) found in macrophages and human B cells that are important in the class II MHC pathway of antigen presentation. The MIIC contains all the components required for formation of peptide–class II MHC molecule complexes, including the enzymes that degrade protein antigens, class II molecules, invariant chain, and HLA-DM.

MHC restriction. The characteristic of T lymphocytes that they recognize a foreign peptide antigen only when it is bound to a particular allelic form of an MHC molecule.

MHC-tetramer. A reagent used to identify and enumerate T cells that specifically recognize a particular MHC-peptide complex. The reagent consists of four recombinant, biotinylated MHC molecules (usually class I) bound to a fluorochrome-labeled avidin molecule and loaded with a peptide. T cells that bind the MHC-tetramer can be detected by flow cytometry.

β_2-**Microglobulin.** The light chain of a class I MHC molecule. β_2-Microglobulin is an extracellular protein encoded by a nonpolymorphic gene outside the MHC, is structurally homologous to an Ig domain, and is invariant among all class I molecules.

Mitogen-activated protein (MAP) kinase cascade. A signal transduction cascade initiated by the active form of the Ras protein and involving the sequential activation of three serine/threonine kinases, the last one being MAP kinase. MAP kinase in turn phosphorylates and activates other enzymes or transcription factors. The MAP kinase pathway is one of several signal pathways activated by antigen binding to the TCR.

Mixed leukocyte reaction (MLR). An *in vitro* reaction of alloreactive T cells from one individual against MHC antigens on blood cells from another individual. The MLR involves proliferation of and cytokine secretion by both CD4+ and CD8+ T cells and is used as a screening test to assess the compatibility of a potential graft recipient with a potential donor.

Molecular mimicry. A postulated mechanism of autoimmunity triggered by infection with a microbe containing antigens that cross-react with self antigens. Immune responses to the microbe result in reactions against self tissues.

Monoclonal antibody. An antibody that is specific for one antigen and is produced by a B cell hybridoma (a cell line derived by the fusion of a single normal B cell and an immortal B cell tumor line). Monoclonal antibodies are widely used in research and clinical diagnosis and therapy.

Monocyte. A type of bone marrow–derived circulating blood cell that is the precursor of tissue macrophages. Monocytes are actively recruited into inflammatory sites, where they differentiate into macrophages.

Monocyte colony-stimulating factor (M-CSF). A cytokine made by activated T cells, macrophages, endothelial cells, and stromal fibroblasts that stimulates the production of monocytes from bone marrow precursor cells.

Monokine. An old name for a cytokine produced by mononuclear phagocytes.

Mononuclear phagocytes. Cells with a common bone marrow lineage whose primary function is phagocytosis. These cells function as accessory cells in the recognition and activation phases of adaptive immune responses and as effector cells in innate and adaptive immunity. Mononuclear phagocytes circulate in the blood in an incompletely differentiated form called monocytes, and once they settle in tissues, they mature into macrophages.

Mucosa-associated lymphoid tissue. Lymphocytes and accessory cells within the mucosa of the gastrointestinal and respiratory tracts that are sites of adaptive immune responses to environmental antigens. Mucosa-associated lymphoid tissues include intraepithelial lymphocytes, mainly T cells, and organized collections of lymphocytes, often rich in B cells, below mucosal epithelia, such as Peyer's patches in the gut or pharyngeal tonsils.

Mucosal immune system. A part of the immune system that responds to and protects against microbes that enter the body through mucosal surfaces, such as the gastrointestinal and respiratory tracts. The mucosal immune system is composed of mucosa-associated lymphoid tissues, which are collections of lymphocytes and accessory cells in the epithelia and lamina propria of mucosal surfaces.

Multiple myeloma. A malignant tumor of antibody-producing B cells that often secretes Igs or parts of Ig molecules. The monoclonal antibodies produced by multiple myelomas were critical for early biochemical analyses of antibody structure.

Mycobacterium. A genus of aerobic bacteria, many species of which can survive within phagocytes and cause disease. The principal host defense against mycobacteria such as *M. tuberculosis* is cell-mediated immunity.

N nucleotides. The name given to nucleotides randomly added to the junctions between V, D, and J gene segments in Ig or TCR genes during lymphocyte development. The addition of up to 20 of these nucleotides, which is mediated by the enzyme terminal deoxyribonucleotidyl transferase, contributes to the diversity of the antibody and TCR repertoires.

Naive lymphocyte. A mature B or T lymphocyte that has not previously encountered antigen, nor is it the progeny of an antigen-stimulated mature lymphocyte. When naive lymphocytes are stimulated by antigen, they differentiate into effector lymphocytes, such as antibody-secreting B cells or helper T cells and CTLs. Naive lymphocytes have surface markers and recirculation patterns that are distinct from those of previously activated lymphocytes. ("Naive" also refers to an unimmunized individual.)

Natural antibodies. IgM antibodies, largely produced by B-1 cells, specific for bacteria that are common in the environment and gastrointestinal tract. Normal individuals contain natural antibodies without any evidence of infection, and these antibodies serve as a preformed defense mechanism against microbes that succeed in penetrating epithelial barriers. Some of these antibodies cross-react with ABO blood group antigens and are responsible for transfusion reactions.

Natural killer (NK) cells. A subset of bone marrow–derived lymphocytes, distinct from B or T cells, that function in innate immune responses to kill microbe-infected cells by direct lytic mechanisms and by secreting IFN-γ. NK cells do not express clonally distributed antigen receptors like Ig receptors or TCRs, and their activation is regulated by a combination of cell surface stimulatory and inhibitory receptors, the latter recognizing self MHC molecules.

Negative selection. The process by which developing lymphocytes that express self-reactive antigen receptors are eliminated, thereby contributing to the maintenance of self-tolerance. Negative selection of developing T lymphocytes (thymocytes) is best understood and involves high-avidity binding of a thymocyte to self MHC molecules with bound peptides on thymic APCs leading to apoptotic death of the thymocyte.

Neonatal Fc receptor (FcRn). An IgG-specific Fc receptor that mediates the transport of maternal IgG across the placenta and the neonatal intestinal epithelium. FcRn resembles a class I MHC molecule. An adult form of this receptor functions to protect plasma IgG antibodies from catabolism.

Neonatal immunity. Passive humoral immunity to infections in mammals in the first months of life, before full development of the immune system. Neonatal immunity is mediated by maternally produced antibodies transported across the placenta into the fetal circulation before birth or derived from ingested milk and transported across the gut epithelium.

Neutrophil (also polymorphonuclear leukocyte, PMN). A phagocytic cell characterized by a segmented lobular nucleus and cytoplasmic granules filled with degradative enzymes. PMNs are the most abundant type of circulating white blood cells and are the major cell type mediating acute inflammatory responses to bacterial infections.

Nitric oxide. A biologic effector molecule with a broad range of activities that in macrophages functions as a potent microbicidal agent to kill ingested organisms.

Nitric oxide synthase. A member of a family of enzymes that synthesize the vasoactive and microbicidal compound nitric oxide from L-arginine. Macrophages express an inducible form of this enzyme on activation by various microbial or cytokine stimuli.

Nuclear factor κB (NF-κB). A family of transcription factors composed of homodimers or heterodimers of proteins homologous to the c-Rel protein. NF-κB proteins are important in the transcription of many genes in both innate and adaptive immune responses.

Nuclear factor of activated T cells (NFAT). A transcription factor required for the expression of IL-2, IL-4, TNF, and other cytokine genes. The four different NFATs are each encoded by separate genes; NFATp and NFATc are found in T cells. Cytoplasmic NFAT is activated by calcium/calmodulin-dependent, calcineurin-mediated dephosphorylation that permits NFAT to translocate into the nucleus and bind to consensus binding sequences in the regulatory regions of IL-2, IL-4, and other cytokine genes, usually in association with other transcription factors such as AP-1.

Nude mouse. A strain of mice that lacks development of the thymus, and therefore T lymphocytes, as well as hair follicles. Nude mice have been used experimentally to define the role of T lymphocytes in immunity and disease.

Oncofetal antigen. Proteins that are expressed at high levels on some types of cancer cells and in normal developing (fetal) but not adult tissues. Antibodies specific for these proteins are often used in histopathologic identification of tumors or to monitor the progression of tumor growth in patients. CEA (CD66) and alpha-fetoprotein are two oncofetal antigens commonly expressed by certain carcinomas.

Opsonin. A macromolecule that becomes attached to the surface of a microbe and can be recognized by surface receptors of neutrophils and macrophages and that increases the efficiency of phagocytosis of the microbe. Opsonins include IgG antibodies, which are recognized by the Fcγ receptor on phagocytes, and fragments of complement proteins, which are recognized by CR1 (CD35) and by the leukocyte integrin Mac-1.

Opsonization. The process of attaching opsonins, such as IgG or complement fragments, to microbial surfaces to target the microbes for phagocytosis.

Oral tolerance. The suppression of systemic humoral and cell-mediated immune responses to an antigen after the oral administration of that antigen as a result of anergy of antigen-specific T cells or the production of immunosuppressive cytokines such as transforming growth factor-β. Oral tolerance is a possible mechanism for preventing immune responses to food antigens and to bacteria that normally reside as commensals in the intestinal lumen.

P nucleotides. Short inverted repeat nucleotide sequences in the VDJ junctions of rearranged Ig and TCR genes that are generated by RAG-1– and RAG-2–

mediated asymmetric cleavage of hairpin DNA intermediates during somatic recombination events. P nucleotides contribute to the junctional diversity of antigen receptors.

Paracrine factor. A molecule that acts on cells in proximity to the cell that produces the factor. Most cytokines act in a paracrine fashion.

Partial agonist. A variant peptide ligand of a TCR that induces only a subset of the functional responses by the T cell or responses entirely different from responses to the unaltered (native) peptide. For instance, a partial agonist may stimulate production of only some of the many cytokines that are induced by the native peptide or quantitatively smaller responses. Partial agonist peptides are usually synthetic peptides in which one or two TCR contact residues have been changed; they are also called APLs.

Passive immunity. The form of immunity to an antigen that is established in one individual by transfer of antibodies or lymphocytes from another individual who is immune to that antigen. The recipient of such a transfer can become immune to the antigen without ever having been exposed to or having responded to the antigen. An example of passive immunity is the transfer of human sera containing antibodies specific for certain microbial toxins or snake venom to a previously unimmunized individual.

Pathogenicity. The ability of a microorganism to cause disease. Multiple mechanisms may contribute to pathogenicity, including production of toxins, stimulation of host inflammatory responses, and perturbation of host cell metabolism.

Pattern recognition receptors. Receptors of the innate immune system that recognize frequently encountered structures called molecular patterns produced by microorganisms and that facilitate innate immune responses against the microorganisms. Examples of pattern recognition receptors include CD14 receptors on macrophages, which bind bacterial endotoxin leading to macrophage activation, and the mannose receptor on phagocytes, which binds microbial glycoproteins or glycolipids.

Pentraxins. A family of plasma proteins that contain five identical globular subunits; includes the acute-phase reactant C-reactive protein.

Peptide-binding cleft. The portion of an MHC molecule that binds peptides for display to T cells. The cleft is composed of paired α-helices resting on a floor made up of an eight-stranded β-pleated sheet. The polymorphic residues, which are the amino acids that vary among different MHC alleles, are located in and around this cleft.

Perforin. A protein, that is homologous to the C9 complement protein, is present as a monomer in the granules of CTLs and NK cells. When perforin is released from the granules of activated CTLs or NK cells, it forms a complex with granzymes and proteoglycans that binds to the target cell plasma membrane and promotes entry of the granzymes into the target cell. This channel can cause osmotic lysis of the target cell and serve as a channel for the influx of enzymes derived from the CTL granules.

Periarteriolar lymphoid sheath (PALS). A cuff of lymphocytes surrounding small arterioles in the spleen, adjacent to lymphoid follicles. A PALS contains mainly T lymphocytes, about two thirds of which are CD4$^+$ and one third CD8$^+$. In humoral immune responses to protein antigens, B lymphocytes are activated at the interface between the PALS and follicles and then migrate into the follicles to form germinal centers.

Peripheral lymphoid organs and tissues. Organized collections of lymphocytes and accessory cells, including the spleen, lymph nodes, and mucosa-associated lymphoid tissues, in which adaptive immune responses are initiated.

Peripheral tolerance. Physiologic unresponsiveness to self antigens that are present in peripheral tissues and not usually in the generative lymphoid organs. Peripheral tolerance is induced by the recognition of antigens without adequate levels of the costimulators required for lymphocyte activation or by persistent and repeated stimulation by these self antigens.

Peyer's patches. Organized lymphoid tissue in the lamina propria of the small intestine in which immune responses to ingested antigens may be initiated. Peyer's patches are composed mostly of B cells, with smaller numbers of T cells and accessory cells, all arranged in follicles similar to those found in lymph nodes, often with germinal centers.

Phagocytosis. The process by which certain cells of the innate immune system, including macrophages and neutrophils, engulf large particles (>0.5 μm in diameter) such as intact microbes. The cell surrounds the particle with extensions of its plasma membrane by an energy- and cytoskeleton-dependent process; this process results in the formation of an intracellular vesicle called a phagosome, which contains the ingested particle.

Phagosome. A membrane-bound intracellular vesicle that contains microbes or particulate material from the extracellular environment. Phagosomes are formed during the process of phagocytosis, and fusion with other vesicular structures such as lysosomes leads to enzymatic degradation of the ingested material.

Phosphatase (protein phosphatase). An enzyme that removes phosphate groups from the side chains of certain amino acid residues of proteins. Protein phosphatases in lymphocytes, such as CD45 or calcineurin, regulate the activity of various signal transduction molecules and transcription factors. Some protein phosphatases may be specific for phosphotyrosine residues and others for phosphoserine and phosphothreonine residues.

Phospholipase Cγ (PLCγ). An enzyme that catalyzes hydrolysis of the plasma membrane phospholipid PIP$_2$ to generate two signaling molecules, IP$_3$ and DAG. PLCγ becomes activated in lymphocytes by antigen binding to the antigen receptor.

Phytohemagglutinin (PHA). A carbohydrate-binding protein, or lectin, produced by plants that cross-links human T cell surface molecules, including the T cell receptor, thereby inducing polyclonal activation and agglutination of T cells. PHA is frequently used in experimental immunology to study T cell activation. In clinical medicine, PHA is used to assess whether a patient's T cells are functional or to induce T cell mitosis for the purpose of generating karyotypic data.

Plasma cell. A terminally differentiated antibody-secreting B lymphocyte with a characteristic histologic appearance, including an oval shape, eccentric nucleus, and perinuclear halo.

Platelet-activating factor (PAF). A lipid mediator derived from membrane phospholipids in several cell types, including mast cells and endothelial cells. PAF can cause bronchoconstriction and vascular dilatation and leak and may be an important mediator in asthma.

Polyclonal activators. Agents that are capable of activating many clones of lymphocytes, regardless of their antigen specificities. Examples of polyclonal activators include anti-IgM antibodies for B cells and anti-CD3 antibodies, bacterial superantigens, and PHA for T cells.

Poly-Ig receptor. An Fc receptor expressed by mucosal epithelial cells that mediates the transport of IgA and IgM through the epithelial cells into the intestinal lumen.

Polymerase chain reaction (PCR). A rapid method of copying and amplifying specific DNA sequences up to about 1 kb in length that is widely used as a preparative and analytical technique in all branches of molecular biology. The method relies on the use of short oligonucleotide primers complementary to the sequences at the ends of the DNA to be amplified and involves repetitive cycles of melting, annealing, and synthesis of DNA.

Polymorphism. The existence of two or more alternative forms, or variants, of a gene that are present at stable frequencies in a population. Each common variant of a polymorphic gene is called an allele, and one individual may carry two different alleles of a gene, each inherited from a different parent. The MHC genes are the most polymorphic genes in the mammalian genome.

Polyvalency. The presence of multiple identical copies of an epitope on a single antigen molecule, cell surface, or particle. Polyvalent antigens, such as bacterial capsular polysaccharides, are often capable of activating B lymphocytes independent of helper T cells.

Positive selection. The process by which developing T cells in the thymus (thymocytes) whose TCRs bind to self MHC molecules are rescued from programmed cell death, whereas thymocytes whose receptors do not recognize self MHC molecules die by default. Positive selection ensures that mature T cells are self MHC restricted and that CD8+ T cells are specific for complexes of peptides with class I MHC molecules and CD4+ T cells for complexes of peptides with class II MHC molecules.

Pre-B cell. A developing B cell present only in hematopoietic tissues that is at a maturational stage characterized by expression of cytoplasmic Ig μ heavy chains and surrogate light chains but not Ig light chains. Pre-B cell receptors composed of μ chains and surrogate light chains deliver signals that stimulate further maturation of the pre-B cell into an immature B cell.

Pre-B cell receptor. A receptor expressed on maturing B lymphocytes at the pre-B cell stage that is composed of an Ig μ heavy chain and an invariant surrogate light chain. The surrogate light chain is composed of two proteins, including the λ5 protein, which is homologous to the λ light chain C domain, and the V pre-B protein, which is homologous to a V domain. The pre-B cell receptor associates with the Igα and Igβ signal transduction proteins to form the pre-B cell receptor complex. Pre-B cell receptors are required for stimulating the proliferation and continued maturation of the developing B cell. It is not known whether the pre-B cell receptor binds a specific ligand.

Pre-cytolytic T lymphocyte (pre-CTL). A mature, naive CD8+ T lymphocyte that cannot perform effector functions but, on activation by antigen and costimulators, will differentiate into a CTL capable of lysing target cells and secreting cytokines.

Pre-T cell. A developing T lymphocyte in the thymus at a maturational stage characterized by expression of the TCR β chain, but not the α chain or CD4 or CD8. In pre-T cells, the TCR β chain is found on the cell surface as part of the pre-T cell receptor.

Pre-T cell receptor. A receptor expressed on the surface of pre-T cells that is composed of the TCR β chain and an invariant pre-Tα protein. This receptor associates with CD3 and ζ molecules to form the pre-T cell receptor complex. The function of this complex is similar to that of the pre-B cell receptor in B cell development, namely, the delivery of signals that stimulate further proliferation, antigen receptor gene rearrangements, and other maturational events. It is not known whether the pre-T cell receptor binds a specific ligand.

Pre-Tα. An invariant transmembrane protein with a single extracellular Ig-like domain that associates with TCR β chain in pre-T cells to form the pre-T cell receptor.

Primary immune response. An adaptive immune response that occurs after the first exposure of an individual to a foreign antigen. Primary responses are characterized by relatively slow kinetics and small magnitude compared with the responses after a second or subsequent exposure.

Primary immunodeficiency. A genetic defect in which an inherited deficiency in some aspect of the innate or adaptive immune system leads to an increased susceptibility to infections. Primary immunodeficiency is frequently manifested early in infancy and childhood but is sometimes clinically detected later in life.

Pro-B cell. A developing B cell in the bone marrow that is the earliest cell committed to the B lymphocyte lineage. Pro-B cells do not produce Ig, but they can be distinguished from other immature cells by the expression of B lineage–restricted surface molecules such as CD19 and CD10.

Professional antigen-presenting cells (professional APCs). APCs for naive helper T lymphocytes, used to refer to dendritic cells, mononuclear phagocytes, and B lymphocytes, all of which are capable of expressing class II MHC molecules and costimulators. The most important professional APCs for initiating primary T cell responses are dendritic cells.

Programmed cell death. A pathway of cell death by apoptosis that occurs in lymphocytes deprived of necessary survival stimuli, such as growth factors or co-stimulators. Programmed cell death, also called death by neglect or passive cell death, is characterized by the release of mitochondrial cytochrome *c* into the cytoplasm, activation of caspase-9, and initiation of the apoptotic pathway.

Promoter. A DNA sequence immediately 5′ to the transcription start site of a gene where the proteins that initiate transcription bind. The term *promoter* is often used to mean the entire 5′ regulatory region of a gene, including enhancers, which are additional sequences that bind transcription factors and interact with the basal transcription complex to increase the rate of transcriptional initiation. Other enhancers may be located at a significant distance from the promoter, either 5′ of the gene, in introns, or 3′ of the gene.

Prostaglandins. A class of lipid inflammatory mediators derived from arachidonic acid in many cell types through the cyclooxygenase pathway. Activated mast cells make prostaglandin D_2 (PGD_2), which binds to receptors on smooth muscle cells and acts as a vasodilator and a bronchoconstrictor. PGD_2 also promotes neutrophil chemotaxis and accumulation at inflammatory sites.

Pro-T cell. A developing T cell in the thymic cortex that is a recent arrival from the bone marrow and does not express TCRs, CD3, ζ chains, or CD4 or CD8 molecules. Pro-T cells are also called double-negative thymocytes.

Protease. An enzyme that cleaves peptide bonds and thereby breaks proteins down into peptides. Different kinds of proteases have different specificities for bonds between particular amino acid residues. Proteases inside phagocytes are important for killing ingested microbes during innate immune responses, and proteases released from phagocytes at inflammatory sites can cause tissue damage. Proteases in APCs are critical for generating peptide fragments of protein antigens that bind to MHC molecules during T cell–mediated immune responses.

Proteasome. A large multiprotein enzyme complex with a broad range of proteolytic activity that is found in the cytoplasm of most cells and generates from cytosolic proteins the peptides that bind to class I MHC molecules. Proteins are targeted for proteasomal degradation by covalent linkage of ubiquitin molecules.

Protein kinase C (PKC). Any of several isoforms of an enzyme that mediates the phosphorylation of serine and threonine residues in many different protein substrates and thereby serves to propagate various signal transduction pathways leading to transcription factor activation. In T and B lymphocytes, PKC is activated by DAG, which is generated in response to antigen receptor ligation.

Protein tyrosine kinases (PTKs). Enzymes that mediate the phosphorylation of tyrosine residues in proteins and thereby promote phosphotyrosine-dependent protein-protein interactions. PTKs are involved in numerous signal transduction pathways in cells of the immune system.

Protozoa. Single-celled eukaryotic organisms, many of which are human parasites and cause diseases. Examples of pathogenic protozoa include *Entamoeba histolytica*, which causes amebic dysentery; *Plasmodium*, which causes malaria; and *Leishmania*, which causes leishmaniasis. Protozoa stimulate both innate and adaptive immune responses. It has proved difficult to develop effective vaccines against many of these organisms.

Provirus. A DNA copy of the genome of a retrovirus that is integrated into the host cell genome and from which viral genes are transcribed and the viral genome is reproduced. HIV proviruses can remain inactive for long periods and thereby represent a latent form of HIV infection that is not accessible to immune defense.

Purified antigen (subunit) vaccine. A vaccine composed of purified antigens or subunits of microbes. Examples of this type of vaccine include diphtheria and tetanus toxoids, pneumococcus and *Haemophilus influenzae* polysaccharide vaccines, and purified polypeptide vaccines against hepatitis B and influenza virus. Purified antigen vaccines may stimulate antibody and helper T cell responses, but they do not generate CTL responses.

Pyogenic bacteria. Bacteria, such as the gram-positive staphylococci and streptococci, that induce inflammatory responses rich in polymorphonuclear leukocytes (giving rise to pus). Antibody responses to these bacteria greatly enhance the efficacy of innate immune effector mechanisms to clear infections.

Rac. A small guanine nucleotide–binding protein that is activated by the GDP-GTP exchange factor Vav during the early events of T cell activation. GTP•Rac triggers a three-step protein kinase cascade that culminates in activation of the stress-activated protein (SAP) kinase, c-Jun N-terminal kinase (JNK), and p38 kinase, which are similar to the MAP kinases.

Radioimmunoassay. A highly sensitive and specific immunologic method of quantifying the concentration of an antigen in a solution that relies on a radioactively labeled antibody specific for the antigen. Usually, two antibodies specific for the antigen are used. The first antibody is unlabeled but attached to a solid support, where it binds and immobilizes the antigen whose concentration is being determined. The amount of the second, labeled antibody that binds to the immobilized antigen, as determined by radioactive decay detectors, is proportional to the concentration of antigen in the test solution.

Ras. A member of a family of 21-kD guanine nucleotide–binding proteins with intrinsic GTPase activity that are involved in many different signal transduction pathways in diverse cell types. Mutated *ras* genes are associated with neoplastic transformation. In T cell activation, Ras is recruited to the plasma membrane by tyrosine-phosphorylated adapter proteins, where it is activated by GDP-GTP exchange factors. GTP•Ras then initiates the MAP kinase cascade, which leads to expression of the *fos* gene and assembly of the AP-1 transcription factor.

Reactive oxygen intermediates (ROIs). Highly reactive metabolites of oxygen, including superoxide anion, hydroxyl radical, and hydrogen peroxide, that are produced by activated phagocytes. ROIs are used by the phagocytes to form oxyhalides that damage ingested bacteria. ROIs may also be released from cells and promote inflammatory responses or cause tissue damage.

Reagin. IgE antibody that mediates an immediate hypersensitivity reaction.

Receptor editing. A process by which some immature B cells that recognize self antigens in the bone marrow may be induced to change their Ig specificities. Receptor editing involves reactivation of the RAG genes, additional light chain VJ recombinations, and new Ig light chain production, which allows the cell to express a different Ig receptor that is not self-reactive.

Recombination-activating gene 1 and 2 (*RAG1* and *RAG2*). The genes encoding RAG-1 and RAG-2 proteins, which are the lymphocyte-specific components of V(D)J recombinase and are expressed in developing B and T cells. RAG proteins bind to recombination recognition sequences and are critical for DNA recombination events that form functional Ig and TCR genes. Therefore, RAG proteins are required for expression of antigen receptors and for the maturation of B and T lymphocytes.

Recombination signal sequences. Specific DNA sequences found adjacent to the V, D, and J segments in the antigen receptor loci and recognized by the RAG-1/RAG-2 component of V(D)J recombinase. The recognition sequences consist of a highly conserved stretch of 7 nucleotides, called the heptamer, located adjacent to the V, D, or J coding sequence, followed by a spacer of exactly 12 or 23 nonconserved nucleotides and a highly conserved stretch of 9 nucleotides, called the nonamer.

Red pulp. An anatomic and functional compartment of the spleen composed of vascular sinusoids, scattered among which are large numbers of erythrocytes, macrophages, dendritic cells, sparse lymphocytes, and plasma cells. Red pulp macrophages clear the blood of microbes, other foreign particles, and damaged red blood cells.

Regulatory T cells. A population of T cells that regulates the activation of other T cells and is necessary to maintain peripheral tolerance to self antigens. Regulatory T cells are CD4+ and many constitutively express CD25, the α chain of the IL-2 receptor.

Respiratory burst. The process by which reactive oxygen intermediates such as superoxide anion, hydroxyl radical, and hydrogen peroxide are produced in macrophages and polymorphonuclear leukocytes. The respiratory burst is mediated by the enzyme phagocyte oxidase and is usually triggered by inflammatory mediators, such as LTB$_4$, PAF, and TNF, or by bacterial products, such as N-formylmethionyl peptides.

Reverse transcriptase. An enzyme encoded by retroviruses, such as HIV, that synthesizes a DNA copy of the viral genome from the RNA genomic template. Purified reverse transcriptase is used widely in molecular biology research for purposes of cloning complementary DNAs encoding a gene of interest from messenger RNA. Reverse transcriptase inhibitors are used as drugs to treat HIV-1 infection.

Reverse transcriptase–polymerase chain reaction (RT-PCR). An adaptation of the polymerase chain reaction (PCR) used to amplify a complementary DNA (cDNA) of a gene of interest. In this method, RNA is isolated from a cell expressing the gene, and cDNAs are synthesized by use of the reverse transcriptase enzyme. The cDNA of interest is then amplified by conventional PCR techniques with gene-specific primers.

Rh blood group antigens. A complex system of protein alloantigens expressed on red blood cell membranes that are the cause of transfusion reactions and hemolytic disease of the newborn. The most clinically important Rh antigen is designated D.

Rheumatoid arthritis. An autoimmune disease characterized primarily by inflammatory damage to joints and sometimes inflammation of blood vessels, lungs, and other tissues. CD4+ T cells, activated B lymphocytes, and plasma cells are found in the inflamed joint lining (synovium), and numerous proinflammatory cytokines, including IL-1 and TNF, are present in the synovial (joint) fluid.

RNase protection assay. A sensitive method of detecting and quantifying messenger RNA (mRNA) copies of particular genes based on hybridization of the mRNA to radiolabeled RNA probes and digestion of unhybridized RNA with the enzyme RNase. The double-stranded RNA duplexes created during the hybridization reaction resist degradation by RNase and are of a particular size determined by the length of the probe. They can be separated by gel electrophoresis and are detected and quantitated by radioautography.

Scavenger receptors. A family of cell surface receptors expressed on macrophages, originally defined as receptors that mediate endocytosis of oxidized or acetylated low-density lipoprotein particles but that also bind and mediate the phagocytosis of a variety of microbes.

SCID mouse. A mouse strain in which B and T cells are absent because of an early block in maturation from bone marrow precursors. SCID mice carry a mutation in a component of the enzyme DNA-dependent protein kinase, which is required for double-stranded DNA break repair. Deficiency of this enzyme results in abnormal joining of Ig and TCR gene segments during recombination and therefore failure to express antigen receptors.

Secondary immune response. An adaptive immune response that occurs on second exposure to an antigen. A secondary response is characterized by more rapid kinetics and greater magnitude relative to the primary immune response, which occurs on first exposure.

Second-set rejection. Allograft rejection in an individual who has previously been sensitized to the donor's tissue alloantigens by having received another graft or transfusion from that donor. In contrast to first-set rejection, which occurs in an individual who has not previously been sensitized to the donor alloantigens,

complexes composed of autoantibodies and their specific antigens, with deposition of these complexes in small blood vessels in various tissues. The underlying mechanism for the breakdown of self-tolerance in SLE is not understood.

T cell receptor (TCR). The clonally distributed antigen receptor on $CD4^+$ and $CD8^+$ T lymphocytes that recognizes complexes of foreign peptides bound to self MHC molecules on the surface of APCs. The most common form of TCR is composed of a heterodimer of two disulfide-linked transmembrane polypeptide chains, designated α and β, each containing one N-terminal Ig-like variable (V) domain, one Ig-like constant (C) domain, a hydrophobic transmembrane region, and a short cytoplasmic region. (Another less common type of TCR, composed of γ and δ chains, is found on a small subset of T cells and recognizes different forms of antigen.)

T cell receptor complex. A multiprotein plasma membrane complex on T lymphocytes that is composed of the highly variable, antigen-binding TCR heterodimer and the invariant signaling proteins CD3 δ, ε, and γ and the ζ chain.

T lymphocyte. The cell type that mediates cell-mediated immune responses in the adaptive immune system. T lymphocytes mature in the thymus, circulate in the blood, populate secondary lymphoid tissues, and are recruited to peripheral sites of antigen exposure. They express antigen receptors (TCRs) that recognize peptide fragments of foreign proteins bound to self MHC molecules. Functional subsets of T lymphocytes include $CD4^+$ helper T cells and $CD8^+$ CTLs.

T-dependent antigen. An antigen that requires both B cells and helper T cells to stimulate an antibody response. T-dependent antigens are protein antigens that contain some epitopes recognized by T cells and other epitopes recognized by B cells. Helper T cells produce cytokines and cell surface molecules that stimulate B cell growth and differentiation into antibody-secreting cells. Humoral immune responses to T-dependent antigens are characterized by isotype switching, affinity maturation, and memory.

T_H1 cells. A functional subset of helper T cells that secrete a particular set of cytokines, including IFN-γ, and whose principal function is to stimulate phagocyte-mediated defense against infections, especially with intracellular microbes.

T_H2 cells. A functional subset of helper T cells that secrete a particular set of cytokines, including IL-4 and IL-5, and whose principal functions are to stimulate IgE and eosinophil/mast cell–mediated immune reactions and to down-regulate T_H1 responses.

Thymic epithelial cells. Epithelial cells abundant in the cortical and medullary stroma of the thymus that play a critical role in T cell development. Thymic epithelial cells secrete factors, such as IL-7, that are required for the early stages of T cell development. In the process of positive selection, maturing T cells must recognize self peptides bound to MHC molecules on the surface of thymic epithelial cells to be rescued from programmed cell death.

Thymocyte. A precursor of a mature T lymphocyte present in the thymus.

Thymus. A bilobed organ situated in the anterior mediastinum that is the site of maturation of T lymphocytes from bone marrow–derived precursors. Thymic tissue is divided into an outer cortex and an inner medulla and contains stromal thymic epithelial cells, macrophages, dendritic cells, and numerous T cell precursors (thymocytes) at various stages of maturation.

T-independent antigen. Nonprotein antigens, such as polysaccharides and lipids, that can stimulate antibody responses without a requirement for antigen-specific helper T lymphocytes. T-independent antigens usually contain multiple identical epitopes that can cross-link membrane Ig on B cells and thereby activate the cells. Humoral immune responses to T-independent antigens show relatively little heavy chain isotype switching or affinity maturation, two processes that require signals from helper T cells.

Tissue typing. The determination of the particular MHC alleles expressed by an individual for the purpose of matching allograft donors and recipients. Tissue typing, also called HLA typing, is usually done by testing whether sera known to be reactive with certain MHC gene products mediate complement-dependent lysis of an individual's lymphocytes. PCR techniques are now also used to determine whether an individual carries a particular MHC allele.

TNF receptor–associated factors (TRAFs). A family of adapter molecules that interact with the cytoplasmic domains of various receptors in the TNF receptor family, including TNF-RII, lymphotoxin (LT)–β receptor, and CD40. Each of these receptors contains a cytoplasmic motif that binds different TRAFs, which in turn engage other signaling molecules leading to activation of the transcription factors AP-1 and NF-κB. A transforming gene product of Epstein-Barr virus encodes a protein with a domain that binds TRAFs, and therefore infection by the virus mimics TNF- or CD40-induced signals.

Tolerance. Unresponsiveness of the adaptive immune system to antigens, as a result of inactivation or death of antigen-specific lymphocytes, induced by exposure to the antigens. Tolerance to self antigens is a normal feature of the adaptive immune system, but tolerance to foreign antigens may be induced under certain conditions of antigen exposure.

Tolerogen. An antigen that induces immunologic tolerance, in contrast to an immunogen, which induces an immune response. Many antigens can be either tolerogens or immunogens, depending on how they are administered. Tolerogenic forms of antigens include large doses of the proteins administered without adjuvants, APLs, and orally administered antigens.

Toll-like receptors. Cell surface molecules on phagocytes and other cell types that are involved in recognition of microbial structures, such as endotoxin, and the generation of signals that lead to the activation of innate immune responses. Toll-like receptors share structural homology and signal transduction pathways with the type I IL-1 receptor.

Toxic shock syndrome. An acute illness characterized by shock, skin exfoliation, conjunctivitis, and diarrhea that is associated with tampon use and caused by a *Staphylococcus aureus* superantigen.

Transforming growth factor-β (TGF-β). A cytokine produced by activated T cells, mononuclear phagocytes, and other cells whose principal actions are to inhibit the proliferation and differentiation of T cells, to inhibit the activation of macrophages, and to counteract the effects of proinflammatory cytokines.

Transfusion. Transplantation of circulating blood cells, platelets, or plasma from one individual to another. Transfusions are performed to treat blood loss from hemorrhage or to treat a deficiency in one or more blood cell types resulting from inadequate production or excess destruction.

Transfusion reactions. An immunologic reaction against transfused blood products, usually mediated by preformed antibodies in the recipient that bind to donor blood cell antigens, such as ABO blood group antigens or histocompatibility antigens. Transfusion reactions can lead to intravascular lysis of red blood cells and, in severe cases, kidney damage, fever, shock, and disseminated intravascular coagulation.

Transgenic mouse. A mouse that expresses an exogenous gene that has been introduced into the genome by injection of a specific DNA sequence into the pronuclei of fertilized mouse eggs. Transgenes insert randomly at chromosomal break points and are subsequently inherited as simple mendelian traits. By the design of transgenes with tissue-specific regulatory sequences, mice can be produced that express a particular gene only in certain tissues. Transgenic mice are used extensively in immunology research to study the functions of various cytokines, cell surface molecules, and intracellular signaling molecules.

Transplantation. The process of transferring cells, tissues, or organs (i.e., grafts) from one individual to another or from one site to another in the same individual. Transplantation is used to treat a variety of diseases in which there is a functional disorder of a tissue or organ. The major barrier to successful transplantation between individuals is immunologic reaction (rejection) to the transplanted graft.

Transporter associated with antigen processing (TAP). An adenosine triphosphate (ATP)–dependent peptide transporter that mediates the active transport of peptides from the cytosol to the site of assembly of class I MHC molecules inside the endoplasmic reticulum. TAP is a heterodimeric molecule composed of TAP-1 and TAP-2 polypeptides, both encoded by genes in the MHC. Because peptides are required for stable assembly of class I MHC molecules, TAP-deficient animals express few cell surface class I MHC molecules, which results in diminished development and activation of $CD8^+$ T cells.

Tumor immunity. Protection against the development of tumors by the immune system. Although immune responses to naturally occurring tumors can frequently be demonstrated, true immunity may occur only in the case of a subset of these tumors that express immunogenic antigens (e.g., tumors that are caused by oncogenic viruses and therefore express viral antigens). Research efforts are under way to enhance weak immune responses to other tumors by a variety of approaches.

Tumor-infiltrating lymphocytes (TILs). Lymphocytes isolated from the inflammatory infiltrates present in and around surgical resection samples of solid tumors that are enriched with tumor-specific CTLs and NK cells. In an experimental mode of cancer treatment, TILs are grown *in vitro* in the presence of high doses of IL-2 and are then adoptively transferred back into patients with the tumor.

Tumor necrosis factor (TNF). A cytokine produced mainly by activated mononuclear phagocytes that functions to stimulate the recruitment of neutrophils and monocytes to sites of infection and to activate these cells to eradicate microbes. TNF stimulates vascular endothelial cells to express new adhesion molecules, induces macrophages and endothelial cells to secrete chemokines, and promotes apoptosis of target cells. In severe infections, TNF is produced in large amounts and has systemic effects, including induction of fever, synthesis of acute-phase proteins by the liver, and cachexia. The production of large amounts of TNF can cause intravascular thrombosis and shock. (TNF-β, or lymphotoxin, is a closely related cytokine with biologic effects identical to those of TNF-α but is produced by T cells.)

Tumor necrosis factor (TNF) receptors. Cell surface receptors for TNF-α and TNF-β (LT), present on most cell types. There are two distinct TNF receptors, TNF-RI and TNF-RII, but most biologic effects of TNF are mediated by TNF-RI. TNF receptors are members of a family of homologous receptors with cysteine-rich extracellular motifs that include Fas and CD40.

Tumor-specific antigen. An antigen whose expression is restricted to a particular tumor and is not expressed by normal cells. Tumor-specific antigens may serve as target antigens for antitumor immune responses.

Tumor-specific transplantation antigen (TSTA). An antigen expressed on experimental animal tumor cells that can be detected by induction of immunologic rejection of tumor transplants. TSTAs were originally defined on chemically induced rodent sarcomas and shown to stimulate CTL-mediated rejection of transplanted tumors.

Two-signal hypothesis. A now proven hypothesis that states that the activation of lymphocytes requires two distinct signals, the first being antigen and the second either microbial products or components of innate immune responses to microbes. The requirement for antigen (so-called signal 1) ensures that the ensuing immune response is specific. The requirement for additional stimuli triggered by microbes or innate immune reactions (signal 2) ensures that immune responses are induced when they are needed, that is, against microbes and other noxious substances and not against harmless substances, including self antigens. Signal 2 is referred to as costimulation and is often mediated by membrane molecules on professional APCs, such as B7 proteins.

Type I cytokine receptors. A family of cytokine receptors, also called hemopoietin receptors, that contain conserved structural motifs in their extracellular domains and bind cytokines that fold into four α-helical strands, including growth hormone, IL-2, IL-3, IL-4, IL-5, IL-6, IL-7, IL-9, IL-11, IL-13, IL-15, GM-CSF, and G-CSF. Some of these receptors consist of a ligand-binding chain and one or more signal-transducing chains, and all of these chains have the same structural motifs. Type I cytokine receptors are dimerized on binding their cytokine ligands, and they signal through JAK/STAT pathways.

Type I interferons (IFN-α, IFN-β). A family of cytokines, including several structurally related IFN-α proteins and a single IFN-β protein, all of which have potent antiviral actions. The major source of IFN-α is mononuclear phagocytes; IFN-β is produced by many cells, including fibroblasts. Both IFN-α and IFN-β bind to the same cell surface receptor and induce similar biologic responses. Type I IFNs inhibit viral replication, increase the lytic potential of NK cells, increase expression of class I MHC molecules on virus-infected cells, and stimulate the development of T_H1 cells, especially in humans.

Ubiquitination. Covalent linkage of several copies of a small polypeptide called ubiquitin to a protein. Ubiquitination serves to target the protein for proteolytic degradation by proteasomes, a critical step in the class I MHC pathway of antigen processing and presentation.

Urticaria. Localized transient swelling and redness of the skin caused by leakage of fluid and plasma proteins from small vessels into the dermis during an immediate hypersensitivity reaction.

V gene segments. A DNA sequence that encodes the variable domain of an Ig heavy chain or light chain or a TCR α, β, γ, or δ chain. Each antigen receptor locus contains many different V gene segments, any one of which may recombine with downstream D or J segments during lymphocyte maturation to form functional antigen receptor genes.

V(D)J recombinase. A collection of enzymes that together mediate the somatic recombination events that form functional antigen receptor genes in developing B and T lymphocytes. Some of the enzymes, such as RAG-1 and RAG-2, are found only in developing lymphocytes, and others are ubiquitous DNA repair enzymes.

Vaccine. A preparation of microbial antigen, often combined with adjuvants, that is administered to individuals to induce protective immunity against microbial infections. The antigen may be in the form of live but avirulent microorganisms, killed microorganisms, purified macromolecular components of a microorganism, or a plasmid that contains a complementary DNA encoding a microbial antigen.

Variable region. The extracellular, N-terminal region of an Ig heavy or light chain or a TCR α, β, γ, or δ chain that contains variable amino acid sequences that differ between every clone of lymphocytes and that are responsible for the specificity for antigen. The antigen-binding variable sequences are localized to extended loop structures or hypervariable segments.

Virus. A primitive obligate intracellular parasitic organism or infectious particle that consists of a simple nucleic acid genome packaged in a protein capsid, sometimes surrounded by a membrane envelope. Many pathogenic animal viruses cause a wide range of diseases. Humoral immune responses to viruses can be effective in blocking infection of cells, and NK cells and CTLs are necessary to kill cells already infected.

Western blot. An immunologic technique to determine the presence of a protein in a biologic sample. The method involves separation of proteins in the sample by electrophoresis, transfer of the protein array from the electrophoresis gel to a support membrane by capillary action (blotting), and finally detection of the protein by binding of an enzymatically or radioactively labeled antibody specific for that protein.

Wheal and flare reaction. Local swelling and redness in the skin at a site of an immediate hypersensitivity reaction. The wheal reflects increased vascular permeability and the flare results from increased local blood flow, both changes resulting from mediators such as histamine released from activated dermal mast cells.

White pulp. The part of the spleen that is composed predominantly of lymphocytes, arranged in periarteriolar lymphoid sheaths, and follicles and other leukocytes. The remainder of the spleen contains sinusoids lined with phagocytic cells and filled with blood, called the **red pulp.**

Wiskott-Aldrich syndrome. An X-linked disease characterized by eczema, thrombocytopenia (reduced blood platelets), and immunodeficiency manifested as susceptibility to bacterial infections. The defective gene encodes a cytosolic protein involved in signaling cascades and regulation of the actin cytoskeleton.

Xenoantigen. An antigen on a graft from another species.

Xenogeneic graft (xenograft). An organ or tissue graft derived from a species different from the recipient. Transplantation of xenogeneic grafts (e.g., from a pig) to humans is not yet practical because of special problems related to immunologic rejection.

Xenoreactive. Describing a T cell or antibody that recognizes and responds to an antigen on a graft from another species (a xenoantigen). The T cell may recognize an intact xenogeneic MHC molecule or a peptide derived from a xenogeneic protein bound to a self MHC molecule.

X-linked agammaglobulinemia. An immunodeficiency disease, also called Bruton's agammaglobulinemia, characterized by a block in early B cell maturation and absence of serum Ig. Patients suffer from pyogenic bacterial infections. The disease is caused by mutations or deletions in the gene encoding Btk, an enzyme involved in signal transduction in developing B cells.

X-linked hyper-IgM syndrome. A rare immunodeficiency disease caused by mutations in the CD40 ligand gene and characterized by failure of B cell heavy chain isotype switching and cell-mediated immunity. Patients suffer from both pyogenic bacterial and protozoal infections.

Zeta-associated protein of 70 kD (ZAP-70). An Src family cytoplasmic protein tyrosine kinase that is critical for early signaling steps in antigen-induced T cell activation. ZAP-70 binds to phosphorylated tyrosines in the cytoplasmic tails of the ζ chain of the TCR complex and in turn phosphorylates adapter proteins that recruit other components of the signaling cascade.

ζ **Chain.** A transmembrane protein expressed in T cells as part of the TCR complex that contains ITAMs in its cytoplasmic tail and binds the ZAP-70 protein tyrosine kinase during T cell activation.

Legends/Credits

Page 7

1, Light micrograph of a lymphocyte in a peripheral blood smear. **2,** Light micrograph of a plasma cell in tissue. **3,** Light micrograph of a monocyte in a peripheral blood smear.

(From Abbas AK, Lichtman AH: Cellular and Molecular Immunology, 5th ed. Philadelphia, WB Saunders, 2003, pp 19, 23, and 25; Figs. 2-2A, 2-5A, and 2-7A.)

Page 9

Light micrograph of a lymph node illustrating the T and B cell zones.

(Courtesy of Dr. James Gulizia, Department of Pathology, Brigham and Women's Hospital, Boston. From Abbas AK, Lichtman AH: Cellular and Molecular Immunology, 5th ed. Philadelphia, WB Saunders, 2003, p 28; Fig. 2-10B.)

Page 17

Structure of an antibody molecule: schematic diagram of a secreted IgG molecule. The antigen-binding sites are formed by the juxtaposition of variable light chain (V_L) and variable heavy chain (V_H) domains. The heavy chain C regions end in tail pieces. The locations of complement- and Fc receptor-binding sites within the heavy chain constant regions are approximations.

(From Abbas AK, Lichtman AH: Cellular and Molecular Immunology, 5th ed. Philadelphia, WB Saunders, 2003, p 48; Fig. 3-1A.)

Page 23

Polymorphic residue of a class I MHC molecule.

(Courtesy of Dr. J. McCluskey, University of Melbourne, Parkville, Australia. From Abbas AK, Lichtman AH: Cellular and Molecular Immunology, 5th ed. Philadelphia, WB Saunders, 2003, p 72; Fig. 4-5.)

Page 28

Light micrograph of cultured dendritic cells derived from bone marrow precursors.

(Courtesy Dr. Y-J. Liu, DNAX, Palo Alto, CA. From Abbas AK, Lichtman AH: Cellular and Molecular Immunology, 5th ed. Philadelphia, WB Saunders, 2003, p 87; Fig. 5-4A.)

Page 34, Top

Structure of the T cell receptor.

(From Abbas AK, Lichtman AH: Cellular and Molecular Immunology, 5th ed. Philadelphia, WB Saunders, 2003, p 108; Fig. 6-3.)

Page 34, Bottom

Components of the TCR complex.

(From Abbas AK, Lichtman AH: Cellular and Molecular Immunology, 5th ed. Philadelphia, WB Saunders, 2003, p 111; Fig. 6-6.)

Page 44

Germline organization of human Ig loci.

(From Abbas AK, Lichtman AH: Cellular and Molecular Immunology, 5th ed. Philadelphia, WB Saunders, 2003, p 136; Fig. 7-4.)

Page 53

Formation of the immunological synapse.

(From Moks CRF, Freiberg BA, Kupfer H, et al: Three-dimensional segregation of supramolecular activation clusters in T cells. Nature 395:82-86, 1998. Copyright Macmillan Magazines Limited. Reprinted in Abbas AK, Lichtman AH: Cellular and Molecular Immunology, 5th ed. Philadelphia, WB Saunders, 2003, p 177; Fig. 8-8B.)

Page 59

Histology of a secondary follicle with a germinal center in a lymph node.

(Courtesy of Dr. James Gulizia, Department of Pathology, Brigham and Women's Hospital, Boston. From Abbas AK, Lichtman AH: Cellular and Molecular Immunology, 5th ed. Philadelphia, WB Saunders, 2003, p 208; Fig. 9-15B.)

Page 81

Role of cytokines in innate immunity to microbes.

(From Abbas AK, Lichtman AH: Cellular and Molecular Immunology, 5th ed. Philadelphia, WB Saunders, 2003, p 263; Fig. 11-9.)

Page 82

Morphology of neutrophils.

(From Abbas AK, Lichtman AH: Basic Immunology, 2nd ed. Philadelphia, WB Saunders, 2003, p 25; Fig. 2-3.)

Page 88

Cell-mediated immunity to *Listeria monocytogenes*.

(From Abbas AK, Lichtman AH: Cellular and Molecular Immunology, 5th ed. Philadelphia, WB Saunders, 2003, p 300; Fig. 13-2.)

Page 89, Left

Delayed-type hypersensitivity reaction.

(Courtesy of Dr. J. Faix, Department of Pathology, Stanford University School of Medicine, Palo Alto, CA. From Abbas AK, Lichtman AH: Cellular and Molecular Immunology, 5th ed. Philadelphia, WB Saunders, 2003, p 310; Fig. 13-12.)

Page 89, Right

Morphology of a delayed-type hypersensitivity reaction.

(Courtesy of Dr. J. Faix, Department of Pathology, Stanford University School of Medicine, Palo Alto, CA. From Abbas AK, Lichtman AH: Cellular and Molecular Immunology, 5th ed. Philadelphia, WB Saunders, 2003, p 311; Fig. 13-13.)

Page 90

Morphologic spectrum of tuberculosis. A characteristic tubercle at low magnification (**A**) and in detail (**B**) illustrates central caseation surrounded by epithelioid and multinucleated giant cells.

(From Kumar V, Abbas AK, Fausto N: Robbins and Cotran Pathologic Basis of Disease, 7th ed. Philadelphia, WB Saunders, 2005, p 385; Fig. 8-31A and B.)

Page 91

Conjugate formation between CTLs and a target cell.

(Courtesy of Dr. P. Peters, Netherlands Cancer Institute, Amsterdam. From Abbas AK, Lichtman AH: Cellular and Molecular Immunology, 5th ed. Philadelphia, WB Saunders, 2003, p 315; Fig. 13-17.)

Page 97

Structure of the MAC in cell membranes.

(From Abbas AK, Lichtman AH: Cellular and Molecular Immunology, 5th ed. Philadelphia, WB Saunders, 2003, p 334; Fig. 14-12A.)

Page 102

Lepromatous leprosy. Acid-fast bacilli ("red snappers") with macrophages.

(From Kumar V, Abbas AK, Fausto N: Robbins and Cotran Pathologic Basis of Disease, 7th ed. Philadelphia, WB Saunders, 2005, p 388; Fig. 8-36.)

Page 103

Histoplasma capsulatum yeast forms fill phagocytes in lymph nodes of patient with disseminated histoplasmosis.

(From Kumar V, Abbas AK, Fausto N: Robbins and Cotran Pathologic Basis of Disease, 7th ed. Philadelphia, WB Saunders, 2005, p 754; Fig. 15-38.)

Page 111, Left

Endomyocardial biopsy showing acute cellular rejection.

(Courtesy of Dr. Richard Mitchell, Department of Pathology, Brigham and Women's Hospital, Boston. From Abbas AK, Lichtman AH: Basic Immunology, 2nd ed. Philadelphia, WB Saunders, 2003, p 293; Fig. A-2.)

Page 111, Right

Coronary artery with transplant-associated arteriosclerosis.

(Courtesy of Dr. Richard Mitchell, Department of Pathology, Brigham and Women's Hospital, Boston. From Abbas AK, Lichtman AH: Basic Immunology, 2nd ed. Philadelphia, WB Saunders, 2003, p 294; Fig. A-3.)

Page 112

Histopathology of acute graft-versus-host disease in the skin.

(Courtesy of Dr. Scott Grantor, Department of Pathology, Brigham and Women's Hospital and Harvard Medical School, Boston. From Abbas AK, Lichtman AH: Cellular and Molecular Immunology, 5th ed. Philadelphia, WB Saunders, 2003, p 388; Fig. 16-10.)

Page 123

Urticaria.

(From Kumar V, Abbas AK, Fausto N: Robbins and Cotran Pathologic Basis of Disease, 7th ed. Philadelphia, WB Saunders, 2005, p 1252; Fig. 25-22.)

Page 124, Top

A patient with hyperthyroidism.

(From Kumar V, Abbas AK, Fausto N: Robbins and Cotran Pathologic Basis of Disease, 7th ed. Philadelphia, WB Saunders, 2005, p 1167; Fig. 24-8.)

Page 124, Bottom

Pathologic features of antibody-mediated glomerulonephritis. Glomerulonephritis induced by antibody against the glomerular basement membrane (Goodpasture's syndrome): the light micrograph shows glomerular inflammation and severe damage, and immunofluorescence shows smooth (linear) deposits of antibody along the basement membrane.

(From Abbas AK, Lichtman AH: Cellular and Molecular Immunology, 5th ed. Philadelphia, WB Saunders, 2003, p 416; Fig. 18-3A.)

Page 125

Morphology of a delayed-type hypersensitivity reaction. At higher magnification, the infiltrate is seen to consist of activated lymphocytes and macrophages surrounding small blood vessels in which the endothelial cells are also activated.

(Courtesy of Dr. J. Faix, Department of Pathology, Stanford University School of Medicine, Palo Alto, CA. From Abbas AK, Lichtman AH: Cellular and Molecular Immunology, 5th ed. Philadelphia, WB Saunders, 2003, p 311; Fig. 13-13B.)

Page 126

Rheumatoid arthritis. More advanced disease with loss of articular cartilage, narrowing joint spaces of virtually all the small joints, and ulnar deviation of the fingers. There is a dislocation of the second, third, and fourth proximal phalanges produced by advanced articular disease.

(Courtesy of Dr. John O'Connor, Boston University Medical Center, Boston. From Kumar V, Abbas AK, Fausto N: Robbins and Cotran Pathologic Basis of Disease, 7th ed. Philadelphia, WB Saunders, 2005, p 1308; Fig. 26-45B.)

Page 127, Top

Megaloblastic anemia.

(Courtesy of Dr. Robert W. McKenna, Department of Pathology, University of Texas Southwestern Medical School, Dallas. From Kumar V, Abbas AK, Fausto N: Robbins and Cotran Pathologic Basis of Disease, 7th ed. Philadelphia, WB Saunders, 2005, p 639; Fig. 13-18.)

Page 127, Bottom

Representative form of systemic medium-sized to small vessel vasculitis: polyarteritis nodosa.

(Courtesy of Dr. Sidney Murphree, Department of Pathology, University of Texas Southwestern Medical School, Dallas. From Kumar V, Abbas AK, Fausto N: Robbins and Cotran Pathologic Basis of Disease, 7th ed. Philadelphia, WB Saunders, 2005, p 540; Fig. 11-26A.)

Page 134, Top

Mast cell activation. These granules are seen in the electron micrograph of a resting mast cell shown in **A**. In contrast, the depleted granules of an activated mast cell are shown in the electron micrograph (**B**).

(Courtesy of Dr. Daniel Friend, Department of Pathology, Brigham and Women's Hospital and Harvard Medical School, Boston, MA. From Abbas AK, Lichtman AH: Cellular and Molecular Immunology, 5th ed. Philadelphia, WB Saunders, 2003, p 438; Fig. 19-3E and F.)

Page 134, Bottom

The wheal and flare reaction in the skin.

(Courtesy of Dr. James D. Faix, Department of Pathology, Stanford University School of Medicine, Palo Alto, CA. From Abbas AK, Lichtman AH: Cellular and Molecular Immunology, 5th ed. Philadelphia, WB Saunders, 2003, p 446; Fig. 19-8A and B.)

Page 135

Histopathologic features of bronchial asthma. The diseased bronchus has excessive mucus production, many submucosal inflammatory cells (including eosinophils), and smooth muscle hypertrophy.

(Courtesy of Dr. James D. Faix, Department of Pathology, Stanford University School of Medicine, Palo Alto, CA. From Abbas AK, Lichtman AH: Cellular and Molecular Immunology, 5th ed. Philadelphia, WB Saunders, 2003, p 449; Fig. 19-9B.)

Page 136

Morphology of basophils and eosinophils.

(Courtesy of Dr. Jonathan Hecht, Department of Pathology, Brigham and Women's Hospital, Boston. From Abbas AK, Lichtman AH: Cellular and Molecular Immunology, 5th ed. Philadelphia, WB Saunders, 2003, p 439; Fig. 19-4A and B.)

Page 143

Clinical course of HIV disease: plasma viremic, blood CD4$^+$ T cell counts, and clinical stages of disease.

(Adapted with permission from Pantaleo G, Graziosi C, Fauci A: The immunopathogenesis of human immunodeficiency virus infection. N Engl J Med 328:327-335, 1993. Copyright 1993 Massachusetts Medical Society. All rights reserved. Reprinted in Abbas AK, Lichtman AH: Cellular and Molecular Immunology, 5th ed. Philadelphia, WB Saunders, 2003, p 470; Fig. 20-8A.)

Page 144

Flow cytometry analysis of HIV-infected patient's CD4$^+$ and CD8$^+$ T cells.

(From Abbas AK, Lichtman AH: Basic Immunology, 2nd ed. Philadelphia, WB Saunders, 2003, p 299; Fig. A-6A and B.)